Tarascon Adult Emergency Pocketbook 4th edition

Tarascon Adult Emergency Pocketbook
Copyright © 2009 by Jones and Bartlett Publishers, LLC

World Headquarters
Jones and Bartlett
  Publishers
40 Tall Pine Drive
Sudbury, MA 01776
978-443-5000
info@jbpub.com
www.jbpub.com

Jones and Bartlett
  Publishers Canada
6339 Ormindale Way
Mississauga, ON L5V 1J2
CANADA

Jones and Bartlett
  Publishers International
Barb House, Barb Mews
London W6 7PA
UK

Printed in the United States of America
12 11 10   10 9 8 7 6 5 4

Adult Basic Resuscitation
(Perform until Advanced Resuscitation Available)

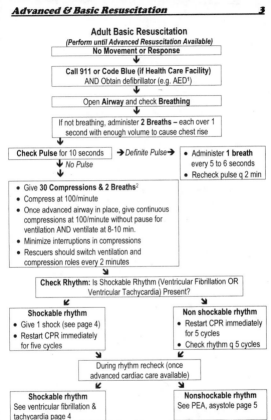

No Movement or Response

↓

Call 911 or Code Blue (if Health Care Facility)
AND Obtain defibrillator (e.g. AED[1])

↓

Open **Airway** and check **Breathing**

↓

If not breathing, administer **2 Breaths** – each over 1 second with enough volume to cause chest rise

↓

Check Pulse for 10 seconds → *Definite Pulse* →
↓ *No Pulse*

- Administer **1 breath** every 5 to 6 seconds
- Recheck pulse q 2 min

- Give **30 Compressions & 2 Breaths**[2]
- Compress at 100/minute
- Once advanced airway in place, give continuous compressions at 100/minute without pause for ventilation AND ventilate at 8-10 min.
- Minimize interruptions in compressions
- Rescuers should switch ventilation and compression roles every 2 minutes

↓

Check Rhythm: Is Shockable Rhythm (Ventricular Fibrillation OR Ventricular Tachycardia) Present?

↙ ↘

Shockable rhythm
- Give 1 shock (see page 4)
- Restart CPR immediately for five cycles

Non shockable rhythm
- Restart CPR immediately for 5 cycles
- Check rhythm q 5 cycles

↘ ↙

During rhythm recheck (once advanced cardiac care available)

↙ ↘

Shockable rhythm
See ventricular fibrillation & tachycardia page 4

Nonshockable rhythm
See PEA, asystole page 5

[1] AED – Automatic External Defibrillator [2] Compressions without breaths may be appropriate for lay people to perform in prehospital setting in cardiac arrest victims.

Adult Advanced Resuscitation
Pulseless Cardiac Arrest/Ventricular Fibrillation & Tachycardia

Pulseless Cardiac Arrest

- See Basic Resuscitation - **Page 3**
- Administer O$_2$, place airway/ventilate, & attach monitor and defibrillator as soon as possible – without delaying compressions

Check Rhythm ↓

Is rhythm SHOCKABLE?: Ventricular Fibrillation (VF) or Ventricular Tachycardia (VT) or **NONSHOCKABLE:** Asystole or Pulseless Electrical Activity (PEA). IF Asystole or PEA occurs at any time – **SEE Page 5** management

VT/VF present ↓

- Administer 1 **Shock**: (1) Manual biphasic @ 120-200 Joules (J) OR (2) AED which delivers device specific shock OR (3) Monophasic shock @ 360 J.
- Resume **CPR** for five cycles, then recheck Rhythm

VT/VF still present ↓

- Continue **CPR** while defibrillator is charging
- Administer 1 **Shock**: (1) manual biphasic (same as first shock [120-200J] or higher OR (2) AED - delivers device specific shock OR (3) Monophasic @ 360 J
- Resume **CPR** immediately after shock
- When Intravenous (IV) line or Intraosseous (IO) needle is available, give **vasopressor** during CPR either before or after the shock. Vasopressors include:
  - ○ **Epinephrine** 1 mg IV or IO (or 2-2.5 mg via endotracheal tube) repeated q 3-5 minutes
  - ○ **Vasopressin** 40 Units IV or IO to replace 1st or 2nd dose of epinephrine.
- Recheck rhythm after 5 cycles of CPR

VT/VF still present ↓

- Continue **CPR** while defibrillator is charging
- Administer 1 **Shock**: (1) manual biphasic (same as first shock [120-200J] or higher OR (2) AED - delivers device specific shock OR (3) Monophasic @ 360 J
- Resume **CPR** immediately after shock
- Consider antiarrhythmics (below) during CPR either before or after the shock.
  - ○ **Amiodarone** - 300 mg IV or IO X 1 dose. May repeat at 150 mg IV or IO X 1
  - ○ **Lidocaine** – 1 to 1.5 mg/kg IV or IO X 1 dose, then 0.5 to 0.75 mg/kg IV or IO every 5-10 minutes to a maximum of 3 doses or 3 mg/kg.
  - ○ **Consider magnesium** – (if Torsades de pointes) – 1-2 g IV/IO over 5-20 min.

↓

- Once return of spontaneous circulation, treat underlying etiology, consider amiodarone infusion 1mg/min X 6 hours plus 0.5 mg/min over 18 hours OR lidocaine 1-4 mg/min (depending upon which antiarrhythmic was used)

Asystole/Pulseless Electrical Activity[1]
(PEA = rhythm on monitor, without detectable pulse)

Pulseless Cardiac Arrest

- See Basic Resuscitation - **Page 3**.
- Administer O_2, place airway/ventilate, & attach monitor and defibrillator as soon as possible – without delaying compressions

Check Rhythm ↓

Ensure SHOCKABLE rhythm is NOT present: Ventricular Fibrillation (VF) or Ventricular Tachycardia (VT) – IF SHOCKABLE RHYTHM, see **Page 4**. If **NONSHOCKABLE:** Asystole or Pulseless Electrical Activity (PEA) see below.

Asystole/PEA ↓

- Resume CPR immediately for 5 cycles
- When Intravenous (IV) line or Intraosseous (IO) needle is available, give **vasopressor** during CPR either before or after the shock. Vasopressors include:
  - o **Epinephrine** - 1 mg IV or IO repeated q 3-5 minutes OR
  - o **Vasopressin** - 40 Units IV or IO to replace 1st or 2nd dose of epinephrine.
  - o **Atropine** – Consider 1 mg IV or IO for asystole or slow PEA rate, repeat every 3-5 minutes up to 3 doses.

Give 5 cycles of CPR ↓

- Recheck rhythm
- **SHOCKABLE** rhythm (VF/pulseless VT), see page 4
- **NONSHOCKABLE** rhythm: If asystole return to box above, If electrical activity, check pulse. If no pulse go to box above.

During Resuscitation ↓

Review for most frequent causes and treat accordingly

• Hypovolemia	• Tablets/toxins (drug OD, ingestion)
• Hypoxia	• Tamponade, cardiac
• Hydrogen ion – acidosis	• Tension pneumothorax
• Hyper/Hypo K+, other metabolic	• Thrombosis, coronary
• Hypoglycemia	• Thrombosis, pulmonary
• Hypothermia	• Trauma

[1] Pacing is not recommended for asystole. Norepinephrine and IV fluids are not recommended for cardiac arrest.

Acid Base Disorders

Anion Gap	• $Na^+ - (Cl^- + HCO_3^-)$ *Normal = 8-16 mEq/L*
Osmolal gap	• measured – calculated osmolality *Normal = 0-10 mOsm/L*
Calculated Osmolality	• $2 \times Na^+ + (glucose/18) + (BUN/2.8) + (ethanol/4.6) + (methanol/2.6) +$ (ethylene glycol/5) + (acetone/5.5) + (isopropanol/5.9)

Causes of ↑Anion Gap		Causes of ↓Anion Gap	Causes of ↑Osmol Gap
Methanol	Lactate[1]	Lithium, bromide	Alcohols (methanol,
Uremia	**E**thanol,ethylene	Multiple myeloma	ethylene glycol,
Diabetes	glycol	Albumin loss in	isopropanol)
Paraldehyde	**S**alicylates,	nephrotic syndrome	Sugar (glycerol,mannitol)
Iron, INH	starvation		Ketones (acetone)

[1]Lactate increased with multiple disorders (shock, seizures, cyanide, cellular toxins)

	Primary Disorder	Normal Compensation
Acid Base Rules of Compensation	Metabolic Acidosis	$PCO_2 = (1.5 \times HCO_3^- + 8) \pm 2$
	Acute Respiratory Acidosis	↑$\Delta HCO_3^- = (0.1 \times \Delta PCO_2$↑)
	Chronic Respiratory Acidosis	↑$\Delta HCO_3^- = (0.4 \times \Delta PCO_2$↑)
	Metabolic Alkalosis	$PCO_2 = (0.9 \times HCO_3^- + 9) \pm 2$
	Acute Respiratory Alkalosis	↓$\Delta HCO_3^- = (0.2 \times \Delta PCO_2$↓)
	Chronic Respiratory Alkalosis	↓$\Delta HCO_3^- = (0.4 \times \Delta PCO_2$↓)

Anaphylaxis

Clinical Criteria for Diagnosis of Anaphylaxis

National Institute of Allergy/Infectious Disease & Food Allergy/Anaphylaxis Network

Anaphylaxis is likely when any 1 of the following three (1, 2, or 3) are met.

1. Acute onset (minutes to hours) with involvement of skin, mucosa or both.
   AND at least one of the following:
   • Respiratory distress (e.g. dyspnea, wheeze, stridor, hypoxia)
   • Hypotension or symptoms of end organ dysfunction (collapse, syncope, incontinence)

2. ≥ 2 of following occur after exposure to likely allergen (minutes to several hours)
   • Skin-mucosa involved (e.g. hives, itch, flushing, swollen tongue/lips/uvula). Skin symptoms may be absent in up to 20% of cases.
   • Respiratory distress (e.g. dyspnea, wheeze, stridor, hypoxia)
   • Hypotension or symptoms of end organ dysfunction (collapse, syncope, incontinence)
   • Persistent GI symptoms (e.g. crampy abdominal pain, vomiting)

3. Hypotension occurring minutes to several hours after exposure to known allergen for a particular patient.
   • Systolic BP < 90 mm Hg or over a 30% ↓ from baseline (adult criteria)

Ann Emerg Med 2006; 47: 373

MANAGEMENT OF ANAPHYLAXIS - National Institute Allergy/Infectious Disease

Airway	Administer 100% O_2 & consider early intubation if airway edema		
Cardiac	Apply cardiac monitor, & pulse oximeter, assess vitals frequently		
Skin	Remove stinger, apply ice to bite, sting sites.		
Drugs	**Dose**	**Route**	**Indications & Detail**
epinephrine	0.01 mg/kg (max 0.5 mg) q5-15 min	IM	Treatment of choice, esp.if any 1 of the 3 clinical criteria (page 6) present. Inject IM into ant. lateral thigh, NOT subcutaneously.
	5-10 mcg (0.2 mcg/kg)	IV[1]	IV epinephrine if severe hypotension or cardiac arrest. Administer 5-10 mcg (0.2 mcg/kg) for hypotension and 0.5 mg IV for cardiac arrest. See IV drip, page 222.
other vasopressors	Consider norepinephrine, vasopressin, or metaraminol if fluids and epinephrine drip fail to maintain systolic BP > 90 mm Hg.		
normal saline	20 ml/kg	IV	Hypotension
Solu-Medrol	1-2 mg/kg	IV	Moderate/severe symptoms
Benadryl	1 mg/kg	IV/IM	moderate/severe symptoms (max 50 mg)
cimetidine	300 mg	IV/IM	H_2 antagonists are unproven in anaphylaxis & may cause wheezing
glucagon	1-5 mg or 5-15 mcg/min	IV	Administer bolus over 5 minutes. Consider if patient taking a β-blocker.
albuterol	2.5 mg	nebulized	Bronchospasm refractory to epinephrine
racemic epi.	guidelines do not recommend use or give parameters for use.		
Patient positioning	Hypotensive patients should be recumbent/supine. Leg elevation (Trendelenberg position) is unproven and potentially detrimental.		
Observation for delayed symptoms	Guidelines recommend observing all anaphylactic patients for 4-6 hours with longer observation for patients with severe or refractory symptoms or with a history of reactive airway disease.		
Follow Up	Prescribe epinephrine auto-injector (e.g. EpiPen, Twinjet [2 doses]) to all patients with cardiovascular or respiratory symptoms.		

[1]Monitor closely as life-threatening complications (e.g. ischemia, arrhythmias) can occur.
2nd Symposium on Definition/Management Anaphylaxis. *Ann Emerg Med* 2006; 47; 373.

Hereditary Angioedema (International Consensus Recommendations)

Autosomal dominant or functional C1 esterase inhibitor deficiency. Features: edema of the airway, face, or extremity edema,abdominal pain, nausea, vomiting, diarrhea. Trauma, stress, and drugs (esp. ACE inhibitors, estrogens) are typical precipitants.

Acute Management: (1) if isolated extremity, truncal edema, wait and see approach with increasing danazol dose in those already taking this agent may abort attack, (2) Otherwise early aggressive therapy with (a) C1-INH concentrate 500 units (if < 50 kg), 1000 units (if 50-100 kg) or 1500 units IV (if > 100 kg) [not available in US as of mid 2008, however, many patients acquire on own and bring with them to hospital], (b) if concentrate unavailable, administer 1-3 units of fresh frozen plasma although attacks may theoretically worsen (c) tranexamic acid (*Cyklokapron*) 25 mg/kg PO or IV up to 1 g q 3-4 h (max 72 mg/kg/day), (d) consider intubation if progressive laryngeal edema), (e) epinephrine (see dosing above) IV or IM may or may not be effective while steroids, and antihistamines are typically not effective.

J Allergy Clin Immunol 2007;102: 941; 2004; 629.

Anesthesia & Airway Management

Mask size	Weight (kg)	LMA length (cm)	LMA cuff volume (ml)	Largest ETT
3	30-60	19	15-20	6
4	60-80	19	25-30	6.5
5	> 80	19	30-40	7

Largest sized ET tube (int. diameter) that can pass through LMA for blind insertion

Rapid Sequence Intubation (RSI) - Preparation

- Ready 2 wall suctions/Yankauer, √ laryngoscope light, ready end tidal CO_2 detector
- select appropriate ET tube (7-7.5 mm internal diameter for adult females and 7.5-8 mm for males) and back-up 1 size smaller with stylet, check ET cuff
- prepare alternate airway plan: (eg. LMA above, bougie, cricothyrotomy)
- ensure pulse oximeter and cardiac monitor attached and working
- specify personnel for (1) cricoid pressure, (2) neck immobilization if trauma, (3) handling ET tube, (4) watching O_2 sat & cardiac monitors, and (5) medications
- position head - sniffing position if no trauma, in-line stabilization if trauma
- draw up all drugs in syringes and ensure secure IV access is available
- preoxygenate with 100% O_2 for at least 3-4 minutes (if possible), avoid bagging if adequate respirations, perform Sellick maneuver (cricoid pressure)

Pre-Medication

- consider lidocaine 1.5 mg/kg IV if head injured to blunt ICP response to laryngoscopy if etomidate or benzodiazepines used for RSI
- defasciculating agent (optional) if succinylcholine given (then wait 1.5-2 min)
- administer sedating, then paralyzing agent IV (see below)

Drugs for Rapid Sequence Intubation

Agent	Dose IV	Onset	Key Properties & Side Effects
Defasciculating drug	*(mg/kg)*	*(min)*	*Defasciculation (optional)*
rocuronium[1]	0.06	2	tachycardia, mild histamine release
succinylcholine	0.1	< 1	↑ICP, GI, and eye pressures
vecuronium	0.01	2.5-5	minimal tachycardia
Sedating drug	*(mg/kg)*	*(min)*	
etomidate[2]	0.3-0.4	1	minimal blood pressure decrease
fentanyl	2-10 mcg/kg	1	↑ICP, chest wall rigidity
ketamine	1-2	< 1	↑BP, ICP, GI, eye pressures
midazolam	0.1-0.3	2	causes hypotension
propofol	1-2.5	< 1	hypotension
thiopental	3-5	< 1	hypotension, bronchospasm
Paralyzing drug	*(mg/kg)*	*(min)*	
succinylcholine[3,4]	1-2	< 1	↑ICP, ↑ K+, ↑ GI and eye pressures
rocuronium[4]	0.6-1.2	2	tachycardia, mild histamine release
vecuronium	0.15 - 0.25	2.5-5	prolonged action

1→2→3 Standard drug sequence if no contraindications.

[4] Avoid succinylcholine (use rocuronium) if open globe, subacute burn, muscle dennervation, renal failure, pacemaker (relative contraindication).

Steps to Perform After Intubation	1. Check tube placement (CO_2 detector, esophageal detector device). Other methods including exam can be inaccurate. 2. Inflate cuff, then release cricoid pressure. 3. Normal depth of ET tube (cm) is ~3 X ET (at incisors) 4. Reassess patient's BP, pulse, and pulse oximetry. 5. Obtain CXR to verify correct ET depth (between T2-T4). 6. Sedate and consider long acting paralytics.

Initial Ventilator Settings for Specific Disorders (See targets below)

	Tidal Volume	FiO_2	Rate	I:E	PEEP
Typical	8-10 ml/kg	100%	10-12/minute	1:2	4 cm H_2O
Asthma/COPD	6	100%	6-8	1:4	4
ARDS	6	100%	10-12	1:2	4-14
Shock	8	100%	10-12	1:2	0-2

Guidelines for Initiating Mechanical Ventilation in Adults

Item	Initial Setting	Comments
Mode	Assist control	Ventilator assists if patient breathes on own
	Controlled	Patient cannot breath on own (e.g. paralyzed)
	IMV, SIMV	Set rate that allows patient to breathe on own
Tidal Volume	8-10 ml/kg	5-7 ml/kg if ↑peak airway pressures (e.g. asthma)
PSV	10 cm H_2O	10-35 CM H_2O – target of spontaneous = set TV
Rate	10-12/minute	
FiO_2	50-100%	Reduce as soon as possible to < 50%
PEEP	0–3 cm H_2O	3-20 cm H_2O if paO_2 < 60 & FiO_2 ≥ 50-60%
I:E	1:2	ARDS, pulmonary edema may require ≥ 2:1
Insp. flow	50-60L/min	If too slow, causes inadequate exhalation
Insp. pause	None	Leads to even ventilation and air trapping
Peak pressure	50 cm H_2O	Start at 20-30 cm if pressure cycled ventilator
Exp. retard	None	May prevent premature collapse of airway

Noninvasive Positive Pressure Ventilation (NPPV) Modes/Parameters

Volume mechanical	Breaths of 250-500 ml (4-8 ml/kg), pressures vary
Pressure mechanical	Pressure support or pressure control at 8-20 cm H_2O, End-expiratory pressure of 0-6 cm H_2O, volumes vary
BiPAP	Inspiratory pressure of 8 (6-14 cm) H_2O, End expiratory pressure of 4 (3-5 cm) H_2O, volumes vary, initial RR = 8
CPAP	5-13 cm H_2O, volumes vary
Weaning parameters for all NPPV modes	• Clinically stable for 4-6 hours • Respiratory rate < 24/minute & Heart rate < 110 • Compensated pH > 7.35, SaO_2 > 90-92%% on ≤ 3L O_2

See indications/contraindications (in COPD), page 151.

New Engl J Med 1997; 337: 1746

Visit (1) www.bt.cdc.gov for updates re: biologic/chemical agents, (2) www.cdc.gov/other.htm#states or www.astho.org/state.htm for state health departments, (3) www.orau.gov/reacts/care.htm or Call (615) 576-1004 re: radiation exposure. CDC Bioterrorism Preparedness and Response Center 1-770-488-7100 **General rules.** Gown, gloves, HEPA filter masks protect vs. most biological agents while soap/water removes most agents from skin. Hypochlorite (0.1%) bleach removes most contaminants from objects (do not use on skin unless VX exposure).

Anthrax – *Incubation* –Skin exposure leads to symptoms in a few days. Inhalation exposure leads to symptoms in < 1 week with possibility of symptoms occurring 2 months after exposure (and theoretically up to 100 days). *Features* – Initially patients develop fever/chills (> 95%), nausea/vomiting (80%), myalgia/headache (50% each), minimally-nonproductive cough (90%), then sweats, chest pain (60%), shortness of breath (80%), abdominal pain (30%), and shock. Rhinorrhea (~10%) & sore throat (20%) are rare. Skin - edema, then pruritic macule/papule, ulcer, painless, depressed eschar, lymphangitis, painful lymphadenopathy, *Diagnosis* – initial CXR-wide mediastinum (~70%) and effusion (~80%), CT chest with mediastinal adenopathy, Wright or Gram stain blood or CSF with gram positive bacilli, positive blood cultures, or ELISA for toxin. *Exposure* – (1) ciprofloxacin 500 mg PO BID X 60 d OR (2) doxycycline 100 mg PO BID X 60 (3) if organism penicillin sensitive, may switch to amoxicillin 500 mg PO TID X 60 d. If extremely high inhalation exposure, the CDC lists alternate options of above antibiotics for total of 100 days with or without vaccination (3 doses over 4 weeks). Ciprofloxacin or amoxicillin is recommended in exposed pregnant women. Switch to penicillin or amoxicillin once sensitivity known. *Disease treatment* for inhalational, GI, or oropharyngeal: (1) ciprofloxacin 400 mg IV q 12 hours. OR (2) doxycycline 100 mg IV q 12 h [do not use if meningitis possible] **PLUS** 1 or 2 of following agents: clindamycin, rifampin, vancomycin, penicillin, ampicillin, chloramphenicol, imipenem, or clarithromycin. Switch to combined [(1) or (2) above plus added agent(s)] oral antibiotics when clinically appropriate and continue antibiotics for total of 60 days (IV and PO combined). Steroids are a recommended option for patients with severe edema or meningitis.

Blistering Agents – Mustard gas - Severe skin, lung, or eye damage with delayed blisters up to 4-12 hours. Mustard passes through clothes without burning & through living tissue without symptoms for hours. Smell - mustard, onion, or garlic. Skin is red & blisters form late and skin initially may only look like 1st or 2nd degree burn. Airway irritation is prominent early. *Treat* First decontaminate and remove all clothing, jewelry. Remove skin droplets by blotting, cleanse with soap and water or chloramine solution. IV N-acetylcysteine may decontaminate systemically. Treat skin injury as chemical burn, with irrigation, topical antibiotics. Mild to moderate eye exposures may irrigate with 2.5% sodium thiosulfate. **Lewisite -** immediate burn eyes, nose, & skin (flushed). Treat by decontaminating & using dimercaprol.

Botulinum – _Onset_ – 1-4 days. *Features* – afebrile, descending symmetric flaccid paralysis starts at cranial nerves. Normal mental status. 4D's: Dry mouth, dysarthria, dysphonia, dysphagia & diplopia are prominent. Respiratory failure ± in 24 hours. _Diagnosis_ – Check gag, cough reflexes, inspiratory force, oxygen saturation. Consult local and state health department (prior page). Nasal swab ELISA or serum, food bioassay. Gastric or stool samples may be tested if airborne or food borne. _Treatment_ – Supportive, wash skin with soap/H_2O. Cleanse objects with 0.1% hypochlorite (bleach) solution. Trivalent (vs. A,B,C) or US Army heptavalent (vs. A to G) antitoxin (equine) may prevent progression. 1st, skin test with 0.2 ml diluted in 2 ml NS SC. If not allergic, dilute 10 ml vial with 90 ml NS and administer slow IV. If allergic, desensitize as per Crotalidae antivenin page 65.

Brucellosis –aerosol or food source *Incubation* – 1-4 weeks. *Features* – fever, headache, fatigue, colitis, hepatitis, arthritis, lymph nodes, osteomyelitis, epididymoorchitis, endocarditis _Diagnosis_ – blood & bone marrow culture, or serology. _Prophylaxis_ – doxycycline 100 mg PO BID OR ciprofloxacin 500 mg PO BID X 3 weeks. _Treatment_ – (1) doxycycline 100 mg PO bid + rifampin 600-1200 mg PO daily X 6 wks OR (2) doxycycline X 6 wks + streptomycin 15 mg/kg IM q day X 3 wks
Cyanide – colorless, inhale > ingest, bitter almond smell. H/A, dyspnea, HTN, ↑ HR then apnea, ↓BP, ↓ HR, seizure, dysrhythmias, cell death. Retinal veins cherry red. Labs – anion gap acidosis (lactate), venous pO_2 > 40 mm Hg. Treat with 100% O_2, (± hyperbaric O2).Two cyanide antidote kits exist(1) *Cyanokit*: hydrocobalamin 5g IV over 15 min, may repeat X1 (2) standard *Cyanide Antidote Kit*: (2a) inhale amyl nitrate 30 sec/min until IV meds ready + (2b) Na⁺ nitrite 300 mg (10 ml of 3% solution) IV over ≥ 5 minutes. Use less if anemic. May ↓BP and induce methemoglobinemia (goal MetHb ≤ 25%) + (2c) Na⁺ thiosulfate 12.5 g (50 ml of 25% solution) IV over 10-20 minutes. Some experts recommend using both kits (in separate IVs) *Ann Emerg Med* 2008; 51: 338.

Nerve Agents – **[GF, Sarin (GB), Soman (GD), Tabun (GA), VX, Substance 33 (V-gas)]** –inhaled & dermally absorbed cholinesterase inhibitors (organophosphates). VX may persist on scene for weeks. Symptoms: CNS Δ (confused, resp depression, seizures), muscarinic (SLUDGE; salivate, lacrimate, urinate, defecation, GI, emesis, & miosis, bronchoconstrict, ↓HR) & nicotinic (muscles weak, HTN, ↑HR, ± mydriasis). Treat (1) decontaminate (wear protection) dermally, soap/H_2O. Since hydrolysis converts VX into longer lasting/toxic metabolic, experts recommend using 0.1% bleach (diluted hypochlorite household sol'n) to topically decontaminate VX. Avoid abrading skin.,(2) resp support (3) ↑dose atropine, (4) pralidoxime (esp. Sarin, VX, not Soman), See page 176. (5) Bispyridinium or H oximes (e.g. obidoxime, HI-6) may reactivate aged cholinesterase that is resistant to pralidoxime. (esp.Soman)
Phosgene – smells like newly mowed hay. Inhalation causes irritation to eyes, nose, skin with tissue damage in minutes. Chest tightness, difficulty breathing & delayed pulmonary edema (2-24 hours). A 24-48 hr latency after initial irritant or asymptomatic phase may occur. Decontaminate skin with water irrigation. Remove clothing. Medical personnel involved in topical decontamination require activated charcoal protective mask. Observe for 6 hours due to latency. Treat supportively.

Phosgene oxime (CX) is a urticariant/nettle gas that is topically absorbed and produces immense dermal pain penetrating to muscle layer. It penetrates garments and rubber acting rapidly. The skin is initially gray, blanched, then severe itching, hives, and blisters. Blanched area forms wheals that turn brown in 24 hours, forming eschar. CX also irritates eyes & lungs (ARDS). Decontaminate skin with water, or M291 military decontamination kit. Otherwise treat supportively.

PFIB (perfluoroisobutylene) gas can be made from heated *Teflon* and causes similar picture/more toxicity than phosgene. Initial eye, airway, chest irritation with early or delayed pulmonary edema after latent period. Shivering, sweating, fever, and tachypnea may occur similar to metal fume fever. Medical personnel require positive pressure air respiratory (charcoal respirator is inadequate). Ventilate with air to decontaminate and DO NOT irrigate with water if PFIB exposure. This results in hydrofluoric acid (HFl) formation which requires intensive burn therapy and IV and local calcium gluconate (contact local poison center if HFl is a concern). Observe 6 hours due to latency. Otherwise, treat supportively.

Plague – *Onset* 1-6 days. *Features* – bubonic (malaise, fever, purulent lymphadenitis), sepsis, or pneumonic (esp. weaponized) plague. Weaponized symptoms – fever, cough, dyspnea, hemoptysis, only rare cervical buboes. GI upset, vomiting, diarrhea common. CXR – patchy/consolidated pneumonia. *Diagnosis* – Wright-Giemsa or gram stain of sputum, node, or blood (gram negative, bipolar/safety pin shaped) or culture of blood, lymph node aspirate or sputum. Specific tests (e.g. PCR) available at state health departments (page 10) *Chemoprophylaxis* (1) doxycycline 100 mg PO BID OR (2) ciprofloxacin 500 mg PO BID X 7 days. *Treatment* – (1) streptomycin 1 g IM q 12 hours [not currently available in US] OR (2) gentamicin 5 mg/kg IV/IM q 24h OR (3) gentamicin 2 mg IV/IM load, then 1.7 mg/kg IV/IM q 8 hours OR (4) doxycycline 100 mg IV q 12 hours OR (5) ciprofloxacin 400 mg IV q 12 hours – continue for 10 days total. Gentamicin dosed as above preferred in pregnant women although doxycycline or ciprofloxacin are alternatives. May switch to oral agents upon clinical improvement.

Q fever – *Coxiella burnetii* *Incubation* 10-40 days, *Features* – influenza-like: fever, atypical pneumonia/hilar nodes, hepatitis. *Diagnosis* – ELISA, *Treatment* – Cipro or doxycycline X 15-21 days [anthrax dose], macrolides also may be effective.

Radiation – *Features* - acute radiation syndrome – 1st nausea, vomiting, diarrhea, fatigue X 1-2 days, ± burns (± 7-10 days to blister) 2nd symptom free latency (absent if > 1000 rads), 3rd overt symptoms: GI (vomiting, diarrhea, bleed, sepsis), CNS (confusion, edema), Heme ($\downarrow$WBC [lymphocytes] Hb & platelets ± delayed 2-3 weeks if low dose) *Treatment* – Protective clothes, radiation monitor for personnel. Treat trauma, externally decontaminate. Admit if ≥ 200 rads. If no symptoms 1st 24 hours, exposure is < 75 rads. CBC& diff. q 6-8 hours. Reverse isolation, anti-emetics, colony stimulation factor, stem cell, platelet & Hb transfusion, tissue & blood typing (family/marrow transplant). Prophylactic antibiotics, antivirals, anti-fungals prn.

Radioactive fallout from radioactive iodine (e.g. nuclear reactor) causes exposure via inhalation, or ingestion (e.g. cow's milk) resulting in cancer (esp. thyroid).
Depending on thyroid exposure (in rads), potassium iodide (KI) is recommended by the CDC.

Population	Predicted thyroid exposure	Daily KI[1] dose
Adults over 40 years	> 500 rad	130 mg
Adults > 18 to 40 years	≥ 10	130 mg
Pregnancy or lactating	≥ 5	130 mg
> 12 to 18 years (if ≥ 70 kg, treat as adult)	≥ 5	65 mg
> 3 to 12 years	≥ 5	65 mg
> 1 mo to 3 years (dilute in milk, formula, H₂0)	≥ 5	32 mg
0-1 months	≥ 5	16 mg

[1]Do not give if known iodine sensitive, dermatitis herpetiformis, or hypocomplementemic vasculitis & use cautiously if thyroid disease. KI protects only thyroid gland from radioiodines, offers no protection from external radiation, does not protect from effect of exposure to other radioactive materials. KI lasts 24 h, use daily until no risk.

www.fda.gov/cder/guidance/index.htm

Ricin (or **Abrin**)– type II ribosome inactivation from castor beans/seeds. *Onset* – 4-8 h after inhaled. *Features* - ingestion - GI distress, necrosis, hepatitis; inhalation – pulm necrosis, shock. Metabolic acidosis, hepatitis, hematuria, renal failure. *Diagnosis* – Serum or resp. secretion ELISA, *Treat*– remove clothes, cleans objects with 0.1% hypochlorite (bleach), wash skin with soap/water, provide supportive care, oral charcoal if PO ingestion. If injected, excision of area may be useful.

Smallpox – orthopox virus. *Incubation* – 7-17 days. *Features* – fever, headache, backache. Maculopapular rash face > mouth/pharynx, mucosa & arms/legs, palms, soles (*Varicella causes rash on trunk > other areas, at different stages, & no palm/sole involvement*). 1-2 days rash is vesicular, then pustular. Round/tense pustules deeply embedded with crusting on 8-9th day. All lesions evolve at same rate. A rapidly progressive form with sepsis, skin petechiae, hemorrhage can occur as well as a malignant form with abrupt onset, with flattened confluent skin lesions never progressing to pustules. *Diagnosis* - Vesicle/pustule fluid or scabs can be examined by electron microscopy. *Prevention* - Vaccine may prevent disease if given within 3-4 days of exposure. Vaccine reactions including generalized or progressive vaccinia, eczema vaccinatum and periocular infections are treated with vaccinia immune globulin 0.6 ml/kg divided over 24-36 hours since volume is 42 ml in a 70 kg adult. May repeat in 2-3 days. *Treatment* – decontaminate surfaces with 0.1% hypochlorite (bleach) or quaternary ammonia. Isolate if ill and provide support.

Staphylococcal enterotoxin B –inhaled or ingested. *Onset* – 1-12 hours *Features* – sudden fever (often ≥ 40°C/104°F) for up to 5 days, headache, chills, dyspnea, vomiting, diarrhea (if swallow aerosol), & cough up to 4 weeks. CXR - normal, ARDS can develop. *Diagnosis* – Abrupt onset of fever, respiratory symptoms in large numbers of exposed presenting at same time, normal CXR, & nonprogression. Toxin - difficult to ID. Nasal swab ELISA in 1st 24 h may be +. *Treat:* supportively

Trichothecene Mycotoxins – fungal toxins (e.g. yellow rain) inhibit protein & DNA synthesis, and destroy cells. <u>Onset</u> – minutes to hours. <u>Features</u> -Skin damage (blisters). Ingestion: vomiting, bloody diarrhea, and GI bleed. Inhalation: acute eye pain/red, tears, bloody rhinorrhea, hemoptysis + skin findings, ARDS, ↓ BP, bone marrow depression and sepsis. <u>Diagnosis</u> – gas liquid chromatography blood, urine, stool, lung washings. <u>Treatment</u> – supportive, ascorbic acid, dexamethasone, GI decontamination/lavage, skin (soap/water), eye (saline irrigation).

Tularemia – *Francisella tularensis* (gram negative bacillus). <u>Incubation</u> – 1-14 days. <u>Features</u> –glandular (nodes without ulcer), ulceroglandular (indurated, punched out ulcers with lymphadenitis, draining nodes with 10-30% pneumonic). Pneumonic & septic tularemia are weaponized forms – influenza-like symptoms without pneumonia or atypical pneumonia, hilar nodes (not generalized mediastinal widening as in anthrax), effusion. Abdominal pain, vomiting, diarrhea predominate early. <u>Diagnosis</u> – gram stain sputum (small gram negative coccobacilli), serology (ELISA), culture sputum, fasting gastric aspirate, pharyngeal washings. <u>Chemoprophylaxis</u> – doxycycline 100 mg PO BID X 14 days OR ciprofloxacin 500 mg PO BID X 14 days. <u>Treatment</u> – (1) gentamicin 5 mg/kg IV/IM q 24 h X 10 days OR (2) streptomycin 1 g IM q 12 hours X 10 days OR (3) doxycycline 100 mg IV q 12 hours X 14-21 days OR (4) ciprofloxacin 400 mg IV q 12 hours X 10 days. Switch to oral medications when clinically improved.

Viral Encephalitides – (Venezuelan equine encephalitis/VEE, eastern/EEE & western equine/WEE) highly infectious by aerosol. <u>Incubation</u> – VEE 2-6 days, EEE/WEE 7-14 days. <u>Features</u> – fever, headache, myalgias. VEE causes symptoms in most. Only 0.5-4 % have neurologic involvement. EEE will kill 50-75%. <u>Diagnosis</u> – ↓ serum WBC count, CSF – pleocytosis/lymphocytosis, acutely serum IgM antibodies, ELISA, & hemagglutination-inhibiting antibodies are positive by 2nd week. <u>Treatment</u> – no person-person transmission, provide supportive care.

Viral Hemorrhagic fevers (VHF) –due to a variety of RNA viruses (e.g. Marburg, Ebola, yellow fever). <u>Incubation</u> – 4-21 days. <u>Features</u> – fever, myalgias, prostration, early conjunctival injection, mild hypotension, flushing, petechial hemorrhages. Variety of skin rashes occur –online pictures are available at www.jama.ama-assn.org/ *JAMA* 2002; 287: 2391. Later jaundice, DIC picture with hepatitis, renal failure and CV collapse. <u>Diagnosis</u> – ↓ WBC count (↑WBCs with Lassa fever), anemia or hemoconcentration,↓ platelets, ↑LFTs,↑PT/PTT, ↓ fibrinogen. Diagnose by ELISA, or PCR state or federal lab. <u>Prophylaxis</u> – yellow fever vaccine is available but disease onset would occur before vaccine becomes effective. Health care workers require personal air purifying respirators or N-95 mask, negative isolation rooms, complete torso, leg, shoe, face coverings, and goggles. All medical equipment should be dedicated to single patient. Disinfect objects with 0.1% hypochlorites (bleach) <u>Treatment</u> –If VHF due to unknown cause, arenavirus, or bunyavirus administer ribavirin 30 mg/kg IV (max 2 g) X1, then 16 mg/kg (max 1 g) IV q 6 hours X 4 days, then 8 mg/kg IV (max 500 mg) q8 hours X 6 days. If mass casualties, load with ribavirin 2000 mg PO, followed by 600 mg PO BID (if > 75 kg) OR [400 mg PO q AM + 600 mg PO q PM (if ≤ 75 kg)] X 10 days. Otherwise, supportive care.

Burns and Burn Therapy

Estimation of Total Body Surface Area Burned (Add 2nd + 3rd degree)

9%

18% front

9%   9%

18% back

1%

18%   18%

Admission and Transfer Criteria for Patients with Significant Burns

Admission Criteria[1]
Burn TBSA ≥ 15% (2nd + 3rd degree)
Burn TBSA ≥ 10% (age > 50 years)
Burn TBSA ≥ 2-5% (3rd degree)
Burns to hands, feet, face, perineum
Minor chemical burn
Associated carbon monoxide poisoning
Inadequate family support or known or suspected abuse
Severe underlying medical disease (e.g. emphysema, coronary artery disease, diabetes, renal insufficiency)

Transfer to Burn Center[1]
Burn TBSA ≥ 25% (2nd + 3rd degree)
Burn TBSA ≥ 20% (age > 50 years)
Burn TBSA ≥ 10% (3rd degree)
3rd degree hands, feet, face, perineum
Major chemical or electrical burn
Respiratory tract injury
Associated major trauma
Circumferential limb burns

[1]TBSA - total body surface area

Fluid Resuscitation in Burn Victims

Parkland formula	• Lactated ringers 4 ml/kg/%burn TBSA[1] in 1st 24 h (after burn) + maintenance fluid, with ½ over 1st 8 h, & ½ over next 16 h
Alternatives	• *Amended Parkland formula*: for ED stays < 8 hours. IV rate over maintenance (ml/h) = [weight(kg) X burn TBSA%] ÷ 4 • *Carvajal's formula*: Carvajal's solution 5,000 ml/m² of burn + maintenance 2000 ml/m² in 24h, with ½ over the 1st 8 hours and ½ over the subsequent 16 hours.

[1]BSA = body surface area. Note: $(n^{1/2}$ = square root of $n)$

BSA (m²) = $([$Height (cm) X Weight (kg)$] ÷ 3600)^{1/2}$ **OR**

BSA (m²) = $([$Height (inches) X Weight (pounds)$] ÷ 3131)^{1/2}$

ECG Diagnosis of Arrhythmia, Blocks, and Medical Disorders

Normal Adult ECG (small box: 1 mm = 0.04 sec; large box: 5 mm = 0.20 sec)
- *P wave* - < 0.10 sec, ↑ in I, II, and ↓ in aVR; *PR interval* - 0.12 - 0.20 sec.
- *QRS complex* - 0.05-0.10 seconds; normally ↑ in I, II, V5, V6; ↓ in aVR,V1; transition zone in V3; ↑ or ↓ in aVL, aVF,III; left chest leads height is < 27 mm.
- *Q wave-* normally < 0.04 seconds, and < 25% height of following R.
- *QT interval* - 0.34-0.42 seconds or 40% of RR interval. (varies with sex)
- *QTc* (corrected QT) = QT interval/square root of R-R. Normal < 0.47 seconds.
- *T wave* - ↑ in I, V6, and ↓ in aVR; Normal ↓ T waves may be found in III, aVL,V1 : Abnormal ↓ T waves may signify LVH (esp. V6), LBBB, ischemia, MI.
- *Axis :* Normal: -30 degrees to +100 degrees. *Left axis deviation* (LAD): -30 to -90 degrees. *Right axis deviation* (RAD): +100 to +180 or -90 to -180 degrees.

Conduction Blocks
- *1st degree AV block* - PR interval > 0.2 seconds, P precedes each QRS.
- *2nd degree AV block* - (type 1/Wenckebach) - increasing PR interval until QRS dropped. (type 2) - QRS dropped without increasing PR interval.
- *3rd degree AV block* - P and QRS are independent. Fixed P-P intervals.
- *Right bundle branch block* (RBBB) (1) QRS ≥ 0.12 sec (± 0.1-0.12 sec) (2) R-R'/R-S-R' in V1/V2 (3) ST-T opposite to terminal QRS (4) S in I, aVL,V5,V6.
- *Left bundle branch block* (LBBB) - (1) QRS ≥ 0.12 sec (2) R or R-R' in I, aVL, or V6; (3) negative wave (rS or QS) in V1, (4) no septal Q wave of 0.01 or 0.02 in I and V6. (5) ST-T waves directed opposite to the terminal 0.04 sec QRS.
- *Anterior Hemiblock* - LAD > - 45, QRS 0.10-0.12 sec, small Q in I, aVL; R in II, III, and aVF; terminal R in aVR.

Posterior Hemiblock - RAD; QRS 0.10-0.12 sec; S in I; Q in II, III, aVF.

Hypertrophy
- *Right Atrial* - P > 2.5 mm in II or large diphasic P in V1 (tall initial phase)
- *Left Atrial* - diphasic P in V1 with large terminal downward phase.
- *Right Ventricular* (RVH) - RAD > 100, incomplete RBBB in V1; R>S - V1; R > 5 mm - V1; decreasing R in V1 to V4; ST depression + flipped T's V1-V3, ± RAH.
- *Left Ventricular* (LVH) – Romhilt and Estes criteria, Cornell criteria below

Romhilt & Estes Criteria for Left Ventricular Hypertrophy[1]	Points
QRS with largest R or S in limb leads ≥ 20 mm **or** S in V1 or V2 ≥ 30 mm **or** R in V5 or V6 ≥ 30 mm	3
ST-T down sloping without digitalis (3 points) or with digitalis (1 point)	1 or 3
Left atrial enlargement	3
Left axis deviation < 30 degrees or more	2
QRS duration > 0.9 seconds	1
Intrinsicoid deflection (onset QRS to apex R) in V5/V6 ≥ 0.05 sec.	1
Total points ≥ 5 = definite LVH, total points = 4 signifies probable LVH	
Cornell Criteria for Diagnosing Left Ventricular Hypertrophy[2,3]	
R in AVL + S in V3 ≥ 2.8 mV (males) & ≥ 2.0 mV (females)	

[1] 40-50% sensitivity, 80-90% specificity, [2] 42% sensitivity, 96% specificity

[3] R in AVL > 1.1 mV is also 97% specific for LVH

Benign Early Repolarization (BER)

Criteria for BER include (1) wide spread ST elevation (90% < 2 mm in precordial leads, and < 0.5 mm in limb leads) with precordial > limb leads, (2) J point elevation, (3) concave initial upsloping of ST segment (4) notching/irregular contour of J point (5) prominent concordant T waves (6) stability of ECG over time

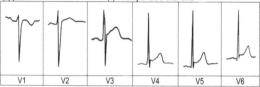

| V1 | V2 | V3 | V4 | V5 | V6 |

ECG Findings in Pericarditis

- ST segment elevation is typically diffuse involving ↑ in I, II, and III or at least 2 bipolar limb leads and precordial leads V1 through V6 or V2 through V6.
- ST depression is common in aVR,+ may occur in II and V1. ST segment ↑ is typically concave upward + ≤ 5 mm height. Pathologic Q waves are rare unless MI. PR segment depression is common inferior + lateral (arrow lead II).
- Sequence of ST-T changes: (1) initial ST ↑, (2) ST returns to baseline before T waves flip (↓) (3) T wave ↓ is usually ≤ 5 mm (4) T waves normalize.
- Low voltage QRS or electrical alternans suggests pericardial fluid.
- ± Height of ST segment/T wave > 0.25 in V5, V6, or I.

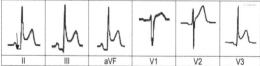

| II | III | aVF | V1 | V2 | V3 |

ECG Findings in Medical Disorders[1] (See ECG examples, page 45, 46)

Disorder	Class ECG Findings (not necessarily most common)
CNS bleed[2]	Diffuse, symmetric deep T wave inversion, U's, prolonged QT
COPD	RAD (negative lead I), overall low voltage, RAH ± RBBB
Pulmonary emboli	ST/T wave changes, RAD, RBBB. large S in I, Q in III, T in III
Hyperkalemia[2]	Peaked T's, wide then flat P's, wide QRS and QT, sine wave
Hypokalemia[2]	Flat T waves, U waves, U > T waves, ST depression
Calcium[2]	High calcium - short QT, low calcium - long QT interval
Digoxin effect	Downward curve of ST segment, flat/inverted T's, shorter QT
Digoxin toxicity	PVC's (60%), AV block (20%), Ectopic SVT (25%), V tach.
Hypothyroidism	Sinus bradycardia, low voltage, ST ↓, flat or inverted T waves

Myocardial injury and ischemia.

Location	ECG ST elevation or Q waves	Coronary Arteries involved
Anterior	V2-V4	Left anterior descending (LAD)
Anteroseptal	V1-V4	LAD
Anterolateral	V1-V6, I, aVL	LAD, diagonal
Inferior	II, III, aVF	Right coronary, circumflex
Lateral	I, aVL, V5, V6	Circumflex, diagonal
Posterior	large R -V1,V2,V3, reciprocal ST ↓	Right coronary artery
Posteriolat.	V6-V9	Right coronary artery

ST ↑ ≥ 1 mm = injury/infarction if found in ≥ 2 contiguous leads. Abnormal Q waves are ≥ 0.04 seconds wide & > ¼ R wave height in same lead (except aVL where Q > ½ R wave height is abnormal).

Typical Sequence of ECG Findings in Acute MI

- An early marked increase in R wave voltage, then prominent (hyperacute) T waves (esp. > 5 mm) - peaked and symmetric ~ church steeple (wider than ↑K).
- ST segment elevation that can be flat, convex, or concave upward.[1]
- Q waves > 0.04 sec other than leads aVR + V1 and T wave flattening/inversion.

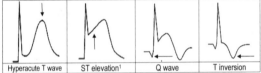

Hyperacute T wave	ST elevation[1]	Q wave	T inversion

[1] While it is often taught that ST elevation during myocardial infarction is typically convex (∩), one author looked at consecutive anterior wall MIs and found horizontal ST (—) elevation was present in 53%, concave ST (∪) elevation in 31% and convex elevation present in 16%. Convex ST elevation patients had a lower ejection fraction and higher CK enzyme elevation. However, patients with Non-MI ST elevation have concave configuration in up to 94%. *Am J Emerg Med* 2002; 20: 609. *Am Heart J* 1999; 137: 522.

Predictive Value of Initial ECG in Acute MI	Sensitivity	Specificity
New Q waves or ST segment elevation	40%	> 90%
Above or ST segment depression	75%	80%
Any of above or prior ischemia/infarction changes	85%	76%
Any of above or nonspecific ST-T changes	90%	65%

Ann Emerg Med 1990; 19: 1359

Diagnosis of Acute MI in Presence of Left Bundle Branch Block

Criteria for Diagnosis of Acute MI (Sgarbossa criteria)	Points
ST segment elevation ≥ 1 mm concordant (same direction) as QRS	5
ST segment depression ≥ 1 mm in leads V1, V2, or V3	3
ST segment elevation ≥ 5 mm and discordant (opposite) with QRS	2

Total ≥ 3 is 36-78% sensitive, 90-96% specific for acute MI. *New Engl J Med* 1996;334: 481.
A new or presumed new LBBB is presumed evidence of MI & need for intervention.

Arrhythmias – Identification – See algorithm page 21

- <u>Multifocal atrial tachycardia</u> - 3 or more different P waves, normal QRS complex - associated with COPD, hypoxia, digoxin or theophylline toxicity, or heart disease.
- <u>Paroxysmal atrial tachycardia</u> - P's occur before each QRS with rate 150-250.
- <u>Paroxysmal supraventricular tachycardia</u> - Rate 120-250, narrow or wide QRS (if Bundle Branch Block or pre-excitation), P waves are visible or hidden in QRS
- <u>Atrial flutter</u> - atrial rate 200-400 saw tooth pattern (esp. leads II and III), common ventricular rate of 150 due to 2:1 block (with atrial rate of 300).
- <u>Atrial fibrillation</u> - highly irregular rhythm, no discernible P waves, ventricular rate may be rapid or slow depending on conduction.
- <u>Ventricular tachycardia</u> - ≥ 3 premature vent. beats in a row, broad QRS rhythm at 100-250/min. Fusion beats, AV dissociation, LAD, precordial concordance.
- <u>Ventricular fibrillation</u> (VF) - irregular chaotic baseline, no beats, no BP.
- <u>Torsades de pointes</u> - twisting QRS, prolonged QT interval, may progress to VF.

Differentiation of Wide Complex SVT from Ventricular Tachycardia

Feature	Suggests SVT	Suggests VT[1]
Age	< 35 years	> 50 years
Prior MI		95% specific for VT
Past Hx	Prior SVT	Angina, Congestive heart failure
Symptoms and BP	Not useful differentiator	Not useful differentiator
AV dissociation	Not applicable (n/a)	specific for VT
QRS duration	n/a	≥ 0.14 seconds (≥ 0.16 if LBBB)
QRS axis	n/a	-90 to ± 180 degrees (NW axis) or concordance in all precordial leads
V1 or V2 if LBBB	n/a	R > .03 sec, or > .07 sec to S nadir
V6 if LBBB	n/a	QR or QS
V1 if RBBB	triphasic QRS or R'>R	Monophasic R, QR, RS
V6 if RBBB	triphasic QRS	R/S < 1, QS, QR

[1] Absence of features suggesting VT DOES NOT imply SVT is more likely. No single feature is 100% accurate at differentiating between VT/SVT. If in doubt, treat as VT.

Synchronized Cardioversion (not for pulseless VT or VF)

If arrhythmia with ventricular rate > 150 (generally not needed ≤ 150), prepare for immediate cardioversion if hypotension, altered mental status, ischemic chest pain, pulmonary edema. May give brief trial of medications based on specific arrhythmia.

⬇

Administer O_2, insert IV, premedicate, and prepare to intubate.

⬇

Synchronized Cardioversion

- **Rhythms** - VT, SVT, atrial fibrillation and flutter
- **Energy levels**– 100J, 200J, 300J, 360 J monophasic energy dose or equivalent biphasic (exception, SVT and atrial flutter – start with 50 joules)
- **If delays** in synchronization & critically ill, go straight to unsynchronized mode

Symptomatic **BRADYCARDIA** Management

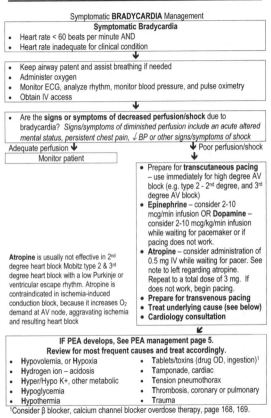

Symptomatic Bradycardia

- Heart rate < 60 beats per minute AND
- Heart rate inadequate for clinical condition

↓

- Keep airway patent and assist breathing if needed
- Administer oxygen
- Monitor ECG, analyze rhythm, monitor blood pressure, and pulse oximetry
- Obtain IV access

↓

- Are the **signs or symptoms of decreased perfusion/shock** due to bradycardia? *Signs/symptoms of diminished perfusion include an acute altered mental status, persistent chest pain, ↓ BP or other signs/symptoms of shock*

Adequate perfusion ↓   ↓ Poor perfusion/shock

| Monitor patient |

Atropine is usually not effective in 2nd degree heart block Mobitz type 2 & 3rd degree heart block with a low Purkinje or ventricular escape rhythm. Atropine is contraindicated in ischemia-induced conduction block, because it increases O_2 demand at AV node, aggravating ischemia and resulting heart block

- Prepare for **transcutaneous pacing** – use immediately for high degree AV block (e.g. type 2 - 2nd degree, and 3rd degree AV block)
- **Epinephrine** – consider 2-10 mcg/min infusion OR **Dopamine** – consider 2-10 mcg/kg/min infusion while waiting for pacemaker or if pacing does not work.
- **Atropine** – consider administration of 0.5 mg IV while waiting for pacer. See note to left regarding atropine. Repeat to a total dose of 3 mg. If does not work, begin pacing.
- **Prepare for transvenous pacing**
- **Treat underlying cause (see below)**
- **Cardiology consultation**

↘

IF PEA develops, See PEA management page 5.
Review for most frequent causes and treat accordingly.

- Hypovolemia, or Hypoxia
- Hydrogen ion – acidosis
- Hyper/Hypo K+, other metabolic
- Hypoglycemia
- Hypothermia
- Tablets/toxins (drug OD, ingestion)[1]
- Tamponade, cardiac
- Tension pneumothorax
- Thrombosis, coronary or pulmonary
- Trauma

[1]Consider β blocker, calcium channel blocker overdose therapy, page 168, 169.

Tachycardia (Narrow & Wide complex) with pulse

- Keep airway patent, assist breathing, and support circulation if needed.
- Administer oxygen, secure airway (intubate if needed) and obtain IV access.
- Monitor ECG, analyze rhythm, monitor blood pressure, and pulse oximetry.
- Diagnose and treat Identified causes (eg. fluids, blood).

- **Is Patient Unstable?** (new altered mentation, persistent chest pain, ↓BP, or other signs of shock). Rate related symptoms are uncommon if HR < 150/min.

Stable ↙	Unstable ↘
• Ensure IV access is present	• Immediately cardiovert-page 19.
• Obtain 12 leak ECG or rhythm strip	• Sedate beforehand if time permits.
• Is the QRS width narrow (QRS < 0.12 seconds)?	• If PEA develops, see page 5.
	• Consider cardiology consult.

Narrow ↓   **(If Wide Complex – See box below) → ↘**

- **Narrow Complex + Regular Rhythm** present - (1) Vagal maneuvers (2) Give adenosine 6 mg IV push, if do not convert, give 12 mg IV q 2 min X 2
  - **If regular rhythm converts –** Reentry SVT was probably present. Observe for recurrence and treat recurrence with adenosine or longer acting AV node blocking drugs (e.g. diltiazem, β blockers)
  - **If regular rhythm does not convert –** Possible atrial flutter, atrial or junctional tachycardia. Control rate (diltiazem or β blockers [caution if CHF or pulmonary disease). Treat underlying cause & consider cardiology consult.
- **Narrow Complex + Irregular Rhythm –** Probable atrial fibrillation or flutter or multifocal atrial tachycardia. Consider expert consultation and control rate using diltiazem or β blockers (see treatment guidelines, page 22-24)

Wide Complex Tachycardia (QRS ≥ 0. 12 seconds)

- **Regular Rhythm –** if ventricular tachycardia or uncertain rhythm (see page 26)
  - **Amiodarone –** 150 mg IV over 10 min, repeat prn to max 2.2 g in 24 hours.
  - **Elective synchronized cardioversion –** page 19.
- **Regular Rhythm –** If SVT with aberrancy, give adenosine (see dosing above)
- **Irregular Rhythm –** If Afib with aberrancy, see guidelines, next page. If pre-excitation atrial fibrillation (WPW), expert consultation advised and avoid AV nodal blocking agent (adenosine, diltiazem, verapamil, digoxin). Consider **amiodarone** 150 mg IV over 10 min or **procainamide** (see next page)
- **If recurrent polymorphic Ventricular Tachycardia[1]** –expert consult, page 26.
- **Torsade de pointes[1] –** magnesium 1-2 g IV in 5-60 min + infusion, see page 26.

[1] See www.qtdrugs.org for agents that prolong QT interval.

American College of Cardiology (ACC)/American Heart Association (AHA) Guidelines for Managing Atrial Fibrillation/Flutter[1]

- <u>History and examination</u> to determine (1) type of AF (1st episode, paroxysmal, persistent or permanent), (2) onset 1st attack or 1st diagnosis, (3) frequency, duration, precipitants, prior methods of terminating, (4) prior response to drugs & (5) presence of other disease (cardiac ischemia, alcoholism, hyperthyroidism)

- <u>ECG</u> to assess arrhythmia, blocks, chamber, preexcitation, prior MI, to measure and follow RR, QRS, and QT intervals, <u>CXR</u>, <u>Echo</u> (inpatient) to evaluate valves, chambers, pericardium, RV pressures, clots, <u>Thyroid function tests</u> for 1st episode when rate difficult to control or if AF reoccurs unexpectedly. <u>Other tests</u> are indicated with specific scenarios: Holter monitor (adequacy of rate control), exercise test (suspected cardiac ischemia or type IC antiarrhythmic planned), transesophageal echo (stroke or systemic embolism), electrophysiologic study (clarify mechanism of wide QRS tachycardia, to identify atrial flutter or paroxysmal SVT, seek sites for ablation of AV conduction block/modification)

- <u>Heart Rate control</u> – (Recommended IV agents)
    - Perform immediate cardioversion (page 19) if acute paroxysmal AF and a rapid ventricular response associated with acute MI, symptomatic hypotension, angina or cardiac failure that does not respond promptly to drug therapy.
    - If congestive heart failure (CHF) is NOT present (and no contraindications) Class I agents for rate control: diltiazem, esmolol, metoprolol, propranolol, and verapamil. Digoxin is recommended Class IIa agent if no CHF.
    - If congestive heart failure (CHF) is present, esmolol and digoxin are Class I agents for heart rate control. If acute pulmonary edema with new onset atrial fibrillation, consider emergent cardioversion. If CHF, diltiazem, metoprolol, propranolol, verapamil are designated as Class IIb. (see pages 23 for dosing)
    - If accessory pathway (e.g. Wolf Parkinson White syndrome) suspected (e.g. wide QRS complex), IV procainamide or ibutilide are Class I recommendations for AF conversion to sinus rhythm. Amiodarone is a class II management alternative. In AF, avoid ß blockers, calcium channel blockers, digoxin if preexcitation (accessory pathway) is suspected.
    - In patients requiring immediate cardioversion (chemical or electrical), administer heparin (or low molecular weight heparin) concurrently if time allows.

- <u>Anticoagulate</u> (inpatient) 1st with heparin (or low molecular weight heparin) all with AF > 48 hours, followed by oral anticoagulation for ≥ 3-4 weeks or longer.

- <u>Rhythm conversion</u> – Other than patients requiring immediate cardioversion, the timing, necessity, and techniques of conversion are complex (and controversial) and are left to consulting/admitting physicians.

    [1] Definition of class recommendations: See page 2

AHA/ACC. *JACC* 2006; 48: 3149.

Rate Control in Atrial Fibrillation (AF)

End points for rate control (NOT necessarily ED goals) include ventricular rates of 60-80 beats/min at rest and 90-115 beats/min during moderate exercise.

Class I (definitely useful): In the absence of preexcitation, IV β blockers (e.g. esmolol, metoprolol, or propranolol) or nondihydropyridine calcium channel blockers (e.g. diltiazem, verapamil) are recommended for rate control during acute AF exercising caution in heart failure or hypotension. IV amiodarone or digoxin is recommended to control heart rate if heart failure is present. However, avoid digoxin if an accessory pathway is present. See pages 36-42 for detailed dosing.

Class IIa (safe accepted): IV amiodarone can be used to control the heart rate when other measures are not useful or do not work. When electrical cardioversion is not necessary in patients with an accessory pathway, IV procainamide or ibitulide can be used. See page 36-42 for detailed dosing. When rate cannot be controlled with medications, or tachycardia mediated cardiomyopathy is suspected, catheter directed ablation of the AV node may be considered to control the heart rate.

Class IIb (safe, optional): IV amiodarone, procainamide, disopyramide, or ibitulide may be considered in patients who are hemodynamically stable with AF involving an accessory pathway.

Class III (DO NOT USE - may be harmful): Digoxin should not be used alone to control the heart rate in paroxysmal AF. In patients with AF and heart failure, calcium channel blockers are not recommended as they may worsen heart failure. IV digoxin or calcium channel blockers are contraindicated in AF with a preexcitation syndrome as they may accelerate the ventricular response.

Agent	Class	IV loading dose	Onset	IV maintenance dose
		Heart Rate Control if Atrial Fibrillation and NO Accessory Pathway and NO Heart Failure[1,2]		
Diltiazem	I	0.25 mg/kg over 2 min	2-7 min	5-15 mg/hour
Esmolol	I	500 mcg/kg over 1 min	5 min	60-200 mcg/kg/min
Metoprolol	I	2.5–5 mg over 2 min, q 5 min X 3 total doses	5 min	None
Verapamil	I	0.075-0.15 mg/kg over 2 minutes	3-5 min	None
Heart Rate Control if Atrial Fibrillation and an Accessory Pathway is present[1]				
Amiodarone	IIa	150 mg over 10 minutes	Days	0.5-1 mg/min
Procainamide	IIb	See dosing detail page 41.		
Heart Rate Control if Atrial Fibrillation with Heart Failure and NO Accessory Pathway[1]				
Digoxin	I	0.25 mg every 2 hours up to 1.5 mg total	≥ 60 min	0.125-0.375 mg IV/PO daily
Amiodarone	IIa	150 mg over 10 minutes	Days	0.5-1 mg/min

[1] More detailed dosing recommendations are listed on pages 36-42.
[2] Do not use IV calcium channel blocker and β blocker together.

AHA/ACC. *JACC* 2006; 48: 3149.

Cardioversion of Atrial Fibrillation (AF)

If hemodynamically <u>stable</u>, cardioversion is <u>not required in the field or ED</u>. The decision of when and how to cardiovert involves consideration of hemodynamic stability, patient symptoms, duration of dysrhythmia, prior conversion attempts, echocardiographic data, coagulation status, and a risk assessment of thromboemboli following cardioversion. Medications are less effective than cardioversion with biphasic shocks. However, anesthesia or sedation is required for direct current (DC) cardioversion. Medications are less effective when AF present > 7 days. There is no evidence thromboembolism risk differs between medical/electric cardioversion.

<u>Class I recommendations (definitely useful):</u> (1) When a rapid ventricular response does not respond promptly to medications in AF patients with ischemia, hypotension, angina, or heart failure, synchronized DC cardioversion is recommended. Immediate DC cardioversion is also recommended for AF patients with preexcitation with very rapid HR or hemodynamic instability. The median successful energy level is 100 J with biphasic waveforms and 200 J with monophasic waveforms. (2) Medication options for pharmacologic cardioversion include flecainide, dofetilide, propafenone, or ibutilide. See page 36-42 for dosing. (3) For patients with ≥ 48 hours of AF, anticoagulation (INR 2-3) is recommended for 3 weeks pre and 4 weeks post cardioversion regardless of cardioversion method. If immediate cardioversion is required, administer heparin (concurrent or immediately after) by IV bolus with continuous infusion and oral anticoagulation for at least 4 weeks (unless there is a contraindication to anticoagulation). (4) IV procainamide or ibutilide is recommended to restore sinus rhythm in patients with WPW in whom AF occurs with a wide QRS complex or with a rapid preexcitent ventricular response.

<u>Class IIa recommendations (safe, accepted):</u> (1) Pretreatment with amiodarone, flecainide, ibutilide, propafenone, or sotalol can enhance the success of DC cardioversion and prevent AF recurrence. (2) Amiodarone alone can be used for cardioversion. Out of hospital recommendations for medical cardioversion are available (http://content.onlinejacc.org/cgi/reprint/48/4/e149) (3) IV flecainide or DC cardioversion can be used when very rapid ventricular rates occur in AF patients who have conduction over an accessory pathway.

<u>Class IIb recommendations (safe, accepted, optional):</u> (1) **Inpatient/NON ED** treatment - quinidine or procainamide although usefulness of these agents is not well established. (2) For persistent AF, consider administration of β blockers, disopyramide, diltiazem, dofetilide, procainamide, or verapamil, although efficacy of these agents to enhance the success of DC cardioversion or to prevent early recurrence of AF is uncertain. (3) The following can be used IV if stable with AF and accessory pathway: quinidine, procainamide, disopyramide, ibutilide, or amiodarone.

<u>Class III recommendations (Do Not Use - may be harmful):</u> (1) Electric cardioversion is contraindicated in digoxin toxicity, hypokalemia, and patients with short periods of sinus rhythm between relapses despite appropriate medications and recurrent electric cardioversion attempts. (2) Digoxin and sotalol may be harmful when used for pharmacological cardioversion of atrial fibrillation and are not recommended.

AHA/ACC. JACC 2006; 48: 3149.

Narrow Complex Supraventricular Tachycardia - Stable

Attempt therapeutic diagnostic maneuver
- Vagal stimulation (Valsalva, carotid massage)
- adenosine 6 mg IV, may repeat 12 mg IV X 2
  (follow adenosine with 20 ml NS bolus)

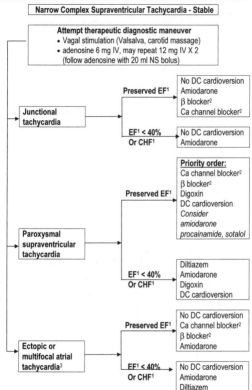

Junctional tachycardia

Preserved EF[1]
- No DC cardioversion
- Amiodarone
- β blocker[2]
- Ca channel blocker[2]

EF[1] < 40% Or CHF[1]
- No DC cardioversion
- Amiodarone

Paroxysmal supraventricular tachycardia

Preserved EF[1]
- **Priority order:**
- Ca channel blocker[2]
- β blocker[2]
- Digoxin
- DC cardioversion
- *Consider amiodarone procainamide, sotalol*

EF[1] < 40% Or CHF[1]
- Diltiazem
- Amiodarone
- Digoxin
- DC cardioversion

Ectopic or multifocal atrial tachycardia[3]

Preserved EF[1]
- No DC cardioversion
- Ca channel blocker[2]
- β blocker[2]
- Amiodarone

EF[1] < 40% Or CHF[1]
- No DC cardioversion
- Amiodarone
- Diltiazem

[1] Preserved – preserved cardiac function, EF – Ejection fraction, CHF – congestive heart failure. See pages 36-42 for drug dosing. [2] Do not use IV β blocker and calcium channel blocker together. [3] MAT – Treat underlying disorder (e.g. bronchospasm)

Ventricular Tachycardia (VT) Management (AHA/ACC *Circulation* 2006; 114: 385)

Rhythm	Class[1]	Specific Recommendation
Sustained Monomorphic (Mono) Ventricular Tachycardia (VT) Sustained - > 30 sec. or need termination in < 30 seconds due to hemodynamic compromise.	I	• Presume all Wide QRS tachycardia is VT if diagnosis unclear. • Cardioversion is recommended at any point in the treatment of VT with hemodynamic compromise.
	IIa	• IV procainamide as initial treatment • IV amiodarone if sustained Mono VT refractory to countershock or procainamide or other agents • Catheter pacer termination if refractory to cardioversion or recurrent despite medications
	IIb	• IV lidocaine initially if stable Mono VT in acute MI
	III	• DO NOT use calcium channel blockers
Repetitive Mono-morphic VT	IIa	• IV amiodarone, β blockers, or procainamide if coronary disease and idiopathic VT
Polymorphic (Poly) VT *with normal repolarization (normal QT) during sinus rhythm. Causes include MI, CHF,and cardiomyopathy*	I	• Cardioversion is recommended at any point in the treatment of VT with hemodynamic compromise. • IV β blockers are useful for recurrent Poly VT esp. if ischemia is suspected or cannot be excluded. • IV loading with amiodarone is useful for recurrent Poly VT in the absence of abnormal repolarization due to congenital or acquired long QT syndrome. • Consider urgent angiography if myocardial ischemia cannot be excluded.
	II	• IV lidocaine for Poly VT associated with myocardial ischemia or infarction
Polymorphic VT due to (LQTS) Long QT Interval Syndrome Or Torsades de pointes (TdP)	I	• Stop offending drugs, correct electrolytes. • Acute + long term pacing is recommended in TdP if heart block or symptomatic bradycardia.
	IIa	• IV magnesium if LQTS • Acute and long term pacing if recurrent pause dependent torsades de pointes • β blockers + pacing if TdP and sinus bradycardia. • Isoproterenol as temporary treatment if recurrent pause dependent TdP and do NOT have congenital prolonged QT syndrome
	IIb	• Correct potassium to 4.5-5 mmol/L • IV lidocaine or oral mexiletine if LQTS type 3
Incessant VT VT storm – very frequent episodes of VT requiring cardioversion	I	• Revascularization and β blockade followed by antiarrhythmics (e.g. procainamide/amiodarone) if recurrent/incessant Poly VT due to ischemia
	IIa	• IV amiodarone or procainamide followed by VT ablation if recurring/incessant Mono VT
	IIb	• IV amiodarone and β blockers if VT storm • Overdrive pacing or general anesthesia

AHA/ACC class of recommendations, see page 2

Myocardial Infarction (MI) & Acute Coronary Syndromes (ACS)
Utility of Various Tests for Diagnosis of Acute MI/ Cardiac Ischemia

Table below details predictive values for diagnosis of Acute Myocardial Infarction if non-italicized and *Acute Cardiac Ischemia (ACI)* if italicized.

Diagnostic Test	Sensitivity	Specificity	PPV[h]	NPV[h]
12 lead ECG (liberal criteria)[a]	94-99	19-27	21	98
12 lead ECG (strict criteria)[b]	38-44	97-98	76	91
15 lead ECG (+V8,V9,V4R)	55-60[f]	97-98		
22 lead ECG (multiple AP thorax leads)	88[f]	---		
Continuous/serial ECG	39	88		
ECG stress test (ACI)	68[g]	77	Data sources:	
CK-MB enzymes over 24 h *(ACI)*	100 *(31)*	98 *(95)*	*Circulation*	
1st CK-MB, pain onset < 4 h prior	41	88	2007;115: 402,	
1st CK-MB, pain onset > 4 h prior	63	90	2006; 114: 1761	
Serial CK-MB isoform, pain = 6 h[c]	96	94	*Ann Emerg Med*	
CK-MB at 0,1,2,3 h after ED arrival[d]	80	94	2007; 49: 125.	
Myoglobin, pain onset = 2 h	89	96	2001; 37: 453.;	
Myoglobin, pain onset 12-24 h prior	59	95	1992; 21: 504.	
Troponin T, pain onset = 3 h	33	100	*Am J Med* 2006;	
Troponin T, pain onset 6 h (12-24 h) prior	78 *(93)*	99 *(99)*	119: 203.	
Stress echocardiography	90	89	*Acad Emerg*	
Sestamibi rest (technetium 99m scan) [f]	74-87	56-85	*Med* 1997;4:13.	
CT angiography multidection 64 slice	86-100%	90-100%	99% NPV	

Coronary artery calcium score: (CACS) A CACS = 0 makes presence of atherosclerotic plaque highly unlikely. A score of 0 also makes the presence of significant luminal obstruction highly unlikely (NPV[k] 95-99%). A positive score (CACS > 0) confirms the presence of coronary artery plaque. A high score (> 100) is consistent with a high risk of a cardiac event within the next 2-5 years (> 2% annual risk). Individuals with a low clinical risk (< 10% over 10 years), and high clinical risk (> 20% over 10 years) do not benefit from CACS. (AHA/ACC Class III recommendation). *Circulation* 2007 (see above)

[a] nonspecific ST segment or T wave changes abnormal but not diagnostic of ischemia; Or ischemia, strain, or infarction known or not known to be old.

[b] ST segment elevation or pathologic Q waves not known to be old.

[c]CK-MB isoforms collected every 30-60 minutes for at least 6 hours after symptom onset when studied. Criteria for AMI diagnosis: MB2 > 1U/L or MB2/MB1 > 1.5.

[d] Sensitivity/specificity if > 6 hours from pain onset. Numbers are lower if < 6 hours.

[e] Must have ongoing chest pain and no nitrate or β blocker administered before test.

[f] Sensitivity using criteria strict ECG above

[g] Sensitivity is higher for three vessel disease and lower if LVH noted on ECG.

[h] NPV - negative predictive value, PPV - positive predictive value

Unstable Angina (US)/Non ST Elevation MI (NSTEMI) Guidelines

Class I Recommendations for Anti-Ischemic Therapy if High Risk Features[1] or Continuing Ischemia[2]

- Bed/chair rest with continuous ECG monitor
- Continuous pulse oximetry, oxygen if arterial saturation < 90%, respiratory distress, or high risk features for hypoxemia
- Aspirin 162-325 mg PO (if unable to take aspirin, take clopidogrel 300 mg PO)
- Nitroglycerin (NTG) SL q 5 min X 3. Assess IV NTG need. See Class III cautions.
- NTG IV for 1st 48 hours for persistent ischemia, heart failure, or hypertension
- Administer β blockers (oral route) within 24 hours unless contraindicated whether or not percutaneous coronary intervention (PCI) is performed.
- If β blockers contraindicated, give nondihydropyridine calcium antagonist (diltiazem, verapamil) unless contraindicated (e.g. severe LV dysfunction)
- Glycoprotein IIb/IIIa inhibitor IV **OR** clopidogrel if angiography/PCI planned.
- Anticoagulants – (1) *invasive strategy*: enoxaparin, unfractionated heparin, bivalirudin, or fondaparinux, (2) *conservative strategy*: enoxaparin, unfractionated heparin, or fondaparinux/F (F preferred if ↑ risk of bleeding)
- (Inpatient) Administer ACE inhibitor (oral) or angiotensin receptor blocker (ARB), if ACE intolerant, within the 1st 24 hours if pulmonary congestion or ejection fraction (EF) < 40% unless contraindication.
- Discontinue nonsteroidal anti-inflammatory medicine (except aspirin).

Class IIa Recommendations for Anti-Ischemic Therapy

- Supplemental oxygen to all patients in the 1st 6 hours.
- Morphine sulfate IV if uncontrolled pain despite NTG, appropriate therapy above.
- IV β blockers unless contraindications (e.g. heart block, shock, asthma)
- Oral long acting nondihydropyridine calcium antagonists for recurrent ischemia in the absence of contraindications after β blockers and NTG fully used.
- Glycoprotein IIb/IIIa inhibitor IV **AND** clopidogrel if angiography/PCI planned.
- Anticoagulants –*conservative strategy*: enoxaparin or fondaparinux is preferred to unfractionated heparin unless CABG planned within 24 hours.
- An ACE inhibitor without heart failure if no contraindications exist. (inpatient)
- Intra-aortic balloon pump if (1) severe ischemia continues/recurs frequently despite intensive medical therapy (2) hemodynamic stability is present before or after coronary angiography or (3) mechanical complications of MI

Class IIb Recommendations for Anti-Ischemic Therapy

- Gp IIb/IIIa inhibitors if PCI NOT planned (eptifibatide or tirofiban only)
- Extended release nondihydropyridine calcium antagonists instead of β blockers.
- Immediate release nondihydropyridine calcium antagonists after adequate β blockade of ongoing ischemia or hypertension.

Unstable Angina (UA)/Non ST Elevation MI (NSTEMI) Guidelines
Continued...

Class III Recommendations for Anti-Ischemic Therapy (DO NOT USE)

- Do not administer nitrates if systolic blood pressure < 90 mm Hg or ≥ 30 mm Hg below baseline, severe bradycardia (< 50 beats/minute), tachycardia [> 100 beats/minute] (in the absence of symptomatic heart failure, or right ventricular infarction), or if patients have used a phosphodiesterase inhibitor for erectile dysfunction in prior 24 hours (if sildenafil/*Viagra*) or prior 48 hours (if tadalafil/*Cialis*), unknown delay needed for vardenafil/*Levitra* use.
- Do not administer immediate release dihydropyridine calcium antagonists in absence of a β blocker.
- Do not administer an IV ACE inhibitor within the 1st 24 hours of UA/NSTEMI due to the increased risk of hypotension.
- IV β blockers may be harmful if contraindication (heart failure, low output state, or other risk factors for cardiogenic shock).
- Do not give nonsteroidal anti-inflammatory (except aspirin) during hospitalization.
- Do not administer abciximab to patients in whom PCI is not already planned.
- Do not administer fibrinolytic therapy to patients without acute ST segment elevation, a true posterior MI, or a presumed new left bundle branch block.
- An early invasive strategy is not recommended if (1) extensive comorbidity (e.g. liver failure, pulmonary failure, cancer) when the risks of revascularization and comorbidity are likely to outweigh the benefits of revascularization, (2) low likelihood of acute coronary syndrome, or (3) in patients who will not consent to revascularization.

[1] High Risk Features: Recurrent angina, ischemia related ECG changes (≥ 0.05 mV ST segment depression or bundle branch block) at rest or with low level activity, ischemia (associated with heart failure, S_3 gallop, or new or worsening mitral regurgitation), hemodynamic instability, serious ventricular arrhythmia, or depressed left ventricular function (EF < 0.4)

[2] See page 2 for definition of Class I-III recommendations

Circulation 2007; 116: e148.

AHA/ACC Guidelines for Invasive vs. Conservative therapy in UA/NSTEMI (Primarily Cardiologist's Decision)

Conservative	• Low Risk Score (e.g. TIMI [www.timi.org], GRACE [www.outcomes-umassmed.org/grace/]), • Physician or patient preference in the absence of high risk factors
Invasive	• Recurrent angina/ischemia at rest of with low level activity despite intensive medical therapy, • Elevated cardiac biomarkers (e.g. TnT or TnI) • New or presumably new ST depression • Signs/symptoms of heart failure or new/worse mitral regurgitation • High risk findings on non-invasive tests • Sustained ventricular tachycardia or hemodynamic instability • Prior CABG or percutaneous coronary intervention (PCI) • High risk score (e.g. TIMI, or GRACE) • Reduced left ventricular function (e.g. ejection fraction < 40%)

Conservative Strategy for Likely or Definite UA/NSTEMI[1]

Administer aspirin or clopidogrel if aspirin intolerant [I]

↓

Initiate anticoagulant [I]: enoxaparin or fondaparinux or unfractionated heparin (enoxaparin or fondaparinux are preferred [IIa])

↓

Start clopidogrel if not already given [I] & consider adding eptifibatide or tirofiban [IIb]

↓

Stress test and echocardiogram:
If EF ≤ 40%, diagnostic angiography [IIb], If stress test not low risk, angiography [I]

↓

If ejection fraction > 0.4 and low risk stress test:
Continue aspirin indefinitely. Continue clopidogrel for 1 month - 1 year.
Discontinue eptifibatide/tirofiban. Discontinue anticoagulant therapy.

[1] Class I, II, recommendations are listed in brackets [ ] (See explanation page 2
[2] If subsequent recurrent symptoms/ischemia, heart failure, or serious arrhythmia consider diagnostic angiography [3] Abciximab should not be administered to patients unless PCI planned.   *Circulation* 2007; 116: e148.

Initial Invasive Strategy for Likely or Definite UA/NSTEMI[1]

Administer aspirin or clopidogrel if aspirin intolerant [I]

↓

Start anticoagulant[I]: enoxaparin, fondaparinux, bivalirudin or unfractionated heparin

↓

Prior to angioplasty start one [I] of clopidogrel or IV GP IIb/IIIa inhibitor[2] or both [IIa].
Consider both agents if delay to angioplasty, high risk, early recurrent ischemia.

↓

Diagnostic angiography

[1] Class I, II, recommendations are listed in brackets [ ]. See explanation page 2.
[2] GP IIb/IIb inhibitors may not be necessary if patient received at least 300 mg clopidogrel at least 6 hours earlier and bivalirudin selected as anticoagulant.
Circulation 2007; 116: e148.

ACC/AHA Recommendations for ST Elevation Myocardial Infarction (STEMI)
Class I Recommendations for STEMI (See page 2 for class definition)[1]

- **ECG:** If possible, perform & interpret ≤ 10 minutes from ED arrival. If ECG is not diagnostic and high suspicion for STEMI, repeat ECG or perform continuous 12 lead ST monitoring. If inferior MI, obtain right sided ECG for RV infarction.

- **Radiography:** Initial CXR - do not delay reperfusion unless contraindication possible (e.g. aortic dissection). High quality CXR, transthoracic or trans-esophageal echo, contrast chest CT, or MRI is used to differentiate STEMI from aortic dissection if diagnosis unclear.

- **Oxygen:** Administer supplemental oxygen if oxygen saturation < 90%.

- **Aspirin** (162-325 mg) chewed if not yet taken. Nonenteric is preferred.

- **β blockers** (oral): Administer if no contraindications regardless of concomitant fibrinolytic therapy or performance of percutaneous coronary intervention/PCI.

- **Clopidogrel:** Add to aspirin 75 mg PO daily ≥ 14 days if STEMI regardless of whether undergo fibrinolysis. If CABG, withhold ≥ 5-7 days pre-procedure.

- **NTG:** If ongoing ischemic pain, administer SL nitroglycerin (NTG) q 5 min X 3. IV NTG is indicated for ongoing pain, hypertension, or pulmonary congestion.

- **Morphine** repeated at 5-15 min. intervals is the analgesic of choice for STEMI.

- **Anticoagulation options – post fibrinolytics:** Administer ≥ 48 hours up to 8 days if undergo fibrinolysis. Use enoxaparin or fondaparinux if administered > 48 hours.
  - **IV heparin** dose if reperfusion with alteplase, reteplase, or tenecteplase: bolus 60 U/kg (max 4000 U) then 12 U/kg/hour (max 1000/hour) adjusted to maintain aPTT at 1.5-2 times control. UFH should be administered IV if treated with nonselective fibrinolytic agents and high risk for systemic emboli (large or anterior MI, Afib, prior embolus, or LV thrombus). Monitor platelet count daily.
  - **Enoxaparin** dose (if creatinine < 2.5 mg/dl in male or < 2 mg/dl in female): If < 75 years old, 30 mg IV, then 15 min later 1 mg/kg SQ q 12h. (some experts administer 0.5 - 0.75 mg/kg SQ pre PCI; *New Engl J Med* 2006; 355: 1006.). If ≥ 75 years, no IV bolus, administer 0.75 mg/kg SQ q 12h. At any age, if creatinine clearance is < 30 ml/min, administer 1 mg/kg SQ q 24 hours. Administer maintenance dose ≤ 8 days.
  - **Fondaparinux** dose (if creatinine is < 3 mg/dl): 2.5 mg IV, then 2.5 mg SQ q 24 hours. Continue during hospitalization up to 8 days. (Due to risk of catheter thrombosis, do not use as sole anticoagulant to support PCI).

- **Anticoagulation – PCI completed:** See guidelines (www.acc.org)

- **Reperfusion choice:** (PCI and fibrinolysis): All require rapid evaluation for reperfusion (i.e. PCI ≤ 90 min. or fibrinolysis ≤ 30 min. of arrival). PCI preferred if skilled PCI lab available (esp. ≤ 90 min. of arrival), high risk STEMI (shock, Killip III/IV), fibrinolysis contraindications, or arrive > 3 h after onset. Fibrinolysis may be preferred if early presenter (< 3 h after onset) esp. if PCI unavailable (or has long transport), difficult vascular access or arrival to PCI time is > 90 min.

Class I Recommendations continued[1]

- <u>Fibrinolysis</u>: STEMI patients at site without PCI available or cannot transfer in ≤90 min. should undergo thrombolysis unless contraindicated. Class I indications –symptoms < 12 hours and ST elevation > 0.1 mV in ≥ 2 contiguous precordial or 2 adjacent limb leads. Perform exam to look for stroke or cognitive deficit pre-administration. Assess for contraindications (page 35). If intracranial bleed (ICH) risk is ≥ 4%, perform PCI - not fibrinolysis. Treat neurologic deterioration as ICH until CT. Consider neurology, neurosurgical consult, FFP, protamine, platelets.

- <u>PCI</u>: Perform in STEMI or MI with new LBBB if can undergo PCI within 12 hours onset (90 min arrival). Primary PCI if < 75 y with STEMI or LBBB and shock within 36 h of MI, & suitable for revascularization. Diagnostic coronary angiography/PCI is performed if (1) PCI candidate, (2) cardiac shock if revascularization candidate and < 75 years old (Class IIa if ≥ 75 years old), (3) candidate for VSD or severe MR repair. (4) persistent electrical instability.

- <u>Insulin</u>: An insulin infusion to normalize blood glucose is recommended for patients with STEMI and complicated courses.

- <u>Intra-aortic balloon pump</u> counterpulsation is recommended for STEMI with cardiogenic shock not quickly reversed with medications to stabilize.

- <u>ACE:</u> (inpatient) Administer ACE inhibitor (oral) within 1st 24 hours of STEMI if anterior MI, pulmonary congestion, or LVEF < 0.4 unless hypotension is present (SBP < 100 mm Hg or ≥ 30 mm Hg below) or contraindicated (e.g. allergy).

- <u>ARB:</u> Administer an angiotensin receptor blocker (ARB) to STEMI patients who are intolerant of ACE inhibitors and who have heart failure or LVEF < 0.4.

Class IIa Recommendations for STEMI[1]

- <u>Radiography</u>: Portable echo is reasonable for clarifying STEMI diagnosis and risk stratify patients who present to the ED, especially if LBBB or pacemaker present, or suspicion of posterior STEMI with anterior ST depression.

- <u>Oxygen</u>: Supplemental O_2 to all uncomplicated STEMI patients in the 1st 6 hours

- <u>Clopidogrel</u> – Administer 300 mg PO if < 75 years old if STEMI regardless of whether or not receive reperfusion therapy. (See CABG caution Class I). Long term (> 1 year), administer 75 mg PO daily for > 1 year if STEMI.

- <u>β blockers</u> It is reasonable to administer IV β blockers to patients at the time of presentation of STEMI who are hypertensive without contraindications (heart failure, low output state, increased risk for cardiogenic shock, or other relative contraindications including PR interval > 0.24 seconds, 2nd or 3rd degree heart block, active asthma, or reactive airway disease).

- <u>CCB</u>: It is reasonable to administer calcium channel blockers/CCB (verapamil or diltiazem) if β blockers are contraindicated for ongoing ischemia, atrial fibrillation /flutter after STEMI in the absence of CHF, LV dysfunction or AV block.

[1]More comprehensive/detailed recommendations are cited within article and online
  Circulation 2008; 117; 296 ; *JACC* 2008; 51: 210 (update 2004 guidelines - *JACC* 2004; 44: 671.)

Class IIa STEMI recommendations continued

- **Glycoprotein IIa/IIIb inhibitors** – Decision to use these agents generally involves cardiologist with consideration of type of intervention. Abciximab before primary PCI in STEMI is Class IIa (tirofiban and eptifibatide are IIb pre primary PCI).
- **Anticoagulation**: If STEMI and no reperfusion+ no contraindications continue LMWH (enoxaparin/ or fondaparinux) for ≥ 48 h up to 8 days (Class I dosing)
- **Primary PCI** if ≥ 75 years with ST elevation or LBBB and develop shock post-fibrinolysis and suitable for revascularization, or hemodynamic/ electrical instability, or persistent ischemia or failed fibrinolysis (ST elevation < 50% resolved 90 min after initiation in lead showing worst elevation with moderate or large area of myocardium at risk [ant. MI, inferior MI with RV involved, or precordial ST depression]).
- **Fibrinolytics** - If no contraindications exist, fibrinolytics are reasonable to give (1) if symptoms began within prior 12 hours and 12 lead ECG shows a true posterior MI or (2) STEMI patients with symptoms onset within prior 12-24 hours if continuing ischemic symptoms are present and there is ST elevation > 0.1 mV in a least 2 contiguous precordial leads or at least 2 adjacent limb leads.
- **Insulin**: During the 1st 24-48 hours of STEMI in patients with hyperglycemia, it is reasonable to administer an insulin infusion to normalize glucose even in patients with uncomplicated courses. After the acute phase of a STEMI, individualize hyperglycemia control with oral agents or insulin.
- **Magnesium (Mg)**: Correct deficits esp. if patients receiving diuretics before onset of STEMI. Treat torsade de pointes VT assoc. with prolonged QT with 1-2 g Mg.
- **ACE**: An ACE inhibitor (oral) administered within the 1st 24 hours of STEMI can be useful in absence of Class I recommendations or contraindications.

Class IIb Recommendations for STEMI

- **Combination abciximab and half dose reteplase** (or tenecteplase) may be considered for prevention of reinfarct and other STEMI if anterior MI, age < 75 years, and no risk factors for bleeding. This combination also may be considered if anterior MI and age < 75 years if early angiography and PCI is planned.
- **Glycoprotein IIa/IIIb inhibitor** – Selection of these agents requires cardiologist and intervention decision. Tirofiban or eptifibatide pre primary PCI in STEMI.
- **Facilitated PCI** (immediate PCI after IIb combination above) might be performed in higher risk patients when PCI is not immediately available & bleeding risk low.
- **UFH**: It may be reasonable to give UFH IV to patients receiving streptokinase.
- **LMWH**: Low molecular weight heparin (LMWH) is alternative to UFH as ancillary therapy for patients < 75 years old receiving fibrinolytics if creatinine < 2.5 mg/dl in men (< 2 mg/dl in women). Enoxaparin (30 mg IV bolus + 1 mg/kg SC q 12 hours until discharge) combined with full dose tenecteplase is most studied
- **PCI Angiography** – No Class I or IIa indications and moderate to high risk patient

[1]More comprehensive/detailed recommendations are cited .   _Circulation_ 2008; 117; 296.

Class III Recommendations for STEMI (DO NOT USE)

- <u>NTG</u>: Do Not administer NTG if SBP < 90 mm Hg or ≥ 30 mm Hg below baseline, severe bradycardia (< 50 beats per min), tachycardia (unless related to heart failure), suspected RV infarction, or to patients with recent phosphodiesterase inhibitor use for erectile dysfunction (e.g. sildenafil/*Viagra* use in prior 24 hours, tadalafil/*Cialis* use in prior 48 hours, unknown delay for vardenafil/*Levitra* use).

- <u>ACE</u>: An IV ACE inhibitor should not be administered within the 1st 24 hours of STEMI except in the setting of refractory hypertension.

- β blockers Do Not administer if signs of CHF, cardiogenic shock risk, low output state, or other relative contraindications (PR > 0.24 sec, 2nd, 3rd degree heart block, active asthma or reactive airway disease).

- <u>Heparin</u>: Do Not use low molecular weight heparin as an alternative to UFH in patients > 75 years old receiving fibrinolytics or in patients < 75 years receiving fibrinolytics with renal dysfunction–creatinine > 2.5 mg/dl in men (> 2 in women).

- <u>Antithrombins</u>: if heparin induced thrombocytopenia, consider bivalirudin as an alternative to heparin used in conjunction with streptokinase. Give 0.25 mg/kg IV bolus, followed by 0.5 mg/kg/hour X 12 hours, then 0.25 mg/kg/hour X 36 hours. Reduce the infusion rate if PTT is above 75 seconds within the 1st 12 hours.

- PCI – Do Not perform in asymptomatic patients > 12 hours after onset of STEMI if hemodynamically and electrically stable. Do not perform PCI without on site cardiac surgery capability or proven plan for rapid transport to cardiac surgery unless appropriate hemodynamic support, capability for rapid transfer. Full dose fibrinolytic therapy followed by immediate PCI may be harmful.

- <u>Fibrinolytics</u> – See recommendations page 35. If ICH occurs, reduce ICP with mannitol, intubation/hyperventilation and consider need for neurosurgery.

- Do not perform <u>coronary angiography</u> in patients with extensive comorbidity in whom risk of revascularization outweighs the benefits.

- <u>Combination therapy with abciximab and half dose reteplase</u> (or tenecteplase) should not be given if > 75 years old.

- <u>CCB</u>: Diltiazem and verapamil are contraindicated in STEMI associated with LV dysfunction or CHF. Nifedipine (immediate release) is contraindicated in STEMI due to reflex tachycardia, sympathetic activation, hypotension.

- <u>Nonsteroidal anti-inflammatory</u> – Do not take during STEMI admit (aspirin is OK)

[1]Rescue PCI , post fibrinolysis PCI, and CABG indications are detailed in cited article and online
Circulation 2008; 117;296.

Absolute Contraindications to Thrombolytic Use	
Prior CNS bleed,	Active internal bleeding (not menses)
CNS structural lesion or neoplasm	Significant head trauma past 3 months
Ischemic stroke in past 3 months	Suspected aortic dissection, pericarditis

Relative Contraindications or Cautions to Thrombolytic Use	
Chronic, severe, poorly controlled HTN	Recent internal bleeding (< 2-4 weeks)
SBP > 180 or DBP > 110 on arrival	Noncompressible vessel puncture
Stroke (< 3-6 mo old), dementia, other	Pregnancy or active peptic ulcer
intracranial pathology not noted above	Current anticoagulants (esp. high INR)
Traumatic or prolonged (> 10 min) CPR	For streptokinase(*Streptase*): prior
Major surgery < 3 weeks ago	exposure or prior allergic reaction to SK

J Am Coll Cardiol 2004; 44: e1.

AHA/ACC Recommendations for Thrombolytic Therapy in Acute MI

Class	Recommendation (See STEMI PCI Recommendations 1st)
I	• Onset ≤ 12 hours AND (1) ST elevation > 0.1 mV in ≥ 2 contiguous leads or (2) new left bundle branch block
II a	• Onset ≤ 12 hours and true posterior MI • STEMI symptoms onset 12-24 hours prior with continuing ischemic symptoms and ST elevation > 0.1 mV in ≥ 2 contiguous leads
III	• ST elevation + time to therapy > 24 h Or ST segment depression only (unless true posterior MI is present)

See page 2 for Definition of Class.   *Cardiol Clin 2006; 24: 37.*

Thrombolytics in STEMI - See Above & page 32, 33 for Indications/Contraindications

Agent	Dose
reteplase (*r-PA, Retavase*)	• 10 units IV over 2 min, repeat dose in 30 min
tenecteplase (*TNK-ase*)	• Single IV bolus over 5 seconds; if < 60 kg (30 mg), 60-69 kg (35 mg), 70-79 kg (40 mg), 80-89 kg (45 mg), ≥ 90 kg (50 mg)
alteplase, (*t-PA, rtPA, Activase*)	• 15 mg bolus + 0.75 mg/kg (max 50 mg) over 30 min + 0.50 mg/kg (max. 35 mg) over 60 min + heparin 60 U/kg bolus + 12 U/kg/h. PTT goal is 1.5-2.0 X control.
streptokinase (*Streptase*)	• 1.5 million U. IV over 1 hour

See heparin recommendations page 33, 34, 40.   *Cardiol Clin 2006; 24: 37.*

Indications for Transcutaneous Patches/Pacing in Acute MI

Hemodynamically unstable bradycardia (< 50 beats/minute)

Mobitz type II 2nd degree AV block, or 3rd degree heart block

Bilateral BBB, Alternating BBB or RBBB and alternating LBBB

Left anterior fascicular block or newly acquired or age-indeterminate LBBB

RBBB or LBBB and 1st degree AV block

In ED, place pads on all, only pace if unstable.   *Circulation 2000: 102: (suppl).*

Select Parenteral Cardiovascular Medications & AHA/ACC Guidelines
[*Circulation* 2008; 117:296; 2002; 106: 1896; *JACC* 2004;44:e1] (www.acc.org)

Abciximab (ReoPro)	• PCI – 0.25 mg/kg IV pre PCI, + 0.125 mcg/kg/min (maximum of 10 mcg/min) X 12 h after PCI **Class I – UA/NSTEMI** –for 12-24 hours if PCI planned next 24 hours **Class IIa – STEMI** reasonable to use as early as possible pre-PCI **Class IIb – STEMI** – combination with half dose reteplase or half dose tenectecplase may be considered for prevention of reinfarct and other STEMI circumstances (per cardiology recommendation) **Class III – UA/NSTEMI** – patients in whom PCI is not planned
ACE inhibitors (e.g. benazepril, captopril,enalopril, fosinopril,lisinopril quinapril, ramipril, trandolapril)	**Class I** – (1) 1st 24 h of acute MI with ST elevation in > 2 ant precordial leads or CHF without ↓ BP or contraindication (2) UA/NSTEMI – hypertension despite NTG & β blocker if LV systolic dysfunction or CHF and in patients with diabetes. **Class IIa** – all other within 24 h of suspected MI. All post acute coronary syndrome patients. **Class IIb** – after MI recovery when normal or mildly abnormal LV function.
Adenosine (Adenocard)	• <u>SVT</u> – 6 mg IV. Repeat 12 mg IV q 2 min X 2 doses. Avoid if: 2nd/3rd degree AV block, sick sinus syndrome, on dipyridamole
Alteplase (t-PA)	• See thrombolytics page 35
Amiodarone (Cordarone)	• <u>VF/pulseless VT</u> – 300 mg IVP • <u>Recurrent VF/Pulseless VT</u> – 150 mg IVP • <u>Ventricular arrhythmias</u> – 150 mg IV over 10 minutes, then 1 mg/min X 6 h (360 mg), then 0.5 mg/min X 18 h (540 mg) **Class I Cardiac arrest** – preferred anti-arrhythmic for VF/VT during cardiac arrest and post VT/VF cardiac arrest **Class I Polymorphic VT** – in absence of abnormal repolarization related to long QT syndromes **Class I STEMI** – (1) sustained monomorphic VT not associated with angina, pulmonary edema or hypotension. As alternate to above regimen may administer 150 mg (or 5 mg/kg) over 10 minutes and repeat same dose q10-15 minutes. Do not exceed 2.2 g in 24 hours.(2) AF in patients with hemodynamic compromise that does not respond to electrical cardioversion **Class IIa** – (1) monomorphic VT that is hemodynamically unstable, refractory to countershock or recurrent despite alternate medication administration (2) Atrial fibrillation/flutter with normal cardiac function (3) VT/pulseless VT refractory to electric shock (4) repetitive monomorphic VT in setting of coronary artery disease (5) incessant VT **Class IIb** – (1) monomorphic VT with impaired cardiac function (2) polymorphic VT (3)VT storm (4) Atrial fibrillation/flutter- impaired cardiac function/underlying WPW
Argatroban (formerly Acova) Use if heparin induced thrombo- cytopenia	• <u>UA/NSTEMI/Pre-PCI</u> – 350 mcg//kg IV over 3-5 minutes plus 25 mcg/kg/min. Check activated clotting time (ACT) 5-10 min. after bolus complete. Therapeutic ACT is 300-450 sec. If ACT < 300 sec., administer 2nd bolus of 150 mcg//kg and ↑ infusion to 30 mcg/kg/min and recheck ACT in 5-10 minutes. If ACT > 450 sec., ↓ infusion to 15 mcg//kg/min and recheck ACT in 5-10 minutes. May take with aspirin.

Aspirin	• <u>Acute MI</u> – 162 – 325 mg PO *Class I – STEMI/UA/NSTEMI – begin immediately* *If allergy, choose clopidogrel over ticlopidine, dipyridamole*
Atenolol (*Tenormin*)	• <u>Acute MI</u> –50 mg/day PO increased to 50 mg PO BID as tolerated. 5 mg IV over 5 minutes, repeat in 10 minutes, *Class I – STEMI/UA/NSTEMI – Oral administration within 12 hr of MI* *or ongoing, recurrent pain.* *Class IIa STEMI – IV administration if no contraindications.* *Class IIb – STEMI –moderate LV failure (bibasilar rales without low* *cardiac output) or other relative contraindications to β blockers,* *provided patients can be monitored closely.* *Class III STEMI/UA/NSTEMI – DO NOT use - severe LV failure, ↓* *HR,or other contraindications*
Atropine	• <u>Asystole</u> – 1 mg IV, repeat q 3-5 minutes (Max 0.04 mg/kg) • <u>Bradycardia</u> 0.5 – 1.0 mg IV q 3-5 minutes (Max 0.04 mg/kg) ET dose is 2-3 mg diluted in 10 ml NS. *Class I – Acute MI – (1) sinus bradycardia with low cardiac output &* *hypoperfusion, or frequent PVCs at onset of acute MI (2) inferior MI* *with type I 2nd or 3rd AV block & ↓BP, ischemic pain or ventricular* *arrhythmias (3) sustained ↓ HR/BP after nitroglycerin (4) nausea and* *vomiting associated with morphine (5) asystole* *Class IIa – Acute MI – symptomatic inferior infarction and type I 2nd or* *3rd degree heart block at AV node (narrow QRS or known BBB)* *Class IIb - Acute MI – (1) administration with morphine in the* *presence of bradycardia (2) asymptomatic with inferior infarction and* *type I 2nd or 3rd degree heart block at the AV node (3) 2nd or 3rd degree* *AV block of uncertain mechanism when pacing unavailable* *Class III – Acute MI - DO NOT use – sinus bradycardia > 40 without* *hypoperfusion or frequent PVCs (2) type II AV block or 3rd degree AV* *block with new wide QRS complex presumed due to MI*
Bivalirudin (*Angiomax*)	• <u>Indication</u>: a direct thrombin inhibitor used if unstable angina and undergoing PCI (if heparin allergy/thrombocytopenia). This agent is an alternative to heparin in STEMI and UA/NSTEMI if heparin induced thrombocytopenia. • **STEMI** - HERO-2 dosing recommended by ACC/AHA. Bolus 0.25 mg/kg then 0.5 mg/kg/hour for 12 hours, then 0.25 mg/kg/hour for 36 hours. Reduce infusion if PTT is > 75 seconds within the 1st 12 hours. • Alternate **UA/NSTEMI/PCI** dosing: (1) 0.75 mg/kg IV bolus pre-procedure1 mg/kg IV bolus prior to PCI, then 1.75 mg/kg/hour during procedure up to 4 hours after procedure (with IIb/IIIa agent).
Bumetanide	• (*Bumex*) 0.5-1.0 mg IV/IM; 1mg *Bumex* ~ 40 mg *Lasix*

Class I-III definitions – see page 2
PCI – procedural coronary intervention, MI – myocardial infarction, UA – unstable angina,
NSTEMI – nonST elevation MI, STEMI – ST elevation MI

Clopidogrel (Plavix)	• 300 mg PO loading dose, then 75 mg PO daily ***Class I – UA/NSTEMI/STEMI** – (1) all patients unable to take aspirin (2) add to aspirin whether or not undergo fibrinolysis (Caution - withhold 5-7 days if elective CABG is planned).* ***Class IIa STEMI** – If < 75 years old, 300 mg PO X 1 (see caution)*
Dalteparin (Fragmin)	• UA/NSTEMI – 120 units/kg SC q 12 h. Max dose 10,000 units
Digoxin (Lanoxin)	• Rapid Afib - 0.25 mg IV q 2 hours up to 1.5 mg. ***Class Ib – Afib** - if congestive heart failure* ***Class IIb – Afib** - rate control if no congestive heart failure*
Diltiazem (Cardizem)	• 20 mg (0.25 mg/kg) IV over 2 min. Repeat 25 mg (0.35 mg/kg) IV 15 min after 1st dose prn. Drip at 5-15 mg/h prn ***Class I – UA/NSTEMI** –continuing or recurring ischemia when β blockers are contraindicated & no contraindications.* ***Class I – Atrial Fib/flutter/SVT** – preserved LV function – rate control* ***Class IIa – UA/NSTEMI** – oral long acting agents if recurrent ischemia in absence of contraindications & β blockers/nitrates are fully used.* ***Class IIb – Atrial Fib/flutter** – if CHF;* ***Class IIb – U/ANSTEMI** – (1) extended release form of non-dihydropyridine calcium antagonist (diltiazem, verapamil) instead of β blocker Or (2) immediate release dihydropyridine calcium antagonist (nifedipine) in presence of a β blocker.* ***Class III – Atrial fibrillation/flutter – DO NOT USE** if preexcitation - WPW*
Dobutamine (Dobutrex)	• 2-20 mcg/kg/min IV; 250 mg in 250 ml NS or D5W = 1 mg/ml
Dopamine (Intropin)	• 2-50 mcg/kg/min IV, Mix 400 mg in 250 ml D5W = 1.6 mg/ml. • 1-5 mcg/kg/min (renal), 5-10 mcg/kg/min (cardiac), > 10 mcg/kg/min (vasoconstriction), > 40 consider norepinephrine
Dofetilide (Tikosyn)	• AF -Specialized dose based on creatinine, body size, and age. ***Class I** – cardioversion if AF of < or > 7 days duration.* May be more effective for atrial flutter than for atrial fibrillation.
Enoxaparin (Lovenox)	• STEMI – (if creatinine [Cr] < 2.5 mg/dl if male, < 2 mg/dl if female). Age < 75 years, 30 mg IV, then 15 min later 1 mg/kg SC q 12 h. If ≥ 75 years, no IV bolus, administer 0.75 mg/kg SC q 12h. If Cr clearance < 30 ml/min, 1 mg/kg SC q 24 hours. (Some experts administer 0.5 - .75 mg/kg IV pre PCI) • UA/NSTEMI/PCI – 1 mg/kg SC q 12 hours (with aspirin) and continued ≥ 2 days until clinically stable. Max single dose is 150 mg SC. Overdose associated with severe bleed may be reversed by slow infusion of protamine sulfate IV (page 42). See heparin for specific AHA/ACC recommendations

Class I-III definitions – see page 2
PCI – procedural coronary intervention, MI – myocardial infarction, UA – unstable angina, NSTEMI – nonST elevation MI, STEMI – ST elevation MI

Epinephrine *(Adrenalin)*	• <u>Cardiac arrest</u> – 1 mg IV q 3-5 min. (10 ml of 1:10,000 followed by 20 ml NS flush). ET dose: 2-2.5 mg • <u>Shock</u> – 2 –10 mcg/min. IV infusion. Mix 1 mg in 500 ml NS and infuse at 1-5 ml/min.
Eptifibatide *(Integrilin)*	• <u>UA/NSTEMI</u> – 180 mcg/kg IV, + 2 mcg/kg/min X 72-96 h. If serum creatinine (Cr) > 2 mg/dl or Cr clearance < 50 ml/min, bolus same amount and decrease infusion to 1 mcg/kg/min. • <u>PCI</u> above dosing or alternate dosing –of 135 mcg/kg IV, plus 0.5mcg/kg/min X 20-24 hours *Class I – UA/NSTEMI –high risk, troponin positive pre PCI* *Class IIa – UA/NSTEMI/STEMI – administered pre PCI* *Class IIb – UA/NSTEMI – if conservative (nonPCI) strategy*
Esmolol *(Brevibloc)*	• SVT/AF/Flutter/(Torsades with normal baseline QT) - Load 500 mcg/kg IV over 1 min, then 50 mcg/kg/min X 4 min. If no response, 500 mcg/kg IV over 1 min, then 100 mcg/kg/min X 4 min. Continue to repeat 500 mcg/kg over 1 min prn while increasing infusion by 50 mcg/kg/min until desired effect achieved or max. of 300 mcg/kg/min. Once adequate response, do not change rate > 25 mcg/kg/min or rebolus. *Class I – Afib – rate control*
Flecainide *(Tambocor)*	• <u>AF</u> – 200-300 mg PO and 1.5-3 mg/kg IV over 10-20 minutes (IV formulation not available in the U.S) *Class I – AF – cardioversion of AF of up to 7 days duration.* *Class IIb – AF – cardioversion of AF of > 7 days duration.* Oral dosing is up to 91% effective for cardioversion at 8 hours. Frequent side effects (IV or PO) include atrial flutter with rapid ventricular rate, bradycardia (after cardioversion), hypotension, and mild neurologic side effects. Avoid if known organic heart disease (esp. if abnormal ventricular function).
Fondaparinux *(Arixtra)*	• <u>STEMI & NSTEMI</u> – 2.5 mg SC daily until hospital discharge or up to 8 days total. Do not use as sole PCI anticoagulant. • <u>DVT/PE</u> – 5 mg SC daily (if < 50 kg), 7.5 mg SC daily (50-100 kg), 10 mg SC daily (if > 100 kg). *Class I – STEMI – (if creatinine < 3 mg/dl), 2.5 mg IV, then 2.5 mg SC q 24hours.* *Class I – UA/NSTEMI – may use as anticoagulant for conservative or invasive strategies (see page 30)*
Furosemide	• *(Lasix)* 0.5-2.0 mg/kg IV
Group IIb/IIIa Inhibitors	see Abciximab *(ReoPro)*, Eptifibatide *(Integrilin)* and Tirofiban *(Aggrastat)*

Heparin *Unfractionated* *See enoxaparin* *& dalteparin for* *low molecular* *heparin options*	• <u>UA/NSTEMI/PCI/PE/DVT</u>- 80 U/kg IV + 18 U/kg/h, titrate to PTT • <u>MI/alteplase use</u> – 60 U/kg IV (max 4,000 U), + 12 U/kg/h [max 1000 U/h] (PTT goal 50-70 sec or 1.5-2.0 X control) • In patients at risk for heparin induced thrombocytopenia consider fondaparinux, bivalirudin or argatroban as an alternative (see page 36, 37, 40). Consult cardiology. ***Class I – STEMI** – Patients undergoing PCI or surgical revascularization (unfractionated heparin/UFH). Administer UFH IV if undergoing reperfusion with alteplase, reteplase, or tenecteplase. If receiving nonselective fibrinolytic, administer UFH IV if at high risk for systemic emboli (large or anterior MI, atrial fibrillation, prior embolism, or known LV thrombus).* ***Class I –UA/NSTEMI** – add to aspirin and clopidogrel* ***Class IIa STEMI** – If no reperfusion, no contraindication continue UFH or LMWH for at least 48 hours or until patient ambulatory.* ***Class IIa –UA/NSTEMI** – Lovenox is preferred over unfractionated heparin in UA/NSTEMI in absence of renal failure unless CABG planned in24 hours.* ***Class IIb – STEMI** – It may be reasonable to give UFH IV to patients receiving streptokinase. LMWH may be considered an acceptable alternative. See indications/contraindications page 38* ***Class IIb UA/NSTEMI** – SC use if non-selective thrombolytics given & low risk for emboli until walking.*
Ibutilide *(Corvert)*	• <u>AF</u> – If > 60 kg, 1 mg IV over 10 minutes. If < 60 kg, 0.01 mg/kg IV over 10 minutes. May repeat initial dose for either weight 10 minutes after completion of either infusion. ***Class I** – AF cardioversion of up to 7 days duration.* ***Class IIb** – AF cardioversion if present > 7 days.* *4% risk of torsades de pointes (esp. if female) usually within 1st hour but occasionally up to 4 hours after use. Avoid if low ejection fraction, CHF, prolonged QT interval, current use of Ia or III anti-arrhythmics. Ensure K, Mg are normal*
Isoproterenol *(Isuprel)*	• <u>Bradycardia</u> – 2 – 10 mcg/min IV (if atropine, dopamine have failed and no pacer) ***Class indeterminate** – polymorphic VT as temporizing measure*
Lidocaine	• <u>Vfib/Pulseless Vtach</u> - 1.0-1.5 mg/kg IV (2-4 mg/kg ET) may repeat 0.5-0.75 mg/kg IV over 3-5 minutes (Max 3 mg/kg) • <u>Vtach</u> – monomorphic, stable, normal cardiac function 1.0-1.5 mg/kg IV q 5-10 min.; <u>Vtach</u> - impaired cardiac function – 0.5 – 0.75 mg/kg IV q 5-10 minutes. (Max 3 mg/kg) • If conversion with lidocaine infuse 1-4 mg/min IV ***Class IIa**– for 24-48 hours after ventricular fibrillation/tachycardia* ***Class IIb**– sustained monomorphic ventricular tachycardia (VT) not associated with angina hypotension or CHF.* ***Class III** – prophylaxis with thrombolytics, isolated PVC's, couplets, accelerated idioventricular rhythm, nonsustained VT* ***Class Indeterminate** – pulseless Vfib/Vtach, (2) monomorphic ventricular tachycardia with impaired cardiac function.*

Magnesium	• <u>Torsades/Various tachyarrhythmias</u> - 2 g IV over 15 minutes ***Class I*** *– no class I recommendations* ***Class IIa*** *– Treating ↓K, ↓Mg, or torsades de pointes (indeterminate)*
Metoprolol *(Lopressor)*	• <u>Acute MI</u> – 25-50 mg PO q6h OR 5 mg IV q 5 min X 3, then 50 mg PO q 12 h X 24 hours, then ↑ to 100 mg q 12 h or 50 mg q 6 h as tolerated • <u>Afib</u>- 2.5-5.0 mg IV (over 2 min) q 5 min, up to 3 doses ***Class I*** *– STEMI/UA/NSTEMI – <12 h of MI or with ongoing, recurrent pain. Class I STEMI – orally administered.* ***Class I*** *– Afib – if no congestive heart failure* ***Class IIa*** *– STEMI – IV administration if no contraindication* ***Class IIb*** *– Afib – if congestive heart failure* ***Class III*** *– heart failure, bradycardia or other contraindication*
Nitroglycerin	• <u>MI/CHF/UA/NSTEMI</u> – Initiate at 10-20 mcg/min IV. Increase 5-20 mcg/min q 3-5 min until desired effect. One study found high dose (200-400 mcg/min) IV effective if pulmonary edema, systolic BP > 160 or MAP > 120. *Ann Emerg Med* 2007; 144 ***Class I*** *– (1) 1ˢᵗ 24 – 48 hours in acute MI with CHF, large anterior infarct, persistent ischemia or hypertension. (2) continued use (> 48 h) if recurrent angina, or persistent pulmonary congestion.* ***Class IIa*** *– (1) 1ˢᵗ 24-48 hours after MI without ↓ BP, ↑HR or ↓ HR (2) continued use (> 48 h) if large or complicated infarction* ***Class III*** *- DO NOT USE – systolic BP < 90 mm Hg or ≥ 30 mm Hg below baseline, or HR < 50, or within 24 hours of sildenafil (Viagra), 48 hours of tadalafil/Cialis use with unknown delay needed for vardenafil*
Norepinephrine *(Levophed)*	• <u>Shock</u> - 0.5-1 mcg/min, ↑1-2 mcg/min q 3-5 min until desired effect. Usual maintenance dose is 2-4 mcg/min, occasionally 8-30 mcg/min is required. Use central line if possible.
Procainamide	• <u>Afib/Flutter,Wide complex tachycardia</u> - 30 mg/min IV (max total dose 17 mg/kg) until (1) ↓BP, (2) QRS complex increases 50%, (3) arrhythmia stops or (4) total 17 mg/kg • <u>VF/pulseless VT</u> –50 mg/min IV (up to max dose 17 mg/min) ***Class IIa*** *– stable SVT/Atrial fib/flutter/ventricular tachycardia.* ***Class IIb*** *– VT/shock refractory VF, polymorphic VT, or Supraventricular tachycardia in WPW*
Propafenone *(Rythmol)*	• <u>AF</u> – 600 mg PO **OR** 1.5-2 mg/kg IV over 10-20 minutes. ***Class I*** *– AF cardioversion if present up to 7 days.* ***Class IIb*** *– AF cardioversion if present > 7 days.* *Adverse effects include rapid atrial flutter, ventricular tachycardia, intraventricular conduction disturbances, hypotension, and bradycardia (after cardioversion). Avoid in patients with heart failure, severe obstructive lung disease, and use cautiously in patients with organic heart disease.*

Class I-III definitions – see page 2
PCI – procedural coronary intervention, MI – myocardial infarction, UA – unstable angina, NSTEMI – nonST elevation MI, STEMI – ST elevation MI

Protamine sulfate	• 1 mg protamine neutralizes 100 units unfractionated heparin, 100 anti-Xa units of dalteparin or tinzaparin, OR 1 mg of enoxaparin (*Lovenox*). If aPTT is still elevated 2-4 hours after initial protamine dose, give 0.5 mg protamine for each 100 anti-Xa units of dalteparin or tinzaparin OR each 1 mg of enoxaparin. Administer by slow IV injection of 1% solution over > 10 minutes. Maximum dose is 50 mg. • Observe for anaphylaxis/hypotension if given too rapidly. Increased risk of allergic reaction if prior exposure (e.g. insulin), fish allergy, vasectomy (anti-protamine antibodies) . • Protamine reverses anti-thrombin activity but only partially reverses anti-Xa activity.
Reteplase	(*r-PA, Retavase*) see thrombolytics page 35
Sodium Nitroprusside	• 0.1 mcg/kg/min IV titrated up q 3-5 minutes to desired effect up to maximum of 10 mcg/kg/min
Sotalol (*Betapace, Betapace AF*)	Maintenance of sinus rhythm in Afib: 80 – 320 mg PO bid. ***Class IIa – Afib/flutter*** - pre-electric cardioversion to prevent recurrence of Afib/flutter. ***Class III*** – DO not use to cardiovert atrial fibrillation/flutter. Note: there is high incidence of torsades if > 320 mg/day administered, female, or heart failure.
Streptokinase	(*Streptase*) see thrombolytics page 35
Tenecteplase	(*TNKase*) see thrombolytics page 35
Thrombolytics	• See page 35
Tirofiban (*Aggrastat*)	• UA/NTSTEMI/PCI – 0.4 mcg/kg/min X 30 min, then 0.1 mcg/kg/min X 48-108 hours or until 24 hours after procedure. ***Class I – UA/NSTEMI*** –high risk, troponin positive pre PCI ***Class IIa – UA/NSTEMI/STEMI*** - administered pre PCI ***Class IIb – UA/NSTEMI*** – if conservative (nonPCI) strategy
Vasopressin	• Vfib/Pulseless Vtach – 40 units IV. No repeat dose. • Asystole – 40 units IV q 3 min X 2. May follow with epi prn.
Verapamil (*Calan*)	• SVT – 2.5-5.0 mg IV over 2 minutes. May repeat 5-10 mg IV over 2 minutes, 15-30 minutes after 1st dose • Afib – 0.075 – 0.15 mg/kg IV over 2 min. ***Class I – Afib*** – no congestive heart failure ***Class IIb – Afib*** – congestive heart failure
Vernakalant (*Cardiome*)	• Atrial fibrillation - 3 mg/kg IV over 10 min. If arrhythmia does not terminate after 15 minutes, administer 2 mg/kg IV. As of publication date, not yet FDA approved.

Class I-III definitions – see page 2
PCI – procedural coronary intervention, MI – myocardial infarction, UA – unstable angina, NSTEMI – nonST elevation MI, STEMI – ST elevation MI

Pulmonary Edema, Hypotension, Cardiogenic Shock Management

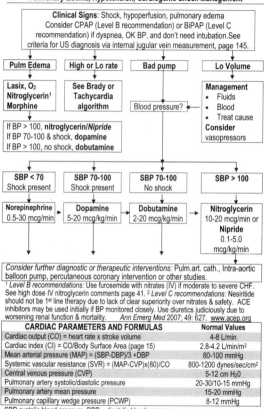

Clinical Signs: Shock, hypoperfusion, pulmonary edema
Consider CPAP (Level B recommendation) or BiPAP (Level C recommendation) if dyspnea, OK BP, and don't need intubation. See criteria for US diagnosis via internal jugular vein measurement, page 145.

Pulm Edema	High or Lo rate	Bad pump	Lo Volume
Lasix, O₂ Nitroglycerin¹ Morphine	**See Brady or Tachycardia algorithm**	Blood pressure?	**Management** • Fluids • Blood • Treat cause **Consider** vasopressors

If BP > 100, **nitroglycerin**/*Nipride*
If BP 70-100 & shock, **dopamine**
If BP > 100, no shock, **dobutamine**

SBP < 70 Shock present	SBP 70-100 Shock present	SBP 70-100 No shock	SBP > 100
Norepinephrine 0.5-30 mcg/min	**Dopamine** 5-20 mcg/kg/min	**Dobutamine** 2-20 mcg/kg/min	**Nitroglycerin** 10-20 mcg/min or **Nipride** 0.1-5.0 mcg/kg/min

Consider further diagnostic or therapeutic interventions: Pulm.art. cath., Intra-aortic balloon pump, percutaneous coronary intervention or other studies.

¹ *Level B recommendations:* Use furosemide with nitrates (IV) if moderate to severe CHF. See high dose IV nitroglycerin comments page 41. ² *Level C recommendations:* Nesiritide should not be 1st line therapy due to lack of clear superiority over nitrates for safety & safety. ACE inhibitors may be used initially if BP monitored closely. Use diuretics judiciously due to worsening renal function and mortality.   *Ann Emerg Med 2007; 49: 627.* www.acep.org

CARDIAC PARAMETERS AND FORMULAS	Normal Values
Cardiac output (CO) = heart rate x stroke volume	4-8 L/min
Cardiac index (CI) = CO/Body Surface Area (page 15)	2.8-4.2 L/min/m²
Mean arterial pressure (MAP) = (SBP-DBP)/3 +DBP	80-100 mmHg
Systemic vascular resistance (SVR) = (MAP-CVP)x(80)/CO	800-1200 dynes/sec/cm²
Central venous pressure (CVP)	5-12 cm H₂0
Pulmonary artery systolic/diastolic pressure	20-30/10-15 mmHg
Pulmonary artery mean pressure	15-20 mmHg
Pulmonary capillary wedge pressure (PCWP)	8-12 mmHg

SBP-systolic blood pressure, DBP – diastolic blood pressure

Abdominal Aortic Aneurysm (AAA)

AAA-diameter ≥1.5X adjacent aorta or ≥ 3cm

Risk factors: male, family history (25% risk if AAA in sibling/parent), ↑ age, smoking, ↑BP peripheral or collagen vascular disease.

Radiologic evaluation: Plain films show calcified aorta in ~ 60%. Angiography can miss AAA with mural thrombus. US detects all AAA but only leakage in 4%. CT identifies 100% of AAA's & > 95% rupture but not aortoenteric or venous fistula, inflammatory AAA. Use MRI.

Management: (1) If rupture and unstable, resuscitate as needed, go to O.R. for repair

Clinical Features of Ruptured AAA	
Abdominal pain	77%
Flank or back pain	60%
Vomiting	25%
Syncope	18%
Hematemesis	5%
Known AAA	5%
Pulsatile mass	40-70%
Abdomen tenderness	41%
Pain, mass, and low BP	30-40%
Absent low ext. pulses	6%
Anuria or abd. bruit	< 1%

(± bedside US-see features page 144). Do not delay repair. (2) If rupture and stable, monitor, O₂, large IV X 2 with NS. ECG, CXR, CBC, electrolytes, renal, function, type & cross ≥ 4-6 units blood. Immediately notify surgeon. CT or MRI

Thoracic Aortic Dissection

	DeBakey Classification			
Classification of Thoracic Aortic Dissection	Type I - Ascending + descending aorta, Type II - Ascending aorta only, Type III - Distal to subclavian artery (IIIa above diaphragm and IIIb below diaphragm)			
	Stanford Classification			
	A – ascending aorta involved, B – only descending aorta			
Clinical Features	Chest or back pain			88-95%
	Aortic regurgitation ± congestive heart failure			50%
	Transitory pulse deficits			50%
	Neurologic deficits, hypotension (each 20%)			20%
	Syncope, tamponade, abdominal pain, GI bleed hematuria, dyspnea, Horner's syndrome, superior vena cava syndrome, and hemoptysis			variable

Diagnosis

CXR Findings		Diagnostic Study	Sensitivity	Specificity
Any abnormality	85%	D-dimer elevation	97-100%	34%
Wide mediastinum	75%	Transthoracic echo.	75%	85-90%
Aortic knob (Ca⁺² rim > 5mm from	-	Angiography	85%	90-95%
knob, bulge, obliterated knob)	66%	Conventional CT	65-85%	95-100%
Irregular aortic contour	38%	Helical CT	95-100%	95-100%
Displaced trachea or NG tube	26%	Transesophageal echo	95-100%	90-97%
Left pleural effusion	27%	MRI	95-100%	95-100%

Thoracic Aortic Dissection - Management

If unstable, resuscitate & prepare for surgery. If stable, consult surgeon, control pain, Control BP & HR. Goal = HR of 60-80 & systolic BP = 90-110 mm Hg.

- Labetalol OR [(Esmolol/*Brevibloc*) + *Nipride*]. (See page 222 for dosing)
- Surgery is indicated for most ascending (Stanford A) dissections. Type B dissections are usually treated medically but occasionally require surgery.

Syncope

Syncope: sudden loss of consciousness with loss of tone/spontaneous recovery. Relatively benign causes include vasodepressor syncope from excess vagal tone, micturation & defecation syncope, orthostasis from dehydration or blood loss and drug induced. Life threats include dysrhythmias, aortic stenosis, MI, pulmonary embolus, vertebrobasilar transient ischemic attacks & cardiac conduction defects.

Cause of Syncope	
Cardiac 9-25%	**Not heart 34-46%**
Vent tachycardia 11%	Orthostasis 10-21%
Sick sinus 3%	Vasovagal 8-9%
Complete heart	Situational 8%
or Mobitz II block 2%	Drugs 2-7%
SVT 2%	TIA 2-4%
Aortic stenosis 2%	Seizure 2-5%
MI, ↓HR -	**Unknown 37-41%**
Carotid sinus -	*NEJM* 2002; 347:
Aortic dissection 1%	878.; *Medicine*
Pulm. embolism 1%	1990; 69: 160

Diagnosis

Evaluation includes complete examination with orthostatic vitals signs, a βhCG in women of child-bearing age, an ECG and pulse oximetry. Further evaluation is guided by the history and physical.

Studies Revealing Syncope Etiology	
History and physical exam	49%
Electrocardiographic monitoring	27%
Electrocardiogram	11%
Cardiac catheterization	7%
Electrophysiologic study	3%
Cerebral angiography, EEG	1-2%

ECG Features of Disorders Causing Syncope/Cardiac Arrest[1]

Disorder	ECG Abnormality[1]
Arrhythmogenic right ventricular cardiomyopathy - Right bundle branch block (RBBB), or in absence of RBBB - QRS > 110 ms in leads V1-V3 with T wave inversion in V2 & V3, LBBB ectopic beats. Epsilon wave[2]	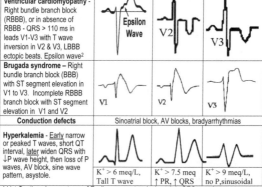

Epsilon Wave — V2 — V3

| **Brugada syndrome** – Right bundle branch block (BBB) with ST segment elevation in V1 to V3. Incomplete RBBB branch block with ST segment elevation in V1 and V2 | V1 — V2 — V3 |

| **Conduction defects** | Sinoatrial block, AV blocks, bradyarrhythmias |

| **Hyperkalemia** - Early narrow or peaked T waves, short QT interval, <u>later</u> widen QRS with ↓P wave height, then loss of P waves, AV block, sine wave pattern, asystole. | K^+ > 6 meq/L, Tall T wave — K^+ > 7.5 meq ↑ PR, ↑ QRS — K^+ > 9 meq/L, no P, sinusoidal |

[1] List Continued on next page [2] Epsilon wave – terminal notch in QRS complex

ECG Features of Disorders Causing Syncope/Cardiac Arrest[1] continued

Hypocalcemia – Classically cause prolonged T waves (*see prolonged QT below*)	Prolongs QT by lengthening ST segment, also ↓ T wave voltage, flat T waves, terminal T wave inversion, or deeply inverted T waves (if severe), rare ST elevation.
Hypokalemia - ST depression flat T waves and prominent U wave (arrow), prolonged QT	U wave

Hypertrophic cardiomyopathy (Idiopathic subaortic stenosis) Nonspecific ST-T wave abnormalities; left ventricular hypertrophy. QRS complexes largest in midprecordial leads; Q waves in inferior (II, III, aV$_F$) or precordial (V$_2$ to V$_6$) leads, or both.

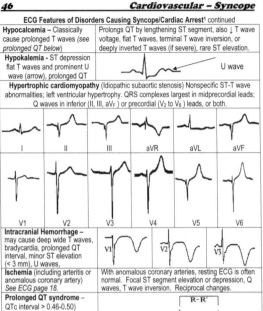

I   II   III   aVR   aVL   aVF

V1   V2   V3   V4   V5   V6

Intracranial Hemorrhage – may cause deep wide T waves, bradycardia, prolonged QT interval, minor ST elevation (< 3 mm), U waves,	V1 V2 V3
Ischemia (including arteritis or anomalous coronary artery) See ECG page 18.	With anomalous coronary arteries, resting ECG is often normal. Focal ST segment elevation or depression, Q waves, T wave inversion. Reciprocal changes.
Prolonged QT syndrome – QTc interval > 0.46-0.50) milliseconds, although may need stress testing to uncover prolongation of QT. Go to www.qtdrugs.org for causes.	R – R′ $$QT_c = \frac{QT}{\sqrt{RR}}$$ QT
Wellens' syndrome – (anterior wall changes due to LAD block) symmetric/deep inverted T waves V2/V3 (±V1-V6) or biphasic T waves in V2, V3, ST elevation usually < 1 mm.	V1 V2 V3
Wolff-Parkinson-White syndrome - Delta wave, wide QRS, short PR interval, wide complex Afib/SVT	Delta Wave

[1] The list is not all inclusive and only describes common ECG findings for listed diseases.

Management: If a cardiac or life-threatening cause is likely, it must be ruled out definitively in the ED or the patient must be admitted (on continuous telemetry). In 2 studies, the Boston Syncope Criteria were 97-100% sensitive in identifying patients requiring intervention within 30 days for serious event. If NO Boston Criteria present there was a 0-1% probability of serious event (99-100% negative predictive value).

Boston Syncope Criteria

Acute Coronary Syndrome Signs and Symptoms	• Chest pain that may be ischemic in origin • ECG with ischemia (ST elevation or > 1 mm ST depression • Other ECGs (VT, VF, SVT, rapid Afib, new ST-T changes) • Complaint of shortness of breath felt to be cardiac
Worrisome cardiac history *(HOCM=hypertrophic obstructive cardiomyopathy)*	• Prior CAD, deep q waves, HOCM or cardiomyopathy • CHF history or LV dysfunction • Prior VT, VF, pacemaker, ICD • Prehospital use of antidysrhythmics (not BB, or CCB)
Family history	• Family history sudden death, HOCM, Brugada, or long QT
Valvular heart disease	• Valvular heart disease or murmur on ED examination
Cardiac conduction defect	• Multiple syncopal episodes prior 6 months, rapid heartbeat by history, syncope during exercise, QT > 500 ms, 2nd or 3rd degree heart block or intraventricular heart block
Volume depletion	• GI bleeding by history or hemoccult positive • Hematocrit < 30% or dehydration not corrected in ED
Vital sign (VS) abnormality persisting in ED	• VS abnormality persisting (> 15 min) in ED without need for oxygen, pressors, temporary pacer. (e.g. RR > 24 breaths/min, O₂ sat. < 90%, HR < 50 or > 100, BP < 90 mm Hg)
Primary CNS event	• Subarachnoid hemorrhage, stroke

J Emerg Med 2007; 33: 233-239; Acad Emerg Med 2007; 14: S47.

American College of Emergency Physicians Syncope Guidelines

Level	Level - Recommendations[1]
History & Physical	• Level A – Use history/physical findings of heart failure to identify patients at risk for adverse outcome • Level B – Older age, structural heart disease, coronary heart disease have ↑adverse outcome. Young patients are at low risk unless exertional syncope, family history sudden death, or comorbidity. • Level C – No recommendations
Testing	• Level A – Obtain a 12 lead ECG.; Level B – No recommendations • Level C – Lab tests, advanced studies (e.g. CT scan, Echo) are not routinely performed unless indicated based on history/physical exam.
Admission	• Level A – No recommendations • Level B – Admit patients with heart failure, coronary artery disease, structural heart disease, older age (> 45-60 years depending upon cardiovascular health), abnormal ECG (ischemia, dysrhythmia, or significant conduction abnormality), hematocrit < 30%, or suspicion of life threatening illness.

Level A, B, C – See definitions page 2.   www.acep.org

Electrolyte Disorders

Criteria for Detecting Significant Electrolyte Abnormalities in ED Patients

Poor oral intake, vomiting	Recent seizures	Altered mental status
Hypertension, diuretic use	Muscle weakness	Prior abnormal electrolytes
Age ≥ 65 years	Alcohol abuse	(e.g. renal disease, diabetes)

≥ 1 criteria had 95% sensitivity, 97% negative predictive value *Ann Emerg Med* 1991;20:16.

CALCIUM

Hypocalcemia - Total calcium < 8.5 mg/dl or ionized Ca^{+2} < 2.0 mEq/L (1.0 mmol/L)

Hypercalcemia - Total calcium > 10.5 mg/dl or ionized Ca^{+2} > 2.7 mEq/L (1.3 mmol/L)

Hypoalbuminemia – a serum albumin ↓of 1 g/dl will↓ total serum Ca^{+2} 0.8 mg/dl

Hypocalcemia – Clinical Features

Symptoms	Physical Findings	Electrocardiogram
Paresthesias, fatigue	Hyperactive reflexes, Low BP	Prolonged QT[2]
Seizures, tetany	Chvostek(C)/Trousseau(T) signs[1]	(esp. Ca^{+2} < 6.0 mg/dl)
Vomiting, weakness	Anterior neck scar (e.g. thyroid)	• Bradycardia
Laryngospasm	Congestive heart failure	• Arrhythmias

[1] C-muscle twitch if tap facial nerve, T-carpal spasm after forearm BP cuff X 3 min
[2] See ECG example and other ECG findings page 46.

Hypocalcemia Evaluation

Ca^{+2} – calcium
Mg^{+2} – magnesium

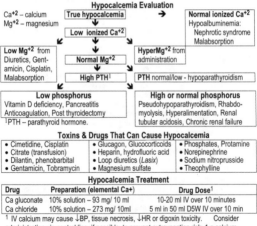

True hypocalcemia	→	Normal ionized Ca^{+2}
↓		Hypoalbuminemia:
Low ionized Ca^{+2}		Nephrotic syndrome
↓		Malabsorption

Low Mg^{+2} from	←	↓	→	HyperMg^{+2} from
Diuretics, Gent-		Normal Mg^{+2}		administration
amicin, Cisplatin,		↓		
Malabsorption		High PTH[1]	→	PTH normal/low - hypoparathyroidism

Low phosphorus	High or normal phosphorus
Vitamin D deficiency, Pancreatitis	Pseudohypoparathyroidism, Rhabdo-
Anticoagulation, Post thyroidectomy	myolysis, Hyperalimentation, Renal
	tubular acidosis, Chronic renal failure

[1] PTH – parathyroid hormone.

Toxins & Drugs That Can Cause Hypocalcemia

• Cimetidine, Cisplatin	• Glucagon, Glucocorticoids	• Phosphates, Protamine
• Citrate (transfusion)	• Heparin, hydrofluoric acid	• Norepinephrine
• Dilantin, phenobarbital	• Loop diuretics (*Lasix*)	• Sodium nitroprusside
• Gentamicin, Tobramycin	• Magnesium sulfate	• Theophylline

Hypocalcemia Treatment

Drug	Preparation (elemental Ca+)	Drug Dose[1]
Ca gluconate	10% solution – 93 mg/ 10 ml	10-20 ml IV over 10 minutes
Ca chloride	10% solution – 273 mg/ 10ml	5 ml in 50 ml D5W IV over 10 min

[1] IV calcium may cause ↓BP, tissue necrosis, ↓HR or digoxin toxicity. Consider administration via central line, if possible, to prevent extravasation risk. 1 g calcium gluconate = 93 mg elemental calcium, 1 g calcium chloride = 273 mg elemental calcium

Hypercalcemia etiology: (PAM P SCHMIDT) HyperParathyroidism, Addison's disease, Milk alkali syndrome, Paget's disease, Sarcoid, Cancer, Hyperthyroidism, Myeloma, Immobilization, Hypervitaminosis D, Thiazides	
Hypercalcemia – Clinical Features	
General	• Weakness, polydipsia, dehydration
Neurologic	• Confusion, lethargy, irritability, hyporeflexia, headache
Skeletal	• Bone pain, fractures
Cardiac	• Hypertension, QT shortening, wide T wave, arrhythmias
GI	• Anorexia, weight loss, constipation, ulcer, pancreatitis
Renal	• Polyuria, renal insufficiency, nephrolithiasis

Hypercalcemia Evaluation

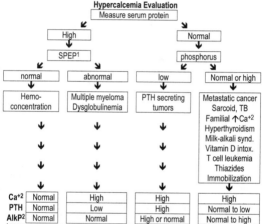

	normal	abnormal	low	Normal or high
	Hemo-concentration	Multiple myeloma Dysglobulinemia	PTH secreting tumors	Metastatic cancer Sarcoid, TB Familial ↑Ca^{+2} Hyperthyroidism Milk-alkali synd. Vitamin D intox. T cell leukemia Thiazides Immobilization
Ca^{+2}	Normal	High	High	High
PTH	Normal	Low	High	Normal to low
AlkP[2]	Normal	Normal	High or normal	Normal to high

[1]SPEP – serum protein electrophoresis; [2]AlkP – alkaline phosphatase

Hypercalcemia Management

- IV NS 1-2 L bolus + 200-500 ml/hr if no heart failure or fluid overload present.
- Furosemide (*Lasix*) 1 mg/kg IV q 2-4 h to keep urine output 200-300 ml/h. Use is controversial as this can release calcium from bone worsening hypercalcemia.
- Follow urine output & magnesium (Mg), and potassium (K$^+$) losses, replacing prn or empirically administering after urine output verified.
- Consider dialysis with calcium free dialysate if renal failure
- Osteoclast inhibition via one of following: bisphosphates (etidronate, pamidronate), plicamycin, calcitonin, hydrocortisone, and gallium nitrate

MAGNESIUM

Hypomagnesemia (<1.5 mEq/L): Due to alcohol, diuretics, aminoglycosides, malnourished. Irritable muscle, tetany, seizures. <u>Treat</u>: MgSO$_4$ 1-2 g IV over 5-20 minutes.

Hypermagnesemia (>2.2 mEq/L) Due to renal failure, excess maternal Mg supplement, or overuse of Mg-containing medicine. Clinical features: weakness, hyporeflexia, paralysis, and ECG with AV block and QT prolongation. <u>Treat</u>: Ca gluconate (10%) 10-20 ml IV.

POTASSIUM

Acute decreases in pH will increase K$^+$ (a $\downarrow$pH of 0.1 will $\uparrow$K$^+$ 0.3-1.3 mEq/L).

Causes of Hypokalemia	
• Decreased K$^+$ intake • Intracellular shift: alkalinia, insulin, β agonists, epinephrine, pseudohypokalemia of leukemia, familial hypo-kalemic periodic paralysis.	• Increased excretion: diuretics, hyper-aldosteronism, penicillins (exchange Na$^+$/K$^+$), sweating, diarrhea (colonic fluid has high K$^+$), vomiting, binding in gut (clay ingestion – e.g. pica)

Hypokalemia Evaluation

Measure blood pH (pH), serum CO$_2$, and Cl$^-$

$\downarrow$CO$_2$, $\uparrow$Cl$^-$		normal CO$_2$, Cl$^-$	$\uparrow$CO$_2$, $\downarrow$Cl$^-$
pH < 7.35 Met acidosis[1]	pH > 7.45 Resp alkalosis[2]	pH 7.35-7.45 Met. Acidosis Resp alkalosis	Normal pH	pH > 7.45 Met. alkalosis
RTA[3] 1 or 2	Diarrhea	Cirrhosis Sepsis Salicylates	Hypokalemic periodic paralysis	Diuretics,$\downarrow$Mg Vomiting Laxative abuse Hyperaldoster-onism Licorice abuse
Urine pH > 6.5 Urine K$^+$ > 30 mM/d	Urine pH < 5.3 Urine K$^+$ < 30 mM/d			

[1]Metabolic acidosis, [2]Respiratory alkalosis, [3]Renal tubular acidosis

Clinical Features of Hypokalemia	Treatment of Hypokalemia
• Lethargy, confusion weakness • Areflexia, difficult respirations • Autonomic instability, Low BP	• Ensure adequate urine output first • Mild hypokalemia, replace orally only • Severe $\downarrow$ K$^+$, use parenteral K$^+$
ECG findings (see page 46)	(e.g. cardiac, or neuromuscular
• K$^+$ ≤ 3.0 mEq/L: low voltage QRS, flat T's, $\downarrow$ST, prominent P & U waves (See example page 46) • K$^+$ ≤ 2.5 mEq/L: prominent U waves • K$^+$ ≤ 2.0 mEq/L: widened QRS	symptoms or DKA). • Correct low magnesium. • Administer K$^+$ at ≤ 10 mEq/h using ≤ 40 mEq/L while on cardiac monitor. • 40 mEq raises serum K$^+$ by 1 mEq/L

Hyperkalemia

Causes of Hyperkalemia

• _Pseudohyperkalemia_ due to blood sampling or hemolysis. • _Exogenous:_ blood, salt substitutes, potassium containing drugs (e.g. penicillin derivatives), acute digoxin toxicity, β blockers, succinylcholine.	• _Endogenous_ – renal failure, acidemia, trauma, burns, rhabdomyolysis, DIC, sickle cell crisis, GI bleed, chemotherapy (destroying tumor mass or tumor lysis syndrome), mineralo-corticoid deficiency), congenital defects (21 hydroxylase deficiency)

Hyperkalemia Evaluation

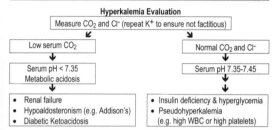

Measure CO_2 and Cl^- (repeat K^+ to ensure not factitious)

Low serum CO_2 → Serum pH < 7.35 Metabolic acidosis →
- Renal failure
- Hypoaldosteronism (e.g. Addison's)
- Diabetic Ketoacidosis

Normal CO_2 and Cl^- → Serum pH 7.35-7.45 →
- Insulin deficiency & hyperglycemia
- Pseudohyperkalemia (e.g. high WBC or high platelets)

Clinical Features of Hyperkalemia	Treatment of Hyperkalemia
• Paresthesias, weakness • Ascending paralysis sparing head, trunk, and respiration.	• Calcium gluconate[1] (10%)–5-30 ml IV over 2-5 min, may repeat **OR** • $CaCl_2$[1] (10%) 5-10 ml IV over 5-10 min • $NaHCO_3$[2] 1 mEq/kg IV, repeat ½ dose q 10 min prn

ECG in Hyperkalemia (K^+ in mEq/L)	
K^+	**ECG findings**
> 5.5-6	Peaked T waves
> 6-6.5	↑ PR and QT intervals
> 6.5-7	flat or isoelectric P waves, ↓ ST segments
> 7-7.5	↑intraventricular conduction
> 7.5-8	↑ QRS, ST&T waves merge
> 10.0	sine wave appearance (See examples page 45)

- Glucose/Insulin – 10 units regular insulin IV + 50 ml D_{50} IV, then 10-20 units regular insulin in 500 ml D_{10}W IV over 1 h if needed, check glucose q h.
- Albuterol nebulizer 10-20 mg over 15 min, may repeat
- Furosemide 40-80 mg IV
- Kayexalate[2] 15-60 g PO or 50 g PR
- Dialysis
- Digibind if digoxin toxic (page 173)

[1] Contraindicated if digoxin toxicity. IV $CaCl_2$ can cause phlebitis.

[2] $NaHCO_3$ is hpertonic and may worsen fluid overload (i.e. congestive heart failure).

SODIUM

FE_{Na} = fraction of Na^+ in urine filtered by the glomerulus and not reabsorbed.

FE_{Na} = 100 x (urine Na^+/plasma Na^+) ÷ (urine creatinine/plasma creatinine)

Hyponatremia

Na^+ = falsely ↓ 1.6 mEq/L for each 100 mg/dL ↑ in glucose over 100 mg/dL.

Clinical Features of Hyponatremia	
• Lethargy, apathy, cerebral edema	• Seizures, hypothermia
• Depressed reflexes, muscle cramps	• Pseudobulbar palsies

Hyponatremia Evaluation

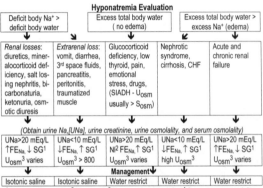

Deficit body Na^+ > deficit body water		Excess total body water (no edema)		Excess total body water > excess Na^+ (edema)
Renal losses: diuretics, mineralocorticoid deficiency, salt losing nephritis, bicarbonaturia, ketonuria, osmotic diuresis	*Extrarenal loss:* vomit, diarrhea, 3rd space fluids, pancreatitis, peritonitis, traumatized muscle	Glucocorticoid deficiency, low thyroid, pain, emotional stress, drugs, (SIADH - U_{osm} usually > S_{osm})	Nephrotic syndrome, cirrhosis, CHF	Acute and chronic renal failure

(Obtain urine Na, [UNa], urine creatinine, urine osmolality, and serum osmolality)

UNa>20 mEq/L ↑FE_{Na}, ↓ SG[1] U_{osm}[3] varies	UNa<10 mEq/L ↓FE_{Na}, ↑ SG[1] U_{osm}[3] > 800	UNa>20 mEq/L NI[2] FE_{Na}, ↑ SG[1] U_{osm}[3] varies	UNa<10 mEq/L ↓FE_{Na}, ↑ SG[1] high U_{osm}[3]	UNa>20 mEq/L ↑FE_{Na}, ↓ SG[1] U_{osm}[3] varies
		Management↓		
Isotonic saline	Isotonic saline	Water restrict	Water restrict	Water restrict

[1] SG – specific gravity, [2] NI- normal, [3] U_{osm} – urine osmolality, [4] S_{osm} -serum osmolality

Hypertonic Saline Administration (3% NaCl = 513 mEq/L)

Indication	• Severe ↓ Na^+ with serious CNS manifestations (e.g. seizures)
Goal	• Only ↑Na^+ to 120-125 mEq/L acutel (maximum of 12 mEq/L/24h).
Formula	• **Na^+ deficit** = weight (kg) X 0.6 X (desired Na^+[~125] − known Na^+) • **Infusion rate (ml/hour)** that will ↑Na^+ 1 mEq/L/hour = (weight [kg] X 0.6) ÷ (0.513 mEq/L X 1 hour)
Rate	• Severe, symptomatic, hyponatremia – empiric dosing for 60 kg adult consists of 300-500 ml 3% NaCl over 1-2 hours or until resolution of seizures or herniation.
Adjuncts	• Furosemide (*Lasix*) – 40 mg IV; remember to check Na^+ q 2 hours

Hypernatremia

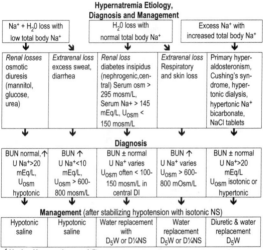

Clinical Features of Hypernatremia	
• Lethargy, irritability, coma	• Doughy skin
• Seizures	• Late preservation of intravascular
• Spasticity, hyperreflexia	volume (and vital signs)

Hypernatremia Etiology, Diagnosis and Management

Na^+ + H_2O loss with low total body Na^+		H_2O loss with normal total body Na^+	Excess Na^+ with increased total body Na^+	
Renal losses osmotic diuresis (mannitol, glucose, urea)	*Extrarenal loss* excess sweat, diarrhea	*Renal loss* diabetes insipidus (nephrogenic,central) Serum osm > 295 mosm/L, Serum Na+ > 145 mEq/L, U_{osm} < 150 mosm/L	*Extrarenal loss* Respiratory and skin loss	Primary hyper-aldosteronism, Cushing's syndrome, hypertonic dialysis, hypertonic Na^+ bicarbonate, NaCl tablets

Diagnosis				
BUN normal, ↑ U Na+>20 mEq/L, U_{osm} hypotonic	BUN ↑ U Na+<10 mEq/L, U_{osm} > 600-800 mosm/L	BUN ± normal U Na+ varies U_{osm} often < 100-150 mosm/L in central DI	BUN ↑ U Na+ varies U_{osm} > 600-800 mOsm/L	BUN ± normal U Na+>20 mEq/L U_{osm} isotonic or hypertonic

Management (after stabilizing hypotension with isotonic NS)				
Hypotonic saline	Hypotonic saline	Water replacement with D_5W or D¼NS	Water replacement D_5W or D¼NS	Diuretic & water replacement D_5W

[1] U-urine, U_{osm} – urine osmolality

Management of Hypernatremia

- Correct hypernatremia slowly over 48 to 72 hours. Over vigorous rehydration can cause cerebral edema, seizures, coma, or death. Lower Na^+ no faster than 1-2 mEq/L/hour.
- With endogenous Na^+ overload, treatment consists of salt restriction and correction of the primary underlying disorder. If there is excess exogenous mineralocorticoid, restrict salt and modify replacement therapy.

Endocrine Disorders

Adrenal Insufficiency

Clinical Features		Adrenal Crisis Therapy
Weakness	99%	• 1-2 Liters NS IV with further IV fluids as needed
↑pigment	92%	• Correct electrolyte abnormalities
Weight loss	97%	• Hydrocortisone (*Solu-Cortef*) 200 mg IV, + 100 mg q8h
Vomiting	70%	or dexamethasone 4 mg IV (will not interfere with ACTH
Anorexia	98%	stimulation testing)
BP < 110/70	85%	• If possible draw & store blood for steroid level analysis
Abdominal		including baseline serum cortisol and ACTH levels.
Pain	34%	• Consider broad spectrum antibiotics (e.g. ceftriaxone 1-
Salt craving	22%	2 g IV) if suspicion of sepsis
Diarrhea	20%	• Perform rapid bedside check of blood sugar
↑ K⁺		• Treat underling precipitants (e.g. sepsis, hypothermia,
↓ Na⁺		MI, ↓glucose, bleeding, trauma, remove meds that
Eosinophilia		↓cortisone: morphine, chlorpromazine, barbiturates)

Diabetes Mellitus

Insulin Regimens - Guidelines

Critically ill patients: blood glucose levels should be kept as close to 110 mg/dl (6.1 mmol/l) as possible generally <180 mg/dl (10 mmol/l), usually with IV regular insulin. *(2008 study found that intensive insulin therapy placed critically ill patients with sepsis at ↑ risk for serious adverse events related to hypoglycemia. N Engl J Med 2008; 358: 125)*

Non–critically ill patients: premeal blood glucose levels should be kept as close as possible to 90–130 mg/dl (5.0–7.2 mmol/l; midpoint of range 110 mg/dl) given the clinical situation and postprandial blood glucose levels <180 mg/dl. Insulin should be used as necessary.

- Monitor blood glucose 30 minutes before meals, if taking PO, and qhs.
- Use correction dose or "supplemental" insulin to correct premeal hyperglycemia in addition to scheduled prandial and basal insulin.
  - Basal/Maintenance insulin:
    - ♦ glargine (*Lantus*) – (1) If no prior insulin use, start 10 units SC/day and adjust accordingly. (2) If switching from NPH to Lantus & NPH is dosed once/day, start a total dose equivalent to the NPH dose. (3) If NPH is dosed twice per day at home, reduce totally daily dose of glargine to 80% of total daily NPH. (4)If switching from premixed insulin (e.g. 70/30), administer 80% of the intermediate acting portion of premixed insulin.
    - ♦ Alternate: NPH insulin (*Novolin N, Humulin N*) – dose at 0.5-1 units/kg/day divided bid with 2/3 given in the AM and 1/3 given in the PM.
  - Sliding scale (SS) insulin (regular or rapid acting/aspart) dosing used alone is NOT recommended by the American Diabetic Association. SS may be used in addition to basal insulin or current oral agents. (See next page)

Sliding Scale Insulin Regimen (Not to be used alone – use with basal dosing)[1]

Glucose (mg/dl)	Low dose insulin (elderly or underweight)	medium dose insulin (average weight patients)	High dose insulin (overweight patients)	Very high dose (steroids or infection)
< 70	Treat hypoglycemia			
70-130	0	0	0	0
131-150	0	0	2 units	3 units
151-200	2 units	4 units	6 units	8 units
201-250	4 units	6 units	8 units	10 units
251-300	6 units	8 units	10 units	12 units
301-350	8 units	10 units	12 units	14 units
351-400	10 units	12 units	14 units	16 units
> 400	12 units[2]	14 units[2]	16 units[2]	18 units[2]

Advance to next higher insulin dose if glucose > 200 mg/dl twice in 24 hours AND all levels > 100 mg/dl in same 24 hours. Decrease to next lower insulin dose if blood glucose < 80 mg/dl at least twice in a 24 hour period.

[1] Regular insulin (30 min premeal) or rapid acting (immediate premeal)
[2] Evaluate for precipitant/complication (infection, acidosis, stroke, other disease)

INSULIN	Preparation	Onset (h)	Peak (h)	Duration (h)
Rapid	aspart (Novolog)	≤ 0.3	1-3	3-5
	glulisine (Apidra)[1]	≤ 0.25	1-1.5	3-5
	lispro	0.25-0.5	0.5-2.5	3-6.5
	regular (Novolin/Humulin R)	0.5-1	1-5	6-10
Intermediate	isophane NPH (Novolin N, Humulin N)	1-2	4-8	10-20
Long	detemir (Levemir)	1-2	6-8	12-20
	Glargine (Lantus)	1-2	prolonged[2]	24

Humulin + Novolin 70/30, 50/50 p = %NPH/%regular insulin, Humalog Mix 75/25, 50/50 = %lispro protamine susp/%lispro, Novolog Mix 70/30 = %aspart protamine susp/%aspart
[1] Can be used in insulin pump
[2] Relatively constant concentration/time profile over 24 h with no pronounced peak.

Diabetic Ketoacidosis (DKA) – Diagnostic Features

	Mild – DKA	Moderate-DKA	Severe-DKA	HHS[1]
Plasma glucose	> 250 mg/dl	> 250	> 250	> 600
Arterial pH	7.25-7.35	7.0-7.24	< 7.0	> 7.3
Serum bicarbonate	15-18 mEq/L	10 to < 15	< 10	> 15
Urine ketones	+	+	+	small
Serum ketones	+	+	+	small
Serum osmolality[2]	Varies	Varies	Varies	> 320 mOsm/kg
Anion gap[3]	> 10	> 12	> 12	Varies
Mentation	Alert	Alert or drowsy	Stupor/coma	Stupor/coma

[1] HHS-Hyperosmolar, Hyperglycemic, Nonketotic State, [2] 2 X (Na) + glucose/18 + BUN/2.8
[3] (Na) – (Cl + HCO_3)

Initial Diabetic Ketoacidosis Management

Initial	• Apply cardiac monitor, administer O_2 if altered mental status/shock • Obtain baseline labs (pH, electrolytes, BUN, creatinine, serum ketones, CBC, UA), baseline ECG (see hyperkalemia ECG page 45), assess for DKA complications & precipitants. • Initially monitor q hourly glucose, q 2-4 h electrolytes, renal function
IV fluids	• IV NS until hypotension, and orthostasis resolve. If no cardiac compromise, administer 1-1.5 L in 1st hour. • If corrected serum sodium (Na) is normal or high, administer ½ NS at 4-14 ml/kg/hour depending on hydration status. • If corrected Na is low, administer NS at 4-14 ml/kg/hour • Corrected Na = Measured serum Na + [(1.6) X (glucose -100 mg/dL)/100] • Add potassium once renal perfusion assured. See below. Fluid replacement should correct estimated fluid deficits within 1st 24 hours. Serum osmolality should not change > 3 mOsm/kg/hour.
Insulin	• Bolus - 0.15 U/kg regular insulin IV (some experts do not bolus). • Infusion - administer 0.1 U/kg/h IV. If serum glucose, does not fall by 50-70 mg/dl in first hour double insulin infusion hourly until glucose falls 50-70 mg/dl in hour. When glucose falls to 250 mg/dl, change IV to D5 ½NS at 150-250 ml/hour with adequate insulin (0.05 – 0.1 U/kg/hour) to keep glucose between 150-200 mg/dl until metabolic control achieved. Change to SC regular insulin once bicarbonate > 15 mEq/L and no anion gap. • Mild DKA option – (definition page 55) consider IM/SC option: bolus 0.4 U/kg (½ IV and ½ IM or SC), then 0.1 U/kg/hour IM or SC. If serum glucose does not fall by 50-70 mg/dl in first hour, give hourly IV insulin bolus (10 units) until glucose falls by 50-70 mg/dl.
Potassium (K)	• Verify renal perfusion, urine output before administration. • If initial K is < 3.3 mEq/L, add 40 mEq to each L (2:1 mix KCL/K_3PO_4). Some experts hold insulin until K is ≥ 3.3 mEq/L. • If initial K is ≥ 3.3 and < 5.0 – administer 20-30 mEq in each L of fluids (2:1 - KCL/K_3PO_4) to keep serum K at 4-5 mEq/L. • If initial K is ≥ 5 mEq/L – do not give K, check K every 2 hours.
Bicarbonate	• Use is controversial. It is primarily indicated for hyperkalemia management, if needed. Guidelines do not recommend if pH > 7.0. • Dosing if used – pH < 6.9: 100 mmol $NaHCO_3$ in 400 ml H_2O, at 200 ml/hour. pH 6.9-7.0: 50 mmol $NaHCO_3$ in 200 ml H_2O, at 200 ml/hour. Repeat q 2 hours until pH > 7, monitor serum K.

Diabetes Care 2004, 27 Suppl 1:S94-102.

Hyperosmolar Hyperglycemic Nonketotic State (HHS)

Diagnosis of HHS	Etiology/Precipitants of HHS	
• Serum osmolarity >320-350 mOsm/L	Renal failure	Pancreatitis
• Glucose > 600 mg/dl (often > 1000)	Pneumonia,Sepsis	Burn
• No ketosis (lactic acidosis ± present)	GI bleed	Heat stroke
• 50-65% have no history of diabetes	MI	Dialysis
• ↑ BUN with BUN/Cr ratio > 30	CNS bleed/stroke	Recent surgery
• ↑ CK due to rhabdomyolysis	Pulmonary emboli	Drugs, Medicines[1]

[1] Calcium channel blockers, β blockers, carbamazepine, chlorthalidone, cimetidine, cocaine/alcohol, diuretics, immunosuppressant, neuroleptics, olanzipine, phenytoin, steroids

History		Physical Exam	
Fever	Polydipsia	↓ consciousness	Hemiparesis
Thirst	Confusion	Tachycardia, ↓ BP	Myoclonus
Polyuria or	Seizures (focal)	Fever	Quadriplegia
Oliguria	Hallucinations	Focal seizure	Nystagmus

Management-Guidelines

- Admit most patients to the ICU, and consider placement of central line if underlying renal or cardiac disease.
- Obtain electrolytes, CBC, CK, UA, CXR, ECG, cultures, ± head CT or spinal tap if suspicion of intracranial disease.
- <u>Fluids</u>- mean fluid deficit is 9 L. Start IV NS until BP & urine output OK. Then, change to ½NS & replace 50% of deficit over 12 h, & 50% over next 12-24 h. The American Diabetic Association guidelines recommend ½ NS at 4-14 ml/kg/hour depending upon hydration state if normal or elevated corrected sodium. If low corrected sodium administration of NS at 4-14 ml/kg/hour.
- Corrected Sodium = Measured serum Sodium + [(1.6) X (glucose -100 mg/dL)/100]
- <u>Add dextrose</u> (D5½NS) once glucose falls ≤ 300 mg/dl.
- <u>Replace potassium</u> (5-10 mEq per h) when level available & OK urine output. If initial serum K is < 3.3 mEq/L add 40 mEq/L/hour. Once urinary output assured and serum K < 5 mEq/L, add 20 mEq to each L of IV fluids. Measure electrolytes and glucose each hour during the 1st 4-6 hours of therapy.
- <u>Insulin</u> may be unnecessary in the ED. Consider beginning once hemodynamic stability is achieved, urine output is adequate, and serum K is ≥ 3.3 mEq/L. Consider 0.1 U/kg/hour IV and modify rate to lower glucose 50-75 dL/hour. Once glucose is ≤ 300 mg/dl, add D$_5$ and decrease insulin to ≤ 0.05 U/kg/hour.
- Empiric phosphate repletion, subcutaneous heparin and broad-spectrum prophylactic antibiotics may be needed depending upon clinical circumstances. Avoid phenytoin for seizures since this agent inhibits the release of exogenous insulin and has been associated with HHS.

Emerg Med Clin North Am 2005; 629; *Diabetes Care* 2004; 27: S94.

Hypoglycemia

Etiology	Clinical Features
Fasting hypoglycemia Symptoms begin 4-6 h after meal. (1) overuse (drugs, insulin, sepsis, tumors, starvation, exercise) or (2) underproduction (alcohol, β blockers, salicylate, hormone deficiency, liver or renal failure, enzyme defects, or substrate defects as in malnutrition). *Reactive hypoglycemia* within 1-2 h of meal & due to impaired GI motility, impaired glucose tolerance (?early diabetes), or enzyme defect.	*Sympathetic response*: ↑HR, hunger, tremors, or sweating. These may be absent if diabetes, alcohol abuse, or β blocker use. *Neuronal dysfunction*: headache, coma, seizures, focal deficits.

Management

- Glucose 1 amp (50 ml) of $D_{50}W$ IV (↑glucose ~ 150 mg/dl) or glucagon 1 mg IM/SC if no IV. IV D_5NS or $D_{10}NS$ to maintain normal blood glucose if needed.
- Diazoxide (*Hyperstat*) 1-2 mg/kg IV if unable to control with IV glucose. This agent is generally used in an ICU setting so that close BP monitoring can occur.
- Octreotide – may be more useful than Diazoxide for sulfonylurea hypoglycemia. Administer via IV infusion or SC dosing. Contact poison center for dosing.
- Hydrocortisone (*Solu-Cortef*) 100 mg IV if possible adrenal insufficiency.
- Thiamine 100 mg IV or IM if malnourished.
- Admit all intentional oral hypoglycemic and most intentional insulin overdoses.
- If mild unintentional insulin overdose, administer D_{50} or oral glucose, feed meal, observe for a short time period and discharge. Admit all long acting intentional or unintentional insulin overdoses due to risk of recurrent prolonged hypoglycemia.
- Admission is generally recommended for sulfonylurea agents due to their long half life. While non-sulfonylurea agents usually do not cause hypoglycemia, any patient who develops hypoglycemia from these agents or acidosis due to biguanide requires admission.

Hyperthyroidism/Thyroid Storm

Underlying Thyroid Disease	Precipitants of Thyroid Storm	
• Grave's disease (most common)	Infection (#1)	Iodine therapy/dye
• Toxic nodular goiter	Pulmonary embolus	Stroke
• Toxic adenoma	DKA, or HHNC	Surgery
• Factitious thyrotoxicosis	Thyroid hormone	Childbirth
• Excess TSH	excess	D&C

Clinical Features of Thyroid Storm (Thyrotoxicosis)

Hyperkinesis	Temperature > 101 F	Psychosis, apathy, coma
Palpable goiter	↑HR + ↑pulse pressure	Tremor, hyperreflexia
Proptosis, lid lag	Arrhythmia (new onset)[2]	Diarrhea, weight loss
Exophthalmos, palsy[1]	Palpitations, dyspnea	Jaundice

[1]Palsy of extraocular muscles, [2]Atrial fibrillation/flutter which may be refractory to digoxin

Laboratory Features of Thyrotoxicosis[1]	• $\uparrow$freeT_4, $\uparrow T_3$, $\downarrow$TSH • $\uparrow T_4$RIA, $\uparrow$FT$_4$I	• $\uparrow$glucose,$\uparrow Ca^{+2}$,$\downarrow$Hb, $\uparrow$WBC,$\downarrow$cholesterol

[1]Laboratory tests can diagnose hyperthyroidism, but thyrotoxicosis is a clinical diagnosis.

Treatment

• Supportive care, O_2,$\checkmark$ glucose, fever control (avoid aspirin) & treat precipitants.

• Inhibit thyroid hormone synthesis: *Propylthiouracil* (PTU) 600-900 mg PO on day 1, then 300-400 mg/d PO X 3-6 weeks. PTU inhibits conversion of T_4 to T_3.

• Inhibit thyroid hormone release: K^+ iodide as *Lugol's solution* (8 mg iodide/drop) - 1 ml or 20 drops PO q 8 h. **OR** *SSKI* (40 mg iodide/drop) 2-10 drops PO daily. **OR** Na^+ *iodide* 1 g IV q 8-12 hours (give over 30 min). **Caution**: Administer iodide $\geq$ 1 h after anti-thyroid medications to prevent use in hormone synthesis.

• Blockade of peripheral effects: Propranolol 1 mg slowly IV q 15 min (Max 5 mg) prn to reduce sympathetic hyperactivity and conversion of T_4 to T_3. Begin propranolol 20-120 mg PO q 6-8 hours when symptoms improve.

• Inhibit conversion of T4 to T3: hydrocortisone (*Solu-Cortef*) 100 mg IV q 8h.

Apathetic Thyrotoxicosis

A rare form of thyrotoxicosis usually occurring in the elderly.

Clinical Features		Management
• Mean age > 60 years • Lethargy, $\downarrow$ mentation • No Grave's eye signs • Smaller goiter • Depression/apathy	• Weak proximal muscles • Mean weight loss > 40 lb. • Atrial fibrillation • Congestive heart failure • Atrial fibrillation/CHF may be refractory to treatment	Treat as thyro-toxicosis but use lower doses & slower rates as side effects are greater in elderly.

Hypothyroidism/Myxedema Coma

Precipitants of Myxedema Coma		Lab tests
Pneumonia, GI bleed CHF, cold exposure,sepsis Stroke, trauma, $\downarrow$glucose $\downarrow pO_2$,$\uparrow pCO_2$, $\downarrow Na^+$	*Drugs* Phenothiazines, lithium, narcotics, sedatives, phenytoin, propranolol	Serum TSH > 60 µU/ml $\downarrow$ total & free T4 $\downarrow$ or $\leftrightarrow$ total & free T3

Clinical Features of Myxedema Coma	
Vitals	• Temperature is often < 90 F, 50% have BP < 100/60
Cardiac	• $\downarrow$HR, heart block, low voltage, ST-T changes, $\uparrow$Q-T, effusion
Pulmonary	• Hypoventilation, $\uparrow pCO_2$, $\downarrow O_2$, pleural effusions
Metabolic	• Hyponatremia, hypoglycemia
Neurologic	• Coma, lethargy, seizures, tremors, ataxia, nystagmus, psychiatric disturbances. Depressed or "hung up" reflexes
GI/GU	• Ileus, ascites, fecal impaction, megacolon, urinary retention
Skin	• Alopecia, loss of lateral 1/3 eyebrows, nonpitting puffiness around eyes, hands, and pretibial region of legs
ENT	• Tongue enlarges, voice deepens and becomes hoarse

Management of Myxedema Coma

- Administer O_2, rewarm and treat cause (e.g. infection, ↓ glucose).
- (Inpatient) Thyroxine – 400-500 mcg slow IV on day 1, + 50-100 mcg IV daily. **CAUTION -** IV thyroxine may cause cardiac arrest. Reduce dose if cardiac ischemia or arrhythmias. Some experts recommend no IV thyroxine for 3-7 days after day 1.
- Start oral thyroxine 100-200 mcg PO daily when possible (after admission).
- Hydrocortisone (*Solu-Cortef*) 100 mg IV q 8h.

Environmental Disorders

Scuba Diving Injuries (Dysbarism)

Dysbaric air embolism (DAE): gas bubbles enter circulation through ruptured pulmonary veins causing symptoms within 10 minutes of surfacing. Symptoms: cardiac arrest, seizure, cardiac ischemia, stroke, and asymmetric multiplegias.
Decompression sickness (DCS): [*Bends*] formation of gas bubbles in blood and body tissues following ↓ in ambient pressure. ↑ risk with old age, obesity, dehydration, alcohol use, exercise, unpressurized flight after dive, prior DCS. Symptoms occur 10 min-6 h (rarely delayed 24-48 h after flying) after ascent and are due to bubbles causing vascular occlusion. Type I DCS involves lymphatics, skin (mottling, itching), musculoskeletal (periarticular joint pain worse with movement).
Type II DCS causes neurologic disruption with spinal cord involvement (low thoracic, lumbar, and sacral primarily) with paraplegia and bladder dysfunction. Pulmonary involvement with pain, dyspnea, and edema may occur.
DCS and DAE Management

- 100% O_2 & IV NS unless contraindicated. Exclude injuries (e.g. pneumothorax).
- Do not place in Trendelenberg. This worsens CNS edema and dyspnea.
- Transport to nearest hyperbaric recompression chamber. If uncertain where nearest facility is call **(919) 684-8111**. Must fly at low altitude < 1000 feet or use aircraft that can pressurize to 1 atmosphere (ATA).

High Altitude Syndromes

Acute Mountain Sickness – AMS

Risk factors: rapid ascent, high sleeping altitudes, 25% > 6900 feet (2000 meters), low vital capacity, low hypoxic ventilatory response (COPD).
Clinical Features: Early: lightheadedness, breathlessness, hangover (headache, anorexia, vomiting, irritable, sleepy), & later dyspnea, oliguria, high altitude cerebral/pulmonary edema (20% local rales), retinal hemorrhages > 5000 meters
Prevention: acetazolamide or dexamethasone 24 h preascent + 2 d after ascent.

Acute Mountain Sickness Management	
•	Stop ascent or descend if worsening, O_2 0.5-1 L/min at night
•	Acetazolamide (*Diamox*) 125-250 mg PO bid
•	Dexamethasone (*Decadron*) 4 mg PO q6h
•	Hyperbaric oxygen therapy (e.g. hyperbaric bag)

High Altitude Syndromes

High Altitude Cerebral Edema - HACE

Progressive neurologic deterioration in someone with HAPE or AMS.
Clinical Features: altered mental status, ataxia, stupor and coma if untreated.
Headache and vomiting are not always present. Focal deficits may occur.

High Altitude Cerebral Edema Management	• Immediate descent or evacuation, supplemental O_2
	• Dexamethasone (*Decadron*) 8 mg PO, IM, or IV then 4 mg q 6h
	• Acetazolamide (*Diamox*) 125 mg PO bid
	• If coma, intubation. Hyperventilation only if acute deterioration
	• Furosemide (*Lasix*) 40-80 mg IV (avoid dehydration, & ↓BP)
	• Hyperbaric oxygen therapy (e.g. hyperbaric bag)

High Altitude Pulmonary Edema - HAPE

Risk factors: male sex, child, exertion, rapid ascent, cold, excess salt, sleeping medications, prior HAPE/AMS. HAPE is a noncardiogenic edema due to exaggerated pulmonary pressor response to hypoxia.
Clinical Features: dry cough, poor exercise, local rales, and later development of tachycardia, tachypnea, dyspnea, cyanosis, generalized rales, and coma. AMS need not be present. A right ventricular heave may be noted. ECG ± right axis deviation, RV strain. CXR may show cephalization or pulmonary edema.

High Altitude Pulmonary Edema Management	• Immediate descent (with minimal exertion), warming, O_2
	• Hyperbarics, morphine 2-5 mg IV, acetazolamide 125 mg PO bid, furosemide (*Lasix*) 40-80 mg IV, CPAP/BiPAP. Sildenafil (*Viagra*) 40 mg PO tid also may be useful.
	• Nifedipine (*Procardia*) 10 mg PO reduces pulmonary artery pressure by 30-50% & ↑O_2 saturation. Nifedipine (extended release) 30 mg PO q8h may prophylax against HAPE.

Hyperthermia and Hypothermia

Minor Heat Illness

- *Heat Syncope*: Postural hypotension from vasodilation, volume depletion, and ↓ vascular tone. Rehydrate, remove from heat, and evaluate for serious disease.
- *Heat cramps*: Painful, contractions of calves, thigh, or shoulders in those who are sweating liberally and drinking hypotonic solutions (e.g. water). Replace fluids: 0.1-0.2% oral solution or IV NS rehydration. Do not use salt tablets.
- *Heat Exhaustion*: Salt and water depletion causing orthostasis, and hyperthermia (usually < 104F). Mental status, and neurologic exam are normal. Lab: high hematocrit, high sodium, or high BUN. Treat with NS 1-2 Liters IV.

Heatstroke

Clinical Features	Risk Factors

• Hyperpyrexia (>104-105.8F/40-41C)
 • Central nervous system dysfunction (seizures, altered mentation, plantar responses, hemiplegia, ataxia)
 • Loss of sweating (variably present)
 • ↓ Na, ↓ Ca, ↓ phosphate, ↓ or ↑ K
 • Rhabdomyolysis, renal/liver failure
	• Old age, skin disorders, obesity
	 • Environmental temperature, humidity
	 • Drugs
	   - amphetamines, anticholinergics
	   - antihypertensive agents
	   - sympathomimetics (e.g. cocaine)
	   - phenothiazines

Management of Heatstroke

- Administer oxygen, protect airway if comatose or seizing. Check blood glucose.
- Measure temperature with continuous rectal probe accurate to high levels.
- Begin IV NS cautiously as pulmonary edema is common and mean fluid requirement is only 1.2 L in first 4 hours.
- Immediate cooling by: (1) *evaporation*: Spray with tepid water and direct fan at patient (0.1 - 0.3C/min temp. drop). For shivering, lorazepam 1-3 mg IV. (2) *ice water (or 60F) tub immersion*: *(controversial)* (temp. drop ~ 0.16C/min). (3) *Ice packs, cooling blankets, peritoneal dialysis, gastric lavage* with cold saline are slow or unproven. (4) Avoid aspirin (hyperpyrexia). Avoid repeated acetaminophen doses (possible liver damage and ineffective in heatstroke).
- Stop above measures at temperature of 102-104°F to avoid over-correction.
- Place Foley catheter to monitor urine output (see rhabdomyolysis below).
- Obtain CBC, electrolytes, renal function, glucose, liver enzymes, LDH/CK, PT, and PTT, arterial blood gas, and fibrin degradation products. ECG and CXR.
- Exclude other fever cause: infection, malignant hyperthermia, thyroid, drugs etc.

Other Heat Related Disorders

- **Malignant hyperthermia (MH)**: Autosomal dominant disorder causing fever, & rigid muscles after anesthetics or succinylcholine is administered.
 Treatment: Stop agent, lower temp. as in heatstroke (avoid phenothiazines), give dantrolene 2-3 mg/kg IV q 6 hours (max cumulative dose is 10 mg/kg).
- **Neuroleptic Malignant Syndrome:** Similar to MH with **FEVER** (**F**ever, **E**ncephalopathy, **V**itals unstable, **E**levated CK enzymes, **R**igid muscles) occurring in anticholinergic agents (e.g. phenothiazines) or psychotropics. *Treatment:* Stop agent, treat heat stroke with cooling. Avoid phenothiazines and administer benzodiazepines IV (e.g. lorazepam). Many authorities recommend (1) dantrolene 2-3 mg/kg IV then continuous infusion until symptoms subside or maximum dose of 10 mg/kg plus (2) bromocriptine 2.5-10 mg PO tid. (However, use of dantrolene and bromocriptine is controversial as one study [20 total patients] found their use prolonged illness and increased adverse sequelae, *Br J Psychiatry* 1991;159:709)

Other Heat Related Disorders Continued

- **Rhabdomyolysis** – Syndrome with release of contents into circulation due to tissue hypoxia, direct injury, exercise, enzyme defects, metabolic disease (DKA, ↓ K, ↓ Na, or ↓ phosphate, thyroid), toxins, infections, heatstroke. *Complications[1]*: renal failure, ↑K^+, ↑Ca^{+2} or↓ Ca^{+2}, ↑or↓phosphate, ↑ uric acid, compartment syndrome, disseminated intravascular coagulation

  Treatment: (1) IV NS to keep urine output > 100-200 ml/hr, (2) NaHCO3 ≥ 50 mEq IV to keep urine pH > 6.5, (3) If poor urine output, administer Mannitol – 25-50 g IV,+ 12.5 g to each L of NS, (4) Dialyze if ↑K^+ or uremia is present

- **Serotonin syndrome** – see page 179

HYPOTHERMIA

Severity	Temp. F (C)	Features
Mild	> 93.2 (>34)	Maximal shivering + slurred speech at 95F
Moderate	86-93 (30-34)	At 89 – altered mental status, mydriasis, shivering ceases, muscles are rigid, incoordination, bradypnea
Severe	< 86 (< 30)	Bradycardia, Osborne waves on ECG, voluntary motion stops, pupils become fixed dilated
	79 (26)	Loss of consciousness, areflexia, no pain response
	77 (25)	No respirations, appear dead, pulmonary edema
	68 (20)	Asystole

Management of Hypothermia

- Evaluate for cause (e.g. sepsis, hypoglycemia, CNS disease, adrenal crisis). Avoid vigorous manipulation (can precipitate ventricular fibrillation)
- **Mild hypothermia (> 34C):** Passive external rewarming, treatment underlying disease only treatment needed. Standard BLS/ACLS if cardiac arrest.
- **Moderate hypothermia** (30-34C): Active external rewarming. Warm humidified O_2, warmed fluids. CPR, & advanced life support prn. *If cardiac arrest*, active internal rewarming, standard ACLS with medications spaced at longer intervals.
- **Severe hypothermia** (< 30 C): Active internal warming. Warm humidified O_2, warm IV fluids. If nonarrested, consider warm peritoneal dialysis (41C dialysate), or pleural irrigation (41C), cardiopulmonary bypass, or extracorporeal membrane oxygenation (ECMO). If signs of life, and non-arrested, avoid CPR, and ACLS. Do not treat atrial arrhythmias. Treat ↓BP with NS 1st. Use pressors cautiously. Consider underlying cause: empiric D50, thiamine 100 mg IV, naloxone 2mg IV, + hydrocortisone 100 mg IV, sepsis treatment. *If cardiac arrest*, perform standard BLS, intubate and attempt defibrillation for shockable rhythm X 1. If no response, defer defibrillation until rewarmed to 30-32C. Withhold drugs until core temperature > 30C. Consider peritoneal/pleural lavage, ECMO, cardiopulmonary bypass.

Circulation 2005; 112: IV136.

Snake Bite Envenomation

(Crotalid) Snakebite Severity Score (for serial snake bite evaluation)

System	Manifestations	Points
Lung	No symptoms/signs	0
	Dyspnea, tight chest, mild discomfort, respiratory rate (RR) 20-25	1
	Moderate distress (RR 26-30, accessory muscle use)	2
	Cyanosis, air hunger, RR > 30, respiratory insufficiency/failure	3
Cardiac	No symptoms/signs	0
	Heart rate (HR) 100-125, palpitations, generally weak, ↑BP	1
	HR 126-175, systolic blood pressure (SBP) > 100 mm Hg	2
	HR > 175, SPB < 100, malignant dysrhythmia, cardiac arrest	3
Wound	No symptoms/signs	0
	Pain, swelling, ecchymosis within 5-7.5 cm of wound	1
	Pain, swelling, ecchymosis < ½ extremity (7.5-50 cm from bite)	2
	Pain, swelling, ecchymosis ½ to all extremity 50-100 cm from bite	3
	Pain, swelling, ecchymosis beyond extremity > 100 cm from bite	4
GI	No symptoms/signs	0
	Pain, tenesmus, or nausea	1
	Vomiting or diarrhea	2
	Repeated vomiting, diarrhea, hematemesis, hematochezia	3
Blood[2]	No symptoms/signs	0
	PT < 20, PTT < 50, Plat. (100-150k), Fibrinogen 100-150 mcg/ml	1
	PT 20-50, PTT 50-75, Plat. (50-100k), Fbg. 50-100 mcg/ml	2
	PT 50-100, PTT 75-100, Plat. (20-50k), Fbg. < 50 mcg/ml	3
	PT/PTT/Fbg unmeasurable, Plat < 20k, serious bleeding risk	4
CNS	No symptoms/signs	0
	Mild apprehension, headache, weak, dizzy, chills, paresthesias	1
	Above plus confusion, or fasciculation in area of bite	2
	Severe confusion, seizure, coma, psychosis, gen. fasciculation	3

Ann Emerg Med 2001; 37: 175; & 1996; 27: 321.

Snakebite Grades (for dosing Polyvalent Equine Crotalid Antivenin)

Grade[1]	Features of Crotalid (Pit viper) envenomation	Dose
None 1.3 ± 0.5	± Fang marks, no pain, erythema or systemic symptoms	None
Mild[2] 2.1 ± 0.2	Fang marks, mild pain/edema, no systemic symptoms	0-5 vials (50 ml)
Moderate 3.2 ± 0.3	Fang marks, severe pain, moderate edema in 1st 12h, mild symptoms (vomiting, paresthesias), mild coagulopathy (without bleeding)	10 vials (100 ml)
Severe 8.5 ± 1.0	Fang marks, severe pain/edema, severe symptoms (hypotension, dyspnea), coagulopathy with bleeding	15-20 vials (150-200 ml)

[1] Correlation of Grade and Snakebite Severity Score [2] Controversial – some experts recommend no antivenin for mild envenomation or for most copperhead bites.

Prehospital Treatment for Crotalid Envenomation

- Decrease patient movement, and transport to nearest medical facility.
- Immobilize extremity in neutral position below level of heart.
- Incision + drainage and tourniquets are unproven and not recommended.

Emergency Treatment for Crotalid Envenomation

- Perform exam, measure envenomation site, and administer fluids, pressors prn.
- If no signs of envenomation, clean wound, administer tetanus and observe for a minimum of 6 hours. Consider antibiotics (e.g. *Augmentin* X 5-10 days).
- If significant envenomation, obtain CBC, electrolytes, renal and liver function tests, PT, PTT, fibrinogen, urinalysis, ECG, and type and cross.
- Ovine Fab Antivenin is preferred over equine. Use equine if Ovine unavailable.

Ovine - Crotalidae Polyvalent Immune Fab Antivenin (FabAV)

- Sheep derived antivenin that is 5X more potent than equine antivenin with less risk of allergy/anaphylaxis.
- If treatment indicated, give initial dose of 6 vials if mild, moderate or severe bite.
- Administer an additional 2 vials at 6, 12, and 18 hours.
- Dilute FabAV to a total of 250 ml in NS & infuse IV over one hour.
- Review package insert for further recommendations *Ann Emerg Med* 2001; 37:181.

Equine - Antivenin Crotalidae Polyvalent Administration - see dose prior page

- Perform skin test only if equine to be administered: 0.2 ml SC (dilute 1:10 with NS) at site distant from bite. Observe for allergy ≥ 10 minutes after injection. Absence of reaction does not exclude allergy.
- Need for antivenin and specific dose is controversial. Prior to administration, obtain consent, administer IV NS, consider premedication with diphenhydramine 1 mg/kg IV, and dilute antivenin in 50-100 ml each vial.
- Reconstitute antivenin in a 1:10 solution with NS or D_5W.
- Administer 5-10 ml over 5 min. If no allergy, increase rate so that infusion takes 1-2 hours. If symptoms progress, additional antivenin may be required.
- If allergic reaction and antivenin is necessary, start arterial line, continue to treat with NS ± albumin, methylprednisolone 125 mg IV, and diphenhydramine 50 mg IV. Hang epinephrine drip in line separate from antivenin (see page 222) and maximally dilute antivenin. Begin antivenin slowly. Begin epi drip at low dose only if needed. Once allergic reaction gone, restart antivenin slowly. Contact poison center.

Elapidae (Coral Snake) Envenomation

This species is found in the southeast US, Texas, and Arizona. They must bite and chew. Symptoms are primarily systemic and not local: altered mentation, cranial nerve or muscle weakness, respiratory failure. Symptoms may be delayed up to 24 h. Admit all for possible respiratory or neurologic deterioration. Experts recommend Wyeth Coral Snake Antivenin for all suspected bites even if symptoms are not yet present. Dose of antivenin: 3-6 vials over 1-2 hours using same delivery instructions as crotalidae antivenin (skin test first). Allergy/serum sickness can occur. Sonoran coral snake (also known as Arizona coral snake) venom is less toxic, no deaths have been reported, and coral snake antivenin is ineffective.

Special Situations

Mojave rattlesnake: May cause muscle weakness, paralysis, or respiratory failure with few local symptoms. Crotalidae Polyvalent Immune Fab (Ovine) is effective, Antivenin Crotalidae Polyvalent is not.

Exotic snakes: Call **(602) 626-6016** for information regarding available anti-venin.

Serum sickness will develop in most receiving > 5 vials of antivenin within 5-20 days causing joint pain, myalgias, and possibly rash. Warn patient and treat with diphenhydramine (*Benadryl*) 25-50 mg PO q4-6 h and prednisone 50 mg PO daily.

Spider Bites

Black Widow Spiders	Features of Black Widow Bites
• Found in all of US, mostly South	• Mild-moderate pain, redness, swelling, cramping at bite which later spreads
• Females average 5 cm with legs	• Abdominal wall pain mimics peritonitis
• Only females are toxic	
• 1/5 have red hour glass on abdomen	• ↓BP, shock, coma, respiratory failure

Management of Black Widow Spider Bites	
• Lorazepam *Ativan* 0.05-0.1 mg/kg IV	**Indications[1] for Admission/Antivenin**
• Consider Antivenin - Dose: 1-2 vials IV in 50-100 ml NS Skin test prior to using	• Respiratory or cardiac symptoms
	• Pregnancy or > 65 y with symptoms
• Allergy & serum sickness can occur	• Severe cramping or pain despite lorazepam and narcotic use
• Calcium is ineffective, use narcotics	• History of ↑ BP or cardiac disease

[1]controversial as no deaths have occurred in 30 years *Emerg Med Clin North Am* 1992; 269

Brown Recluse Spiders	Management
• Live mostly in southern US, and dark places. Bites are mild or painless.	• Wound care, tetanus
• At 1st lesions are red and blanch	• Consider referral to plastic surgeon for possible excision if > 2 cm & well-circumscribed border (usually 2 to 3 weeks after bite)
• Later a macule, ulcer or blister	
• Arthralgias, GI upset, DIC, or shock	• ± Dapsone 50-200 mg/day PO
• Hemoglobinuria (renal failure)	• ± Hyperbaric oxygen (controversial)

Marine Envenomation

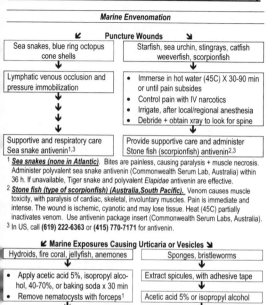

Puncture Wounds

Sea snakes, blue ring octopus cone shells	Starfish, sea urchin, stingrays, catfish weeverfish, scorpionfish
↓	↓
Lymphatic venous occlusion and pressure immobilization	• Immerse in hot water (45C) X 30-90 min or until pain subsides • Control pain with IV narcotics • Irrigate, after local/regional anesthesia • Debride + obtain xray to look for spine
↓	↓
Supportive and respiratory care Sea snake antivenin[1,3]	Provide supportive care and administer Stone fish (scorpionfish) antivenin[2,3]

[1] **Sea snakes (none in Atlantic)**. Bites are painless, causing paralysis + muscle necrosis. Administer polyvalent sea snake antivenin (Commonwealth Serum Lab, Australia) within 36 h. If unavailable, Tiger snake and polyvalent *Elapidae* antivenin are effective.

[2] **Stone fish (type of scorpionfish) (Australia, South Pacific)**. Venom causes muscle toxicity, with paralysis of cardiac, skeletal, involuntary muscles. Pain is immediate and intense. The wound is ischemic, cyanotic and may lose tissue. Heat (45C) partially inactivates venom. Use antivenin package insert (Commonwealth Serum Labs, Australia).

[3] In US, call **(619) 222-6363** or **(415) 770-7171** for antivenin.

Marine Exposures Causing Urticaria or Vesicles

Hydroids, fire coral, jellyfish, anemones	Sponges, bristleworms
↓	↓
• Apply acetic acid 5%, isopropyl alcohol, 40-70%, or baking soda x 30 min • Remove nematocysts with forceps[1]	Extract spicules, with adhesive tape
	↓
	Acetic acid 5% or isopropyl alcohol
↓	↓
• Supportive care (e.g. narcotics) • Antivenin for box jellyfish, *C. fleckeri* • Consider systemic steroids	• Topical steroids if mild reaction • Treat for allergic reactions

[1] Do not rinse in fresh water.

Marine Infections

- Organisms causing soft tissue infection: *Aeromonas hydrophilia, B. fragilis, E. coli, Pseudomonas, Salmonella, Vibrio, Staph./Strep.* species, *C. perfringens*.
- Irrigate, debride, explore, and obtain x-rays to exclude foreign bodies
- Antibiotic agents for treating soft tissue infection or prophylaxis:
  <u>Parenteral agents</u> - 3rd generation cephalosporin and/or an aminoglycoside
  <u>Oral agents</u> –*Septra, Bactrim*, doxycycline, cefuroxime, or ciprofloxacin

Gastrointestinal (GI) Bleeding

Testing gastric aspirate/stool for blood.

- Use gastroccult to test for gastric blood as hemoccult tests are inaccurate at low pH. Up to 20% with upper GI bleed have negative NG aspirates.
- False positive hemoccult/gastroccult - bromides, hypochlorites, iodine, iron, specific vegetables (artichokes, bananas, bean sprouts, broccoli, cantaloupes, cauliflower, grapes, horseradish, oranges, radishes, turnips), rare meat.
- False negative hemoccult/gastroccult antacid, barium, bile, charcoal, chili powder, jello, red wine, rifampin, simethicone, sucralfate, vitamin C (e.g. fruits).

Blatchford Upper GI Bleed Risk Score[1,2]

	Points		Points
BUN (mg/dl)		Systolic blood pressure (mm Hg)	
≥ 18.2 to < 22.4	2	≥ 100 to < 109	1
≥ 22.4 to < 28	3	≥ 90 to < 99	2
≥ 28 to < 70	4	< 90	3
≥ 70	6	Other risk markers	
Hemoglobin (Men) [g/dl]		Heart rate ≥ 100 beats/minute	1
≥ 12 to < 13	1	Melena	1
≥ 10 to < 12	3	Syncope	2
< 10	6	Liver disease	2
Hemoglobin (Women) [g/dl]		Heart failure	2
≥ 10 to < 12	1		
< 10	6		

[1] A Blatchford score > 0 is considered high risk. In study with 354 patients with non-variceal upper GI bleeding, this cutoff was 100% sensitive at identifying patients who died, rebled, or required blood (i.e. no patient with a score of 0 rebled, died, or required transfusion)
[2] All patients were treated with a proton pump inhibitor (omeprazole, pantoprazole)
[3] **ED discharge** can be considered for patients with score of 0, no comorbidities, & closely arranged follow up. *Am J Emerg Med* 2007; 25: 774, *Lancet* 2000; 356; 1318.

Clinical Differentiation of Upper vs. Lower Gastrointestinal Bleeding

Upper GI source features	Lower GI source features.
• Visible upper bleed (hematemesis)	• Bright red blood can be lower source or massive upper GI source
• NG tube with blood/coffee grounds (no blood found in 20% with UGI source)	• Age > 60-painless bleed (diverticular)
• Melena is found in 70% of upper but also 30% of lower GI bleeding	• Weight loss (colon > gastric cancer)
• BUN/creatinine ratio > 30 is > 95% specific (70% sensitive) for upper	• Aortic stenosis (AV malformation)
• Peptic ulcer (aspirin, NSAID, tobacco)	• Rectal pain/mass (hemorrhoids)
• Mallory Weiss tear (vomiting, retching)	• Aortic aneurysm repair (aortoenteric fistula)
	• Inflammatory bowel disease

Management of Moderate-Severe GI Bleeding

Initial Resuscitation	• Apply cardiac monitor, administer O_2, place ≥ 2 large bore IVs. • Administer 20 ml/kg NS IV and repeat X 1-2 to correct hypotension or shock. Administer packed red blood cells if still hypotensive. Goal: stabilized vitals, Hct > 10 g/dl in elderly, lower in young. • Draw blood for CBC, electrolytes, liver/renal function, coagulation studies, type & cross 2-6 units PRBCs if significant bleeding. • Obtain ECG & consider cardiac enzymes - 10-25% of Upper GI bleeds admitted to ICU have MI (often silent). Risk factors for silent MI: age > 75 years, severe coronary artery disease, systolic BP < 110 mm Hg, diastolic BP < 85 mm Hg, hematocrit < 30%, BUN/Creatinine > 30. (*Am J Emerg Med* 2007; 25: 406) • Consider NG if uncertain source (upper vs. lower) for bleeding. NG may not reveal blood in up to 20% with upper source. Gastric lavage & standard NG are not useful in treating upper GI bleed.
Medical Therapy Adjuncts	• <u>Coagulopathy & thrombocytopenia</u> - see warfarin guidelines page 73, platelets (if < 50,000/mm³) - dosing page 74. Fresh frozen plasma 10-15 ml/kg may be required if unknown coagulopathy. • <u>Peptic ulcer</u>–Proton pump inhibitors ↓ rebleeding & surgery rate (e.g. omeprazole/*Prilosec* or pantoprazole/*Protonix* 80 mg PO/IV). • <u>Renal failure</u> – (1) DDAVP - 0.3 mg/kg IV in 50 ml NS or same dose SC or intranasal (2) estrogen – 0.6 mg/kg IV q 24 h X 5 days OR 25 mg PO X 3-5 days OR transdermal 50-100 mcg/day X 3 days [caution, multiple side effects) (3) cryoprecipitate (page 74) • <u>Variceal bleed</u> - (1) *Octreotide*– lowers portal venous pressure *Octreotide* dose: 50 mcg bolus + 50 mcg/h IV. **OR** (2) Vasopressin (*Pitressin*) - <u>Dose</u>: Start 0.4 units/min, gradual ↑ to max 0.9 units /minute IV. Side effects: ↑ BP, bowel ischemia, MI, skin necrosis. Add nitroglycerin IV (20-200 mcg/min) to limit these effects.
Indications for Surgical Consult	• Suspected surgical disorder: aortoenteric fistula, bowel perforation, obstruction, or ischemia, esophageal tear (Boerhaves) • Variceal bleed • Upper/lower source with continued instability or ≥ 4-5 units transfused in 24 hours • Massive lower bleeding or recurrent diverticular bleed • <u>Endoscopic criteria</u>: active or recurrent upper bleed not controlled after 2 endoscopies OR upper endoscopy with > 2 cm ulcer or stigmata of high rebleed risk (visible vessel, adherent clot)

Upper GI Bleeding Evaluation

• <u>High risk patient OR more than minimal bleeding</u> – urgent or emergent endoscopy. Emergency endoscopy (EGD): hematemesis + hemodynamic instability, massive upper bleed, suspected varices. (1) *Ulcer* – active bleed or visible vessel (± adherent clot) - endoscopic therapy + IV proton pump inhibitor. If rebleed repeat EGD or surgery. (2) *Esophageal varices* – meds above + sclerotherapy or band ligation. If rebleed, EGD or transjugular intrahepatic portosystemic shunt (TIPS).
• <u>Low risk patient with minimal bleed</u> – may undergo elective EGD, upper GI series or empirical outpatient therapy. See Blatchfield score prior page.

Lower GI Bleeding Evaluation

- <u>Massive bleed</u> – (1) surgical consult, (2) angiography with embolization if site identified. If unsuccessful, surgery required.
- <u>Intermediate bleed or uncertain source</u> – (1) if positive NG aspirate OR risk factors for upper GI source, 1st perform EGD. (2) Perform colonoscopy if no upper GI source found or no suspicion of upper source (3) if diverticulosis or AVM found, observation if bleeding stops. Endoscopic therapy may be attempted for active bleeding. If unsuccessful, angiography (can detect bleed rates of > 0.5-1 ml/min) with embolization. If persistent bleeding, surgery may be required. (4) if <u>unable to visualize colon</u> due to bleeding see massive bleed above (5) <u>if no source found</u> on colonoscopy consider slower bleeding scan (tagged red blood cells) which detects bleeding at > 0.1 ml/minute. If this is negative, evaluate stomach and small bowel via EGD & consider repeat colonoscopy.
- <u>Minimal bright blood</u> – consider anoscopy ± sigmoidoscopy in ED

Anemia

Anemia Differential Diagnosis

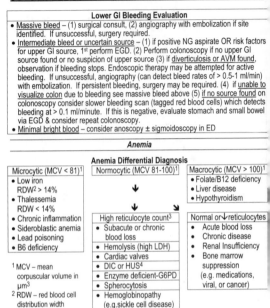

Microcytic (MCV < 81)[1]
- Low iron   RDW[2] > 14%
- Thalessemia   RDW < 14%
- Chronic inflammation
- Sideroblastic anemia
- Lead poisoning
- B6 deficiency

[1] MCV – mean corpuscular volume in µm³

[2] RDW – red blood cell distribution width

Normocytic (MCV 81-100)[1]
↓
↓   ↘

High reticulocyte count[3]
- Subacute or chronic blood loss
- Hemolysis (high LDH)
- Cardiac valves
- DIC or HUS[4]
- Enzyme deficient-G6PD
- Spherocytosis
- Hemoglobinopathy (e.g.sickle cell disease)

Macrocytic (MCV > 100)[1]
- Folate/B12 deficiency
- Liver disease
- Hypothyroidism

Normal or ↓ reticulocytes
- Acute blood loss
- Chronic disease
- Renal Insufficiency
- Bone marrow suppression (e.g. medications, viral, or cancer)

[3] reticulocyte count X (Hct measured/Normal Hct)

[4] DIC – disseminated intravascular coagulation, HUS – hemolytic uremic syndrome

---

Sickle Cell Anemia

Diagnostic Studies in Sickle Cell Disease

- A routine Hb is recommended in most to assess severity or change of anemia.
- A white blood cell count often will be elevated due to sickle crisis alone.
- Obtain a CXR and pulse oximetry if cough, shortness of breath, or fever.
- Evaluate for crisis precipitant (e.g., infection, or dehydration).
- Consider a reticulocyte count if aplastic crisis suspected (rare in adults)
- Urine specific gravity is not a useful test for dehydration, as it may be low from isosthenuria (inability to concentrate urine).

Admission Criteria for Sickle Cell Disease

- Acute chest syndrome –pain/pulmonary infiltrate from infection or pulm. infarct
- Stroke, priapism, serious bacterial infection, aplastic crisis, hypoxia, acidosis
- Unable to take fluids orally or inadequate pain control, abnormal vital signs
- Consider if pregnant (with crisis), or uncertain diagnosis in SCD

Management of Sickle (SS) Cell Complications

Abdominal pain	• Patients with SS have ↑ risk for developing cholecystitis, mesenteric ischemia, or a perforated viscus. Splenic sequestration is rare in adults. Consider CT, ultrasound and surgical consultation (esp. if pain not typical of normal crisis).
Aplastic crisis	• Exclude reversible cause (medications) and transfuse for severe anemia (Hb < 6-7 g/dl) or cardiopulmonary distress.
Pain crisis	• Consider O_2 at 2-4 Liters (esp. if hypoxic). If used for several days, O_2 may inhibit erythropoesis and worsen anemia. • IV ½NS at 150-200 ml/h (if mild pain, ± PO hydration) • IV narcotics titrated to pain relief (PO narcotics if mild pain)
Priapism	• Treat as pain crisis above. • Exchange transfusion to keep Hb S < 30% before surgery • Urology consultation for aspiration or alternate procedure.
Acute chest syndrome	• Admit all patients with a pulmonary infiltrate to the hospital. • Pulmonary infarct from vaso-occlusion ± with pneumonia • Treat as pain crisis with IV antibiotics.
Sepsis	• Admit all patients with invasive bacterial infections.
Sickle cell stroke	• Obtain CT ± spinal tap if uncertain diagnosis, Administer IV NS. • Exchange transfusion – keep HbS <30% total blood volume

---

Bleeding Disorders

Platelet and *capillary* disorders cause mucous membrane bleeds (GI, epistaxis, ↑ bleed with cuts, petechiae (↑bleeding time and abnormal platelets). *Coagulation* disorders cause hemorrhage of deep muscle, CNS, hemarthrosis, and ↑PT/PTT.

Factor VIII and IX Deficiency (Hemophilia A and B)
Severity of Bleeding and Dose of Factor VIII and IX

Severity	Specific Injury	Desired activity	Dose Factor 8	Dose Factor 9
Severe	CNS, GI bleed, major trauma, retroperitoneal or retropharyngeal bleed, pending surgery	80-100%	40-50 Units/kg	80-100 Units/kg
Moderate	Mild head trauma, deep muscle bleed, hip or groin injury, mouth or dental bleed, hematuria	40-50%	15-25 Units/kg	40-50 Units/kg
Mild	Laceration, common joint bleed, tissue or muscle bleed	20-40%	10-15 Units/kg	20-40 Units/kg

Medications used for Hemophilia (H) & Von Willibrand's Disease (vW)

Medication	Dose
amino-caproic acid	• Primary use to prepare for dental procedures (H, vW) • (*Amicar*) 25-100 mg/kg PO q 6 hours for 6 days
DDAVP *Desmo-pressin*	• 0.3 mcg/kg in 50 ml NS IV over 30 minutes or 0.3 mcg/kg SC • Possibly effective via nasal spray or SC injection. (H, vW) • Use for mild bleed, menorrhagia, minor procedures. (H, vW)
Factor VIII (H)	• [desired activity level (%) – baseline activity level (%)] ÷2 • 1 unit/kg factor 8 will ↑ activity level 2% (T½ = 12 hours)[1]
Factor IX (H)	• desired activity level (%) - baseline activity level (%) • 1 unit/kg factor 9 will ↑ activity level 1% (T½ = 24 hours) [1]
Anti-inhibitor Coagulant Complex	• Used in Hemophilia with factor VIII inhibitors (esp. if > 5-10 B.U.) or ↑ INR reversal. (e.g. *FEIBA VH*) • 50-100 units/kg IV q 12 hours.
Humate P Used for von Willibrand's	• 50 units/kg of vWf:RCof (von Willebrand factor: Ristocetin Cofactor) every 8-12 hours for von Willebrand disease if severe bleeding or major surgery.
prednisone	• 2 mg/kg/day PO x 2 days is useful if mild hematuria (H)
Thrombin *ThrombinJMI* *ThrombiPad* *Thrombostat*	• Bovine derived topical thrombin may stop bleeding from venules, capillaries. Bovine thrombin can cause allergic reactions or lead to development of factor V antibodies. Recombinant thrombin (*Recothrom*) may be available in future.

[1]T½ = half life and dosing frequency

Causes of Abnormal Bleeding Tests [1,2]

Lab Value	Causes
thrombocytopenia ↓ platelet count (<150,000/ml)	Heparin, ↓ platelet production, splenic sequestration, platelet destruction (drugs, collagen vascular disease, ITP, DIC, TTP, HUS)
↑ BT (> 9 minutes)	Platelet disorders, DIC, ITP, uremia, liver failure, aspirin
platelet function analysis (PFA)	PFA and bleeding time (BT) give equivalent results in 75% of cases. Aspirin and vWD are most common causes for abnormal PFA with normal BT. For this reason, the PFA has largely replaced the BT.
↑ PTT (> 35 sec)	Coagulation pathway defects (common factors 2, 5, 10, intrinsic 8, 9, 11, 12), DIC, liver failure, heparin
↑ PT (> 12-13 sec)	Coagulation pathway defects (common factors 2, 5, 10, extrinsic 7) DIC, liver failure, warfarin
↑ TT (> 8-10 sec)	DIC, liver failure or uremia, heparin
↓ fibrinogen, ↑ FSP	ITP, liver failure, DIC

[1] BT-bleeding time, TT-Thrombin time, PTT-partial thromboplastin time, PT-prothrombin time, DIC-disseminated intravascular coagulopathy, ITP-idiopathic thrombocytopenic purpura, TTP-thrombotic thrombocytopenic purpura, HUS-hemolytic uremic syndrome.

[2] See page 74 for use/dosing platelets, red blood cells, cryoprecipitate, fresh frozen plasma

Managing Patients with High INR[1] Values[2, 3]

INR > therapeutic , < 5.0 and no significant bleeding (2c)	Lower or omit next dose. Resume therapy at a lower dose when INR is therapeutic. If INR is only slightly above therapeutic, dose reduction may not be needed.
INR ≥ 5.0 but < 9.0; no significant bleeding (Grade 2c)	(1) Omit next dose or two, monitor INR more frequently, & resume therapy at lower dose when INR is therapeutic. (2) Alternatively, omit a dose and give vitamin K₁ (≤ 5 mg orally) (esp. if patient at increased risk for bleeding) (3) Patients requiring more rapid reversal before urgent surgery: vitamin K₁ (2 to 4 mg PO) can be given with the expectation that reduction of INR will occur in 24 hours; if INR remains high at 24 h: add vitamin K₁ dose (1-2 mg PO)
INR ≥ 9.0; no significant bleeding (Grade 2c)	Omit warfarin; give vitamin K₁ (5 to 10 mg PO) with expectation that INR will be substantially reduced in 24-48 hours; closely monitor INR; if INR is not substantially reduced in 24-48 h, monitor INR more often, giving additional vitamin K₁, if necessary. Resume therapy at lower dose when INR is therapeutic.
Serious bleeding at any INR elevation (Grade 1c)	Omit warfarin, give vitamin K₁ (10 mg, slow IV), supplement with fresh frozen plasma (4-6 units) or prothrombin complex concentrate [e.g.FEIBA, see dose page 72] or recombinant factor VIIa (as alternative to PCC), depending on urgency. Vitamin K₁ injections can be repeated q 12 h
Life-threatening bleeding (Grade 1c)	Omit warfarin; administer vitamin K₁ (10 mg by slow IV infusion) and prothrombin complex concentrate [e.g. FEIBA, see dosing page 72] (or recombinant factor VIIa); repeat prn, depending on INR. If prothrombin complex concentrate or factor VIIa unavailable, use fresh frozen plasma (4-6 units).

[1] INR – International Normalized Ratio

[2] If continuing warfarin therapy indicated after high doses of vitamin K₁, heparin or low molecular weight heparin may be administered until the effects of vitamin K₁ are reversed and the patient becomes responsive to warfarin.

[3] Grade 1c – Benefit is clearly greater than risk, evidence is from observational studies, recommendation strength is intermediate and may change with stronger evidence Grade 2c – Risk to benefit ratio is unclear, supporting evidence is derived from observational studies and (3) the strength of the recommendation is very weak and other alternatives may be equally reasonable.

7th Am Coll Chest Phys Consensus Conference *Chest* 2004; 126: 204S-233S.

Management of Bleeding in the Dialysis Patient

- Direct pressure in bleeding from shunt (dialysis unit will have "shunt clamps")
- DDAVP 0.3 mcg/kg in 50 ml NS IV over 30 minutes
- Consider protamine IV if recent dialysis (see dosing page 42)

BLOOD/HEMATOLOGY PRODUCTS

Cryoprecipitate	
Features	• 1 bag (10 ml) has 50-100 units of factor 8 activity. There are 10 donors/bag. It has fibrinogen, von Willibrand's factor, factor 8 + 13.
Indications	• Hypofibrinogenemia if fibrinogen < 100 mg/dl. • Von Willebrand's (vW) disease & active bleeding - if DDAVP is unavailable or factor 8 concentrate with vW factor is unavailable. • Hemophilia A + unavailable monoclonal or viral inactivated factor 8 • Fibronectin replacement for healing in trauma, burns, or sepsis
Dose	• 2-4 bags for every 10 kg of bodyweight or 10-20 bags at a time

Fresh frozen plasma (FFP)	
Features	• Contains all coagulation factors. 40 ml/kg raises activity of any factor to 100%. This may cause fluid overload. ABO compatibility is mandatory although cross matching prior to transfusion is not.
Indications	• Coagulation protein deficiency if factor concentrates unavailable • Reversal of warfarin toxicity or active bleed with liver disease • Bleeding and coagulopathy with unknown cause
Dose	• If bleeding from vitamin K deficiency (liver disease) administer 10-25 ml/kg. 10-15 ml/kg will raise factor 8 levels 15-20%.

Packed Red Blood Cells (PRBC's)	
Features	• Fewer antigens are present in PRBC's compared to whole blood. • *Leukocyte poor* – use if transplant recipient or candidate, or 2 febrile non-hemolytic reaction • *Washed* – use if prior anaphylaxis due to IgA or other proteins. • *Frozen deglycerolized* - purest RBC product, use if reaction to washed RBC's or a transfusion reaction from Anti-IgA antibodies
Indications	• Acute hemorrhage or chronic anemia with hemoglobin < 7-8 g/dl • Symptomatic anemia or cardiopulmonary disease + Hb < 8-10 g/dl
Dose	• One unit raises hemoglobin by 1g/dl or hematocrit by 3%. • ≥ 2 units are needed in most circumstances.

Platelet concentrate	
Features	• 1 unit (pack) = 5-10,000 platelets. Platelets are not refrigerated & survive 7 days. ABO cross-match is not necessary, but preferred.
Indications	• Level < 10,000/µL unless antiplatelet antibodies • Level < 50,000/µL if major surgery, significant bleed, major trauma • Level - 10,000-50,000/µL if concurrent liver or renal disease that is causing platelet dysfunction
Dose	• 6 platelet packs (250-300 ml) or one plateletpheresis pack should raise platelet count by 50,000-60,000/uL.

Transfusion Reactions

Crossmatching and ordering blood products:

- Type-specific non-crossmatched blood causes fatality in 1 in 30 million transfusions (usually due to labeling, clerical, or patient identification error).
- Non-ABO antibodies occur in 0.04% of non-transfused and 0.3% of previously transfused.

Hemolytic transfusion reactions

- Occur in 1/40,000 transfusions and are usually due to ABO incompatibility.
- _Clinical Features_ - palpitations, abdominal and back pain, syncope, and a sensation of doom. Consider in those with a temperature rise of $\geq 2C$.
- _Management_ - Immediately stop transfusion, and look for hemoglobinemia and hemoglobinuria. Perform direct antiglobulin (Coomb's test), haptoglobin, peripheral smear, serum bilirubin, and repeat antibody screen and crossmatch. Keep urine output at 100 ml/hour and consider alkalization of the urine to limit acute renal failure. Mannitol is not helpful, as it increases urine flow by decreasing tubular reabsorption without improving renal perfusion.

Anaphylactic reaction

- Almost exclusively occurs in those with Anti-IgA antibodies (1/70 people).
- _Clinical Features_ - It usually begins after the first few ml of blood with afebrile flushing, wheezing, cramps, vomiting, diarrhea, and hypotension.
- _Management_ - stop transfusion, treat with _Benadryl_, epinephrine & steroids.

Febrile non-hemolytic reaction

- _Clinical Features_ - occurs during or soon after starting 3-4% of transfusions, most common if multiply transfused or multiparous with anti-leukocyte antibodies.
- _Management_ - Stop transfusion and treat as transfusion reaction.

Urticarial reactions

- _Clinical Features_ - causes local erythema, hives and itching.
- _Management_ - Further evaluation unnecessary unless fever, chills, or other adverse effects are present. This is the only type of transfusion reaction in which the infusion can continue.

Hyperviscosity Syndrome

Etiology	Diagnosis
↑serum proteins with sludging & ↓ circulation. Common causes: macroglobulinemia, myeloma and CML.	• WBC (esp. blasts)>100,000 cells/mm^3 • ↑serum viscosity -Ostwald viscometer • Serum protein electrophoresis
Clinical Features	**Management**
• Fatigue, headache, somnolence • ↓vision, seizure, deafness, MI, CHF • Retinal bleed and exudates	• IV NS, plasmapheresis • 2 unit phlebotomy with NS, and packed red blood cell replacement

Spinal Cord Compression

Most often due to lymphoma, lung, breast or prostate cancer. 68% are thoracic, 19% lumbosacral, and 15% cervical spine.

Clinical Features		Diagnosis
Back pain	95%	• Plain films are abnormal in 60-90%
Weakness (usually symmetric)	75%	• MRI or CT or myelography
Autonomic or sensory symptoms	50%	Management[1]
Inability to walk	50%	• Dexamethasone 25 mg IV q 6 hours
Flaccidity, hyporeflexia (early) or	-	• Radiation therapy
Spasticity, hyperreflexia (late)	-	• Surgery may be needed for epidural
Bowel/bladder incontinence	-	abscess/bleed, or disc herniation

[1] Steroid and radiation may be indicated if cancer is cause of compression.

Superior Vena Cava Syndrome

Occurs in 3-8% with lung cancer & lymphoma. Symptoms are due to venous hypertension in areas drained by superior vena cava. Death occurs from cerebral edema, airway compromise, or cardiac compromise.

Clinical Features		Diagnosis
Thoracic or neck vein distention	65%	• CXR shows mediastinal mass or
Shortness of breath	50%	parenchymal lung mass in 10%
Tachypnea	40%	• CT is diagnostic
Upper trunk or extremity edema	40%	Management
Cough/dysphagia/chest pain	20%	• Furosemide 40 mg IV
Periorbital or facial edema	-	• Methylprednisolone 1-2 mg/kg mg IV
Stoke's sign (tight shirt collar)	-	• Mediastinal radiation

Tumor Lysis Syndrome

Occurs within 1-2 days of starting chemotherapy or radiation for rapidly growing tumors (esp. leukemias and lymphomas).

Clinical features are due to hyperuricemia (renal failure), $\uparrow K^+$ (arrhythmias), $\uparrow$phosphate (renal failure), and $\downarrow Ca^{+2}$ (cramping, tetany, confusion, seizures).

Management	Criteria for Hemodialysis
• Hydration with NS	• K^+ > 6 mEq/L
• Allopurinol 100-200 mg PO/day	• Significant renal insufficiency
• Alkalinize <u>serum</u> with $NaHCO_3$ to	• Uric acid > 10 mg/dl
<u>urine</u> pH $\geq$ 7.0	• Symptomatic hypocalcemia
• Treat hyperkalemia (page 51)	• Serum phosphorus > 10 mg/dl
• Dialysis	

Hypertension, Asymptomatic, Urgencies & Emergencies

Asymptomatic Hypertension – ACEP Clinical Policy (*Ann Emerg Med* 2006; 47; 237)
Level B recommendations: Initiating treatment for asymptomatic hypertension (HTN) in the ED is NOT necessary when patients have follow-up. Rapidly lowering BP in asymptomatic patients in the ED is UNNECESSARY and may be harmful in some patients. When ED treatment for asymptomatic HTN is started, an attempt should be made to gradually lower the BP and NOT to normalize the BP in the ED.
Hypertensive urgency – Debate exists as to whether such an entity occurs. Experts have described this entity as an elevated BP that may potentially be harmful if sustained (usually diastolic BP > 115 mm Hg) without end-organ damage. Treatment goal is to reduce pressure gradually within days to weeks to normal for patient. The 7th Joint National Committee on HTN recommends
(1) combination oral antihypertensive therapy (see chart above),
(2) evaluation for heart or renal damage due to HTN and reversible causes of HTN (e.g. non-compliance, sleep apnea, drug induced, chronic renal disease, renovascular disease, aldosteronism, chronic steroid use/Cushing's syndrome, coarctation of the aorta, pheochromocytoma, thyroid or parathyroid disease)

7th Joint National Committee on Hypertension Recommendations
Classification of HTN is based on measurements obtained in $\geq$ 2 physician visits.

Class	SBP/DBP[1]	Management[2,3]	If compelling indications[2,3]
Normal	< 120/80	Lifestyle modification for all classes	Renal disease, diabetes cut-off goal is < 130/80
PreHTN	120-139/80-89		
Stage 1 PreHTN	140-159/90-99	Thiazides for most, may consider [2] below	See drugs listed with underling disease risk below. Add second drug as needed.
Stage 2 HTN	160/100	2 drugs for most – thiazide and any from [2] below[4]	

Underlying disease risk	Diuretic	BB[2]	ACEI[2]	ARB[2]	CCB[2]	AldAnt[2]
Heart failure[5]	+	+	+	+		+
Post myocardial infarct[5]		+	+			+
High coronary risk[5]	+	+	+		+	
Diabetes	+	+	+	+	+	
Chronic renal disease			+	+		
Prevent recurrent stroke	+		+			

[1]SBP systolic blood pressure in mm Hg; DBP-diastolic blood pressure in mm Hg; to classify, choose SBP or DBP that places patient into highest stage/class
[2] ACEI - angiotensin converting enzyme inhibitor, ARB - angiotensin receptor blocker, BB - beta-blocker, CCB - calcium channel blocker, AldAnt - aldosterone antagonist
[3] Routine tests before starting drugs: ECG, urinalysis, glucose, Hb, K+, Creatinine, lipids. Consider other tests if non-response to therapy or other disease suspected.
[4] Initiate combination therapy cautiously (esp. in those at risk for orthostatic hypotension)
[5] See page 78 for **American Heart Assoc**. recommendations. *7th Joint Nat. Comm. on HTN*

American Heart Association Hypertension Recommendations[1,2,3]

Risk	BP target	Medications	Comments
CAD prevention	< 140/90	ACEI or ARB or CCB or thiazide or combo	Start 2 drugs if SBP ≥ 160 or DBP ≥ 100 mm Hg
Hi risk CAD[4]	< 130/80	See CAD prevention	See CAD prevention
Stable angina	< 130/80	β blocker (or if contraindicated substitute diltiazem or verapamil) AND (ACEI or ARB),	Do not use (diltiazem/verapamil) if bradycardia or LVD. A dihydropyridine CCB (not diltiazem or verapamil) or thiazide can be added to β blocker
UA/NSTEMI	< 130/80	See stable angina	See stable angina comments
STEMI	< 130/80	See stable angina	See stable angina comments
Left heart failure[5]	< 120/80	β blocker + (ACEI or ARB) + (thiazide or loop diuretic) + aldosterone antagonist[6]	Contraindicated agents include: verapamil, diltiazem, clonidine, moxonidine (not available in US), α blockers

[1] Targets are for long term control of BP (in mm Hg) and not necessarily ED goals.
[2] ACEI – angiotensin converting enzyme inhibitor, ARB – angiotensin receptor blocker, CAD – coronary artery disease, CCB – calcium channel blocker, DBP – diastolic blood pressure, NSTEMI – non ST elevation MI, SBP – systolic blood pressure, STEMI – ST elevation myocardial infarction, US – unstable angina
[3] Weight loss, healthy diet, smoking cessation, alcohol moderation recommended for all
[4] Diabetes, chronic renal disease, known CAD, or carotid/peripheral artery disease, abd. aneurysm or Framingham ris ≥ 10%(www.nhlbi.nih.gov/guidelines/cholesterol/risk_tbl.htm)
[5] Avoid verapamil, diltiazem, clonidine, α blockers. If African American and NY Heart class III/IV heart failure, consider adding hydralazine/isosorbide dinitrate.
[6] Use if NY Heart Class III/IV or if clinical heart failure and LV ejection fraction < 40%.
Circulation; 115: 2761.

Hypertensive Emergencies (Specific agents listed on next page)

- *Defined* - an elevated BP with end-organ damage or dysfunction.
- **Treatment goal** is to reduce **MAP** [Mean Arterial Pressure (MAP)] = diastolic BP (DBP) + 1/3 pulse pressure (SBP-DBP)] by **20-25%** % in 30-60 min.
- *Catecholamine-induced Hypertension* - Acute ↑catecholamines with acute sympathetic overactivity and hypertension due to pheochromocytomas, monoamine oxidase inhibitors, sympathomimetics, clonidine or β blocker withdrawal. Treat with labetalol or α-blockers (e.g. phentolamine).
- *Left Ventricular Failure and Coronary Insufficiency* - ↑ afterload can lead to pulmonary edema, and myocardial ischemia. Nitroglycerin IV is the drug of choice. See page 43 for recommendations for treating acute pulmonary edema.
- *Hypertensive Encephalopathy* - headache, vomit, & confusion due to loss of cerebral flow autoregulation. Treat with nicardipine (*Cardene*), nitroprusside (*Nipride*), or labetalol (*Normodyne*). Do not lower MAP to < 120 mm Hg.
- *Pregnancy-induced Hypertension* or *Pre-eclampsia*- see page 132.
- *Renal Failure* - ↓ renal function due to ↑ BP is a hypertensive emergency. Proteinuria, red cells, red cell casts and ↑ BUN/creatinine occur. Page 222.
- *Thoracic dissection* – Treat with labetalol or (*Nipride* + esmolol). Page 222.

Drugs in Hypertensive Emergencies

Drug	Dose and route	Mechanism	Onset	Duration	Features
enalapril (*Vasotec*)	1.25-5 mg IV over 5 min, administered q 6 h	ACE inhibitor	15 min	6 hours (h)	Avoid in renal artery stenosis and avoid in acute MI
esmolol (*Brevibloc*)	250-500 mcg/kg IV over 1st min, then titrate 50-100 mcg/kg/min	β-blockade	1-2 min (half life 9 min)	10-30 min	May either repeat recommended bolus q 5 min or increase infusion to 300 mcg/min
fenoldopam (*Corlopam*)	0.1-0.3 mcg/kg/min IV ± ↑ up to 1.6 mcg/kg/min	Dopamine-1 receptor agonist	< 5 min	30 min	↑ renal flow, & Na+ excretion, esp. useful if ↓ renal function
hydralazine (*Apresoline*)	10-20 mg IV q30-60 min or 10-40 mg IM	Arteriolar dilator	10-30 min	1-4 h (IV) 4-6 h (IM)	Causes tachycardia, headache
labetalol (*Normodyne*)	20-80 mg IV q 10 min then 0.5-2 mg/min	α and β blockade in 1:7 ratio	5-10 min	3-6 h	Worsens bronchospasm, heart blocks, & congestive heart failure
nicardipine (*Cardene*)	Start 5 mg/h IV, ↑2.5 mg/h q15 min. Max dose 15mg/h	Calcium channel blocker	1-5 min	20 min	Rarely precipitates angina, ↑HR and ↑ICP
nitroglycerin	5-100 mcg/min	Vasodilator	2-5 min	5-10 min	May ↑heart rate, and ↓BP
propranolol (*Inderal*)	1 mg IV over 1 min q 5 min up to Max of 6-8 mg	β-blockade	seconds	up to 8 h	Worsens bronchospasm, heart blocks, & CHF
phentolamine (*Regitine*)	5-15 mg IV q 5-15 min	α-blocker	1-2 min	30-60 min	tachycardia in pheochromocytoma
sodium nitroprusside (*Nipride*)	0.25-10 mcg/kg/min IV	Arterial and venous dilator	seconds	1-3 min	no ↓cardiac output, possible cyanide toxicity and ↑ICP

Nonoccupational Exposure to Human Immunodeficiency Virus (HIV)

Management Algorithm - if Exposed and Negative Rapid Test (www.cdc.gov)

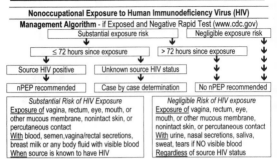

| Substantial exposure risk | Negligible exposure risk |

≤ 72 hours since exposure → > 72 hours since exposure ↓

Source HIV positive → Unknown source HIV status ↓

nPEP recommended | Case by case determination | No nPEP recommended

Substantial Risk of HIV Exposure	*Negligible Risk of HIV exposure*
<u>Exposure of</u> vagina, rectum, eye, mouth, or other mucous membrane, nonintact skin, or percutaneous contact	<u>Exposure of</u> vagina, rectum, eye, mouth, or other mucous membrane, nonintact skin, or percutaneous contact
<u>With</u> blood, semen, vagina/rectal secretions, breast milk or any body fluid with visible blood	<u>With</u> urine, nasal secretions, saliva, sweat, tears if NO visible blood
<u>When</u> source is known to have HIV	<u>Regardless</u> of source HIV status

Drug Regimens for Nonoccupational Postexposure Prophylaxis (nPEP) to HIV

A 28 day regimen of 1 of following category of drugs (•) is recommended. *Test source* for HIV, sexually transmitted disease (STD), Hepatitis B/C, viral load, HIV resistance, CD4 count. Prior to treatment obtain pregnancy test, CBC, liver + renal function tests, tests for STDs, Hepatitis B/C, + rapid HIV test on exposed patient. Renal/liver function CBC require ongoing monitoring. Avoid pregnancy + add barrier contraception (to oral contraceptive).

Non-nucleoside Reverse transcriptase Inhibitor (NNRTI) based	• Efavirenz/*Sustiva* 600 mg PO qhs + (lamivudine/*Epivir* 150 mg PO bid or 300 mg PO daily or emtricitabine/*Emtriva* 200 mg PO daily) + (zidovudine/*AZT* 200 mg PO tid or 300 mg PO bid or tenofovir/*Viread* 300 mg PO daily) **OR** • Efavirenz + (lamivudine 150 mg PO bid or 300 mg PO daily or emtricitabine 200 mg PO daily) + (abacavir/ *Ziagen* 300 mg PO bid (or 600 mg daily) or didanosine/*Videx* [< 60 kg 125 g PO bid, > 60 kg 200 mg PO bid or 400 mg PO daily, or if tenofovir also used 250 mg PO bid] or stavudine/*Zerit* [< 60 kg – 30 mg PO bid; > 60 kg – 40 mg PO daily]) *Combivir* = lamivudine 150 mg + zidovudine 300 mg *Truvada* = 200 mg emtricitabine + 300 mg tenofovir
Protease Inhibitor (PI) based	• Lopinavir/ritonavir (*Kaletra*) 3 tablets (400mg/100 mg each) bid + (lamivudine or emtricitabine) + zidovudine (see NNRTI regimen dosing) • See www.cdc.gov/mmwr/preview/mmwrhtml/rr5402a1.htm for alternate PI based regimens
Nucleoside reverse transcriptase inhibitor (triple NRTI)	• Use only if NNRTI or PI based regimen cannot be used • Abacavir 300 mg PO bid (or 600 mg daily) + lamivudine + zidovudine (see NNRTI dosing) **OR** *Trizivir* 1 tab PO bid (abacavir 300mg+ lamivudine 150mg + zidovudine 300mg)

Contact information: (1) Treatment information: http://aidsinfo.nih.gov/ (2) PEPline at www.ucsf.edu/hivcntr/Hotlines/PEPline 888-448-4911; (3) CDC: 800-893-0485; (4) HIV Antiretroviral Pregnancy Registry at www.apregistry.com/index.htm; 800-258-4263

Health Care Worker Human Immunodeficiency Virus Post Exposure Prophylaxis (PEP) Start as soon As possible (hours not days) - potentially up to 72 hours after exposure.

Percutaneous (P) and mucous membrane/nonintact skin exposure (MN) recommendations

Exposure[1]	HIV class I[1]	HIV class II[1]	Unknown source or HIV status
P-less severe	2 drug PEP	2 drug PEP	consider 2 drug PEP if HIV risks
P-severe	3 drug PEP	≥ 3 drug PEP	consider 2 drug PEP if HIV risks
MN-small vol[2]	± 2 drug PEP	2 drug PEP	No PEP
MN-large vol[2]	2 drug PEP	≥ 2 drug PEP	consider 2 drug PEP if HIV risks

[1] Class I – asymptomatic or viral load < 1500/ml, Class II – symptomatic, AIDS, acute seroconversion, high viral load. Less severe – solid needle, superficial injury, More severe – hollow needle, deep puncture, visible blood, needle inserted into vein or artery.
[2] vol – volume, small volume = a few drops, large volume = splash. Sources of concern include blood, semen, vaginal secretions, CSF, synovial, pleural, peritoneal, pericardial, amniotic fluid or the following only if they contain visible blood: feces, nasal secretions, saliva, sputum, sweat, tears, urine, vomitus. (MMWR 2005: 54[RR09]1-17)

Regimens and Drug Choices for Adult HIV PEP[1] (MMWR 2005: 54[RR09]1-17)

♦ Draw HIV, CBC, liver+renal function, βhCG ± hepatitis exposure work up (pg 82)
♦ Repeat CBC, liver + renal tests at 2 weeks, and HIV at 6 and 12 weeks, + 12 mo.
♦ Treat for 28 days or until source verified to be HIV negative

2 drug regimen	(3TC or emtricitabine/FTC) AND (ZDV or d4T or tenofovir)
≥ 3 drug regimen	2 drug regimen above AND (Kaletra (LPV/RTV) or (ATV±RTV) or (FOSAPV±RTV) or (IDV±RTV) or (SQV±RTV) or (NFV or EFV))

Antiretroviral PEP Drug Dosing[1]

atazanavir (*ATV/Reyataz*) – 400 mg PO daily (altered dosing if used with TDF)

Combivir (ZDV/300 mg + 3TC/150 mg) – 1 PO bid

didanosine (*ddI/Videx*) – 200 mg PO bid OR 400 mg PO daily (1/2 dose if < 60 kg)

efavirenz (*EFV/Sustiva*) – 600 mg PO qhs

emtricitabine (*FTC/Emtriva*) – 200 mg PO daily

fosamprenavir (*FOSAPV/Lexiva*) – 1.4 g PO bid (alone), 700 mg bid if RTV 100 mg bid, 1.4 g daily if RTV 200 mg daily

indinavir (*IDV/Crixivan*) – 800 mg PO bid (use with RTV 100 mg bid)

Kaletra (lopinavir/ritonavir: *LPV/RTV*: 200/50) – 2 PO bid OR 4 PO daily(with food)

lamivudine (*3TC/Epivir*) – 150 mg PO bid OR 300 mg PO daily

nelfinavir (*NFV/Viracept*) – 1.25 g PO bid (with meal)

ritonavir (*RTV/Norvir*) – 100-200 mg PO daily, OR 100 mg PO bid

saquinavir (*SQV/Invirase*) – 1 g PO bid (used with RTV 100 mg PO bid)

stavudine (*d4T/Zerit*) – 40 mg PO bid OR 30 mg bid < 60 kg OR 20-30 mg bid if toxicity

tenofovir (*TDF/Viread*) – 150 mg PO bid OR 300 mg PO daily

Truvada (TDF/300 mg + FTC/200 mg) – 1 PO daily

zidovudine (*AZT/ZDV/Retrovir*) – 300 mg PO bid OR 200 mg PO tid (with food)

[1] Drug dosing &choice is based on type of exposure, risk of resistance, compliance, toxicity assessment. Consider contacting local or national experts (1-888-448-4911) for advice if > 24-36h (but < 72h) from exposure, unknown source, pregnancy/breastfeed,source resistance, or toxicity of initial PEP regimen. See additional contact information page 80

Hepatitis B (HB) Exposure

Exposed Person	Source of Exposure		
	HB Surface (HBs) Antigen (Ag) positive	HB Surface (HBs) Antigen (Ag) negative	Source not known or not available
Unvaccinated	HBIG[1] x 1 and HB vaccine series[1]	Begin HB vaccine series[1]	Begin HB vaccine series[1]
Vaccinated Known responder[2]	No treatment	No treatment	No treatment
Vaccinated Known non-responder	HBIG[1] x 2 or HBIG[1] x 1 & initiate revaccination	No treatment	If high-risk source, treat as if source were HBs Ag positive
Vaccinated Response unknown	Test exposed for anti-HBs[2] (1) If adequate, no treatment. (2) If inadequate HBIG x 1 plus vaccine booster	No treatment	Test exposed person for Anti-HBs[2] If inadequate, HB vaccine booster and recheck titer in 1-2 months.

[1] _HBIG dose_ – 0.06 ml/kg IM, _HB vaccine_ – 1 ml IM deltoid, repeat in 1 & 6 months
[2] _Known responder_ - Adequate anti-HBs = ≥ 10 mIU/ml
Hepatitis A: ISG 0.02 ml/kg IM for exposure via close personal contact, employee at day care center, contaminated food within 2 wks. _Hepatitis C_: No post-exposure prophylaxis.

Tetanus Immunization

Prior immunization	Tetanus prone wound	Non tetanus prone wound
Uncertain or <3	Td[1], TIG[2]	Td[1]
3 or more	Td[1] if >5y since last dose	Td[1] if >10y since last dose

[1] Use Tdap (_Adacel_) for 1st dose if no prior Tdap & 18-64 yo. Td is preferred in pregnancy although Tdap is not contraindicated. If given, administration 2nd, 3rd trimester is preferred.
[2] Tetanus immune globulin. Dose of TIG – 250 units IM at site other than for Td/Tdap.

Postexposure Rabies Prophylaxis (_Ann Emerg Med_ 1999; 33: 590.)

Rabies prophylaxis only indicated if bite or salivary exposure from bat (treat inhalation exposure, e.g. bat found in bedroom) or mammalian carnivore. No prophylaxis is needed if nonsalivary or if bird, reptile, or rodent (rare cases). If questions arise regarding prophylaxis and local/state health department unavailable call CDC at **404-639-1050** (days), **404-639-2888** (nights & weekends)
(1) Rabies vaccine - 1 ml IM, on day 0, 3, 7, 14, & 28. Give in deltoid, not buttock.
PLUS (2) RIG (rabies immune globulin) - 20 IU/kg infiltrated SC around wound (if possible) and remainder IM distal to site of vaccine administration.

		Animal is Cat or Dog	Not Cat or Dog
Was animal captured?	NO, escaped	Give RIG & vaccine only if rabies risk for species in area.	Treat with RIG and full course of vaccine
	YES, captured	Observe animal for 10 days. If abnormal behavior, sacrifice and treat patient with RIG & vaccine. Discontinue treatment if animal pathology negative for rabies.	Sacrifice animal and begin RIG and vaccine. Discontinue treatment if pathology negative for rabies.

Cardiac Conditions Requiring Infective Endocarditis (IE) Prophylaxis[1,2,3]

Prior Infectious Endocarditis or any Prosthetic Cardiac Valve
Congenital Heart Disease (CHD) – only CHD categories below require prophylaxis • Unrepaired CHD including those who have had shunts for palliation • Repaired CHD with residual defects at or adjacent to site of a prosthetic path or device • During 1st 6 months post operative: Completely repaired congenital defects with prosthetic grafts or devices.
Post cardiac transplantation if develop cardiac valvulopathy

[1] Prophylaxis only required before dental procedures, or if invasive respiratory tract procedure with incision or biopsy of respiratory mucosa. [2] Prophylaxis is no longer recommended prior to GU or GI procedures. [3] See page 94 for antibiotic regimens.

Circulation 2007; 116; 1736.

Fever and Neutropenia

Fever – a single oral temp. ≥ 38.3°C (101°F) or ≥ 38.0°C (100.4°F) for ≥ 1 hour
Neutropenia –< 500 neutrophils(NP)/mm³ or < 1000 NP/mm³ + predict ↓ to < 500 NP/mm³

Identification of High vs. Low Risk Patients with Neutropenia	
High Risk (if any factor below present)	*Low Risk (No high risk & most of below)*
• Outpatient at onset of fever • Significant medical illness • Anticipated long severe neutropenia (≤100 cells/mcl for ≥ 7 days) • Hepatic disease (LFTs ≥ 5 X normal) • Renal disease (CrCl < 30 ml.min) • Uncontrolled/progressive cancer • Pneumonia/complex infections • Alemtuzumab use • Mucositis grade 3 – 4 • MASCC risk index < 21 (below)	• Outpatient at onset of fever • No comorbid illness requiring admit • Anticipated short duration neutropenia (≤ 100 cell/mcl for < 7 days) • Good performance status (ECOG 0-1 = full active at predisease performance or restricted in physically strenuous activity but ambulatory + able to carry out work of light or sedentary nature) • No hepatic/renal insufficiency • MASCC ≥ 21 (below)

www.nccn.org

MASCC (Multinational Association for Supportive Care in Cancer) Risk Index

Characteristic	Points	Characteristic	Points
Burden of illness		Solid tumor or heme malignancy	
No or mild symptoms	5	with no prior fungal infection	4
Moderate symptoms	3	No dehydration	3
No hypotension	5	Outpatient status	3
No COPD	4	Age < 60 years	2

MASCC risk < 21 – high risk, MASCC ≥ 21 – low risk in neutropenic fever

Initial Evaluation & Management of Patients with Neutropenic Fever

History	• In addition to standard present & past history ask: time of prior chemotherapy, prior infections, HIV status, current meds, infectious exposures (e.g. TB), recent blood products, pets, and travel history.
Physical Exam	• In addition to head to toe physical examination, examine the groin, perivaginal and perirectal regions for signs of occult infection.
Labs & Xray	• CBC, platelets, renal/liver function, electrolytes, urinalysis with culture, oximetry, CXR (esp. if any respiratory symptoms), blood cultures X 2 (peripheral and/or catheter), if signs or symptoms add viral cultures (nasopharynx for influenza or vesicles for HSV), stool culture/*C. difficile* assay/parasite testing. Other lab testing may be required depending upon signs & symptoms. • If abdomen, pelvic, or perirectal pain - CT scan usually required. • If neurologic symptoms, CT, MRI, lumbar puncture may be required. • If sinus/nasal disease, consider CT/MRI orbit/sinus, ENT consult.
Empiric Anti- microbials If pneumonia SEE <u>Pneumonia</u> & <u>Adjunct Therapy</u> Below Discuss Outpatient Option with Oncologist	<u>Monotherapy options</u>: cefepime 2 g IV q 8h [See cefepime caution page 88] **OR** imipenem 500 mg IV q 6h **OR** meropenem 1g IV q 8h (2g q 8h if meningitis) **OR** *Zosyn* 4.5 g IV q 6h **OR** ceftazidime 2 g IV q 8h
	<u>Combination options</u>: (1) aminoglycoside [dose page 113] + antipseudo-monal penicillin with β lactamase inhibitor [*Zosyn* 4.5 g IV q 6h or *Timentin* 3.1 g IV q 4-6h] or cefepime or ceftazidime 2 g IV q 8h) **OR** (2) ciprofloxacin 400 mg IV q 8-12h + antipseudomonal penicillin (above)
	<u>Staphylococcus aureus coverage</u> – consider only add this coverage if suspected MRSA, clinically apparent serious catheter infection, gram positive on blood culture, known colonization with MRSA or resistant pneumococci, hypotension, shock, soft tissue infection (including periorbital cellulitis), risk factors for viridians strep. (bacteremia, severe mucositis, use of quinolone or TMP-SMX [*Septra/Bactrim*] prophylaxis): vancomycin 15 mg/kg IV q 12 h **OR** linezolid 600 mg IV/PO q 12h **OR** daptomycin 4-6 mg/kg IV q 24h **OR** *Synercid* 7.5 mg IV q 8h.
	<u>Pneumonia</u>: **ADD** *Zithromax* or *Avelox* or *Levaquin* to above regimens. If Intermediate/High risk consider antifungal, antiviral (oseltamivir for influenza outbreak), *Septra/Bactrim* if Pneumocystis, or MRSA coverage
	<u>Antivirals/Antifungals/Antiparasitics</u> : See www.nccn.org website
	<u>Outpatient option</u> for Low Risk patients (prior page) & good support – DO NOT use this regimen if quinolone prophylaxis has been used: (1) *Cipro* 500 mg PO tid (note higher than normal frequency) **AND** (2) *Augmentin* 500 mg PO tid or clindamycin 150-450 mg PO qid
Adjunct Therapy Discuss with Oncologist	• G-CSF (filgrastim/*Neupogen*)/GM-CSF (sargramostim/*Leukine*) con--sider if pneumonia, invasive fungal infection, progressive infection • Granulocyte transfusions may be beneficial if invasive fungal infection, gram negative rod infection unresponsive to antibiotics • IV immunoglobulin in (1) combination with ganciclovir for CMV pneumonia or (2) patients with profound hypogammaglobulinemia.

Fever and Rash

Causes of Petechial Rash and Fever

Infectious		Noninfectious
Endocarditis	Enterovirus	Allergy, thrombocytopenia
Meningococcemia	Hemorrhagic viruses	Scurvy, Lupus
Gonococcemia	Hepatitis B	Henoch Schonlein purpura
Other pathogenic bacteria	Rubella, Epstein Barr	Hypersensitivity vasculitis
(e.g. Gram neg. enterics)	Rat bite fever	Rheumatic fever
Rickettsia (RMSF)	Epidemic typhus	Amyloidosis

Causes of Maculopapular Rash and Fever

Infectious		Noninfectious
Typhoid fever/typhus	ParvovirusB19/5th disease	Allergy, serum sickness
Secondary syphilis, Lyme	Human herpesvirus 6	Erythema multiforme
Meningococcemia	Rubeola/Rubella/Arbovirus	Erythema marginatum
Mycoplasma, Psittacosis	Epstein Barr virus	Lupus, Dermatomyositis
Rickettsia, Leptospirosis	Adenovirus, Primary HIV	Sweet's syndrome
Ehrlichiosis, Enterovirus	Streptobacillus moniliformis	Acroderm. enteropathica

Causes of Vesico-Bullous Rash and Fever

Infectious		Noninfectious
Staphylococcemia	Folliculitis (Staph,Candida	Allergy, Plant dermatitis
Gonococcemia, Rickettsia	Pseudomonas)	Eczema vaccinatum
Herpes/Varicella	Enterovirus, 5th disease	Erythema multiforme
Vibrio vulnificans	ParvovirusB19, HIV	bullosum

Causes of Erythematous Rash and Fever

Infectious		Noninfectious
Staph/Strep infection	C. haemolyticum	Allergy, Vasodilation,
(toxic shock, scarlet fever)	Kawasaki's disease	Eczema, Psoriasis,
Ehrlichiosis	Enterovirus	Lymphoma, Pityriasis
Strep. viridans		rubra, Sezary syndrome

Causes of Urticarial Rash and Fever

Infectious		Noninfectious
Mycoplasma	Adenovirus, Epstein Barr	Allergy
Lyme disease	Strongyloides, Trichinosis	Vasculitis
Enterovirus	Schistosomiasis,	Malignancy
HIV, Hepatitis B	Onchocerciasis, Loiasis	Idiopathic

Human Immunodeficiency Virus

Correlation of HIV Associated Disease and CD4 Counts

CD4	Infection or Other Complication
> 500 cells/mm³	Acute retroviral syndrome, general lymphadenopathy, Candida vaginitis, Guillain Barre, aseptic meningitis
200 – 500	Sinusitis, bacterial pneumonia (pneumococcus), pulmonary TB (up to 40% - normal CXR), Herpes simplex/zoster, Candida esophagitis and thrush, Kaposi's, Cryptosporidiosis, B-cell lymphoma, cervical neoplasia & cancer, anemia, mononeuronal multiplex, ITP, Hodgkins, interstitial pneumonitis
< 200	*Pneumocystis jiroveci* pneumonia, Disseminated herpes, Toxoplasmosis, Cryptococcus, Histoplasmosis, and Coccidiodomycosis, Microspiridiosis, TB (extrapulmonary and miliary), HIV dementia, cardiomyopathy, Non-Hodgkins lymphoma, vacuolar myelopathy, peripheral neuropathy
< 100	Disseminated herpes simplex, Toxoplasmosis, Cryptosporidiosis, Microsporidiosis, Kaposi's (visceral and pulmonary)
< 50	Disseminated CMV & *Mycobacterium avium*, CNS lymphomas

CD4 count indicates health of immune system and risk of certain infections, while the viral load indicates how active HIV is in the patient's system.   *Acta Clinica Belgica* 2002;57.

Diagnostic Evaluation of Acute Fever in HIV

- **If localized signs or symptoms** evaluate & treat source.
- **If central line, neutropenia, sepsis, IV drug use** – empiric IV antibiotics
- **If no local signs or symptoms** obtain following tests and (*manage as indicated*) - CXR/ABG (if +*treat for Pneumocystis, TB, or fungi*), Urinalysis, Stool (*for bacterial culture, C. difficile, parasitic evaluation*), CBC, LFTs (if + *US or CT abdomen and consider liver biopsy*), LDH (*if + with pulmonary symptoms treat Pneumocystis even if negative CXR*), serum cryptococcal antigen/Toxoplasma IgG/IgM, blood cultures (*culture for Mycobacteria & fungi*), serum VDRL
- **If above negative & CD 4 < 200** consider (1) drug fever, (2) sputum/urine for TB (3) CT to exclude lymphoma (4) asymptomatic sinusitis – CT (5) dental source (6) spinal tap (bacterial, viral, parasitic, fungal evaluation), (7) mycobacterial blood cultures (8) bone marrow

Sepsis

Systemic Inflammatory Response Syndrome/SIRS (≥ 2 of following)

• Temp > 38°C(100.4°F) or < 36°(96.8°)	• Heart rate > 90 beats/minute
• Resp rate > 20 breaths per minute or PaCO₂ < 32 mm Hg	• WBC > 12,000 cells/mm³, < 4000 or > 10% bands

Early Goal Directed Therapy in Severe Sepsis and Septic Shock
Eligibility[1] - 2 of 4 SIRS criteria prior page **AND** (Systolic BP ≤ 90 mm Hg or MAP < 70 mm Hg after one 20-30 ml/kg NS challenge or lactate ≥ 4 mmol/L)

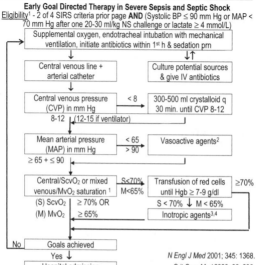

N Engl J Med 2001; 345: 1368.
Crit Care Med 2008; 36: 296.

[1] Original exclusion criteria (some are now relative contraindications) – age < 18 years, acute stroke, pulmonary edema, status asthmaticus, acute coronary syndrome, primary arrhythmia, active GI bleed, seizure, drug overdose, burn or trauma, uncured cancer, immunosuppressed, contraindication to central line, acute surgery needed, DNR status

[2] Vasopressors (dopamine or norepinephrine, then epinephrine if poorly responsive to 1st agent chosen) are given to increase MAP ≥ 65 mm Hg. If MAP > 90 mm Hg. Vasodilators (e.g. sodium nitroprusside, nitroglycerin) are given to lower MAP to ≤ 90 mm Hg.

[3] Inotropes – Initiate dobutamine at 2.5 mcg/kg/min. Increase dose by 2.5 mcg/kg/min every 30 minutes until ScvO2 is ≥ 70% or maximum dose of 20 mcg/kg/min is given. Decrease dobutamine dose or discontinue if MAP < 65 mm Hg or heart rate > 120 beats/min.

[4] Consider IV hydrocortisone (< 300 mg/d) if BP poor response to fluids/vasopressors (Caution – 2008 study found that hydrocortisone did not improve survival or reversal of shock in patients with septic shock, either overall or in patients who did not have a response to corticotropin. N Engl J Med 2008; 358: 111) Consider human activated protein C. (see dose, indications page 108). Keep glucose < 150 mg/dl [Caution – 2008 study found that intensive insulin therapy placed critically ill patients with sepsis at ↑ risk for serious adverse events related to hypoglycemia.N Engl J Med 2008; 358: 125] (see insulin page 54-56). No evidence supports bicarbonate to treat lactic academia in sepsis (esp. if pH ≥ 7.15).

Antimicrobial Therapy for Sepsis/SIRS

Possible Source	Antimicrobial Agents
UNKNOWN	• cenftriaxone 2 g IV q 24 h **AND** vancomycin 1 g IV q 12h **AND** levofloxacin 750 mg IV q 24h
Abdominal Consult surgery	• Zosyn 4.5 g IV q 8 h **AND** aminoglycoside (AG). See IDSA recommendations for intra-abdominal infections below.
Abscess or Cellulitis	• (Imipenem 0.5 g IV q 6h **OR** meropenem 1 g IV q8h **OR** Zosyn 4.5 IV q 6h) **AND** MRSA treatment (see page 101)
Necrotizing fasciitis, Consult surgery	• (Zosyn 4.5 g IV q 8h or imipenem 0.5-1.0 g IV q 6h or meropenem 1 g IV q8) **AND** (vancomycin 1 g IV q 12h or linezolid [*Zyvox*] 600 mg IV q 12h) **AND** clindamycin 900 mg IV q 8h
Pelvic - septic thrombophlebitis	• (Flagyl 1g IV) **AND** (antipseudomonal Cp[3], *Unasyn* 3g IV, *Zosyn* 4.5 g IV, **OR** *Timentin* 3.1)
Pneumonia	• See pneumonia page 104-106
Urinary	• Zosyn 4.5 g IV q 8h **AND** gentamicin (see dosing page 113)
Wounds or	• (or vascular catheter) See UNKNOWN regimen above

[1] **AG** – aminoglycoside (see dosing page 113); amikacin - least *Pseudomonas* resistance, tobramycin most intrinsic activity, & gentamicin - most *Pseudomonas* resistance.
[2] **APP** – Antipseudomonal penicillins (piperacillin 4-6 g IV q6-8h, ticarcillin 3-4 g IV q 4-6h);
[3] **Cp** – cephalosporins; Antipseudomonal Cps include – ceftazidime 2g IV q6h, cefoperazone 2-3 g IV q6h, cefepime 2 g IV q12: **Caution:** cefepime may carry increased mortality compared to other β lactam, Consider risks and benefits before administration.
[4] **FQ** – fluoroquinolone. 2nd generation [effective vs. *Chlamydia, Legionella, Mycoplasma, Pseudomonas*, not strep]: lomefloxacin (*Maxaquin*), *Noroxin, Floxin,* [*Cipro* 400 mg IV q8-12h] 3rd generation – levofloxacin (*Levaquin*), (gram +activity), 4th generation (enhanced anerobic, gram positive coverage) moxifloxacin (*Avelox*), gemifloxacin (*Factive*); [*Cipro* best anti-Pseudomonal activity]

Infect Dis Clin North Am 2008; 22:1. Med Clin North Am 2000/2001

Antibiotics for Complicated[1] Intra-abdominal Infections –
Infectious Disease Society of America (see www.idsociety.org/ for updates)

Severity	Antimicrobial Agents
Mild to Moderate	• <u>Single agent regimen</u> – Ampicillin/sulbactam (*Unasyn*) 1.5-3.0 g IV q6h **OR** ticarcillin/clavulanic acid (*Timentin*) 3.1 g IV q4-6h **OR** ertapenem (*Invanz*) 1 g IM or IV q24h **OR** tigecycline (*Tygacil*) 100 mg IV 1st dose, then 50 mg IV q 12 h • <u>Combination regimen</u> - metronidazole (*Flagyl*) 15 mg/kg [max 1g] IV + 7.5 mg/kg [max 500mg] IV q6h] plus any one of: cefazolin 1-1.5 g IV q6h or cefuroxime 1.5 g IV q 6-8 h or *Cipro* 400 mg IV q 12h or (*Levaquin* 500mg or *Avelox* 400mg)
Severe See cefepime caution under sepsis above	• <u>Single agent regimen</u> – piperacillin/tazobactam (*Zosyn*) 3.375-4.5 g IV q8h **OR** imipenem/cilastin (*Primaxin*) 0.5-1.0 g IV q6-8h **OR** meropenem (*Merrem*) 1 g IV q8h • <u>Combination regimen</u> - metronidazole (*Flagyl*) 15 mg/kg [max 1g] IV + 7.5 mg/kg [max 500mg] IV q6h] plus any one of: *Cipro* 400 mg IV q12h, or aztreonam (*Azactam*) 2 g IV q 8h, or ceftriaxone 1-2 g IV q24h or ceftazidime 2 g IV q8h or cefepime 2 g IV q12h

[1] Avoid ampicillin in areas with increasing *E. coli* resistance.   *Clin Infect Dis 2003; 37: 997*

Therapy - Empiric Antimicrobial Coverage & Specific Infections in Adults[1]

Infection	Treatment
Abdomen	• See IDSA abdominal infection guidelines (pg 88)
Abortion – septic	• See chorioamnionitis page 92
Abscess	• Drainage required, see specific site in text for antibiotics (e.g. brain, breast, parapharyngeal). *See methicillin resistant* Staph. aureus (MRSA) if skin.
Acne vulgaris	• Mild inflammation: tretinoin (*Retin A*) 0.025-0.1% cream **OR** tazarotene (*Tazorac*) 0.1% cream **OR** adapalene (*Differin*) 0.1% cream/gel applied qhs • Moderate: (*Eryderm/Erygel* 2-3% or *Cleocin T* gel bid) **AND** [benzoyl peroxide (*Benzyl, Desquam*) gel/cream daily-bid or *Benzamycin Pak* (benzoyl peroxide 5% gel + erythromycin 3%) bid or *Benza-Clin* (benzoyl peroxide 5% + clindamycin 1% gel) • Severe: doxycycline 100 mg PO bid **OR** azithromycin 500 mg PO daily X 4days/mo X 4 mo **OR** clindamycin 300-450 mg PO qid
Aeromonas	• Diarrhea – ciprofloxacin 500 mg PO bid **OR** *Septra* DS (or *Bactrim*) one PO bid X 3 days
Amebiasis	• See *Entamoeba histolytica*
Ancyclostoma braziliense	• See cutaneous larval migrans
Ancyclostoma duodenalae	• See hookworms
Anthrax	• (Exposure and disease treatment) See page 10.
Appendicitis *Non-surgical option* **ONLY** *if surgical facility & surgeon unavailable or at direction of surgeon*	• See IDSA abdominal infection guidelines (pg 88) • Single study found the following equal to surgery (with 12% requiring surgery if not better in 24 h and 24% recurrence): (cefotaxime 2 g IV q 12h **AND** tinidazole 800 mg IV q 24 h X 2 days) then (ofloxacin 200 mg PO bid **AND** tinidazole 500 mg PO bid X 10 days). *World J Surg* 2006; 30: 1033.
Arthritis – septic	• See Septic Arthritis
Ascaris lumbricoides roundworm	• mebendazole (*Vermox*) 100 mg PO bid X 3 days **OR** albendazole (*Albenza*) 400 mg PO X 1 **OR** pyrantel (*Pin-X, Antiminth*) 11 mg/kg (max 1 g) X 1. • Obstruction: In addition to NG, IV fluids & surgery, piperazine (75 mg/kg/day – max 3.5 g/day, NOT available in US) per NG causes worm paralysis & may relieve worm induced intestinal obstruction.

See further antibiotic categories, detail, & caveats page 113.

Avian "flu"	• See influenzae
Balanitis - Candida	• See vaginitis Candida ± cover strep. or Trichomonas
Bartonella henselae	• See cat scratch
Bite infection – _dog or cat or rat_	• _Augmentin_ 875 mg PO bid X 10 d (1st line listed bites) **OR** cat – _Ceftin_ 500 mg PO bid **OR** dog – _Cleocin_ 300 mg PO qid + _Cipro_ 500 mg PO bid **OR** rat/cat/dog – doxycycline 100 mg PO bid X 10 days • See human bite infection for IV regimens • See methicillin resistant _S. aureus_ if MRSA possible
Bite infection - human	• Oral - _Augmentin_ 875 mg PO bid **OR** (penicillin + cephalosporin) X 10-14 days (shorter if prophylaxis) • IV - _Unasyn_ 3 g IV q6h **OR** _Mefoxin_ 2 g IV q8h **OR** _Timentin_ 3.1 g IV q6h **OR** _Zosyn_ 3.375-4.5 g IV q8h **OR** _Cleocin_ 600-900 mg IV q8h + _Cipro_ 400 mg IV q12h • See methicillin resistant _S. aureus_ if MRSA possible
Blastocystis hominis	• Treatment not always indicated, experts recommend looking for other causes of gastro-intestinal symptoms even if _B. hominis_ in stool. • nitazoxanide (_Alinia_) 500 mg PO bid X 3 days **OR** metronidazole (_Flagyl_) 1.5 g PO daily X 10 days
Botulism	• See biologic exposures page 11
Bowel perforation	• See appendicitis regimens
Brain abscess	• Primary – (cefotaxime 2 g IV q 4h or ceftriaxone 2 g IV q12h) **AND** metronidazole 7.5 mg/kg IV q6h • ADD vancomycin if related to trauma, surgery or recent admission (methicillin resistance suspected)
Breast abscess Incision & drainage required	• Lactating (_S. aureus_)– (nafcillin or oxacillin) 2 g IV q4 h **OR** cefazolin (_Ancef_) 1 g IV q8h • Not lactating (usually anaerobic) – Clindamycin 300 mg IV/PO q6h **OR** [lactating regimen above + metronidazole (_Flagyl_) 7.5 mg/kg q6h] • See methicillin resistant _S. aureus_ if MRSA possible
Breast infection	• See Mastitis page 99
Bronchitis – _antibiotics ONLY indicated in chronic lung disease, cystic fibrosis and not in healthy individuals_	• amoxicillin-clavulante (_Augmentin_) 500-875 mg PO bid (bid or tid if 500 mg) X 7-10 d **OR** azithromycin (_Zithromax_) 500 mg PO daily X 3 **OR** clarithromycin (_Biaxin_) 500 mg PO bid X 7-14 days **OR** Biaxin XL 1 g PO daily X 7 days **OR** flouroquinolone

Brucellosis	• (Exposure and disease treatment) See page 11.
Bubonic plague	• See page 12 for detail re: exposure, disease.
Campylobacter jejuni diarrhea	• azithromycin (*Zithromax*) 500 mg PO daily X 3 d **OR** erythromycin 250-500 mg PO qid X 5 d
Candida	• Oropharyngeal/esophageal – (1) fluconazole (*Diflucan*) 200 mg PO/IV on day 1, then 100 mg PO/IV daily (<u>oropharynx</u> X 14 days or <u>esophageal</u> X 3 weeks & 2 weeks post symptoms) **OR** (2) itraconazole (*Sporanox*) <u>oropharynx</u> – 200 mg swish & swallow X 1-2 weeks or <u>esophageal</u> 100-200 mg swish/swallow X 3 wk & 2 wk post-symptom
	• <u>Vaginitis</u> - miconazole topically bid X 2 weeks **OR** fluconazole (*Diflucan*) 150 mg PO X 1 dose **OR** itraconazole (*Sporanox*) 200 mg PO bid X 1 day
Cat scratch disease *Mild disease resolves without treatment*	• azithromycin 500 mg PO X 1, + 250 mg PO X 4d **OR** *Septra DS* 1 PO bid **OR** ciprofloxacin 400 mg IV q 12h, or gentamicin (see dosing page 113)
Cellulitis – *uncomplicated* Consider possibility of <u>methicillin resistant</u> *Staphylococcus aureus* (MRSA)	• <u>Oral</u> – dicloxacillin or cephalexin (*Keflex*) 250-500 mg PO qid X 10d **OR** azithromycin (*Zithromax*) 500 mg PO X 1 day, 250 mg PO X 4 days **OR** clarithromycin (*Biaxin*) 500 mg PO bid X 10 days
	• <u>IV</u> – nafcillin 1-1.5 g IV q 4-6 h **OR** *Ancef* 1 g IV q8h
	• See <u>methicillin resistant</u> *S. aureus* if MRSA possible
Cellulitis – *diabetic, alcohol,* Consider possibility of <u>methicillin resistant</u> *Staphylococcus aureus* (MRSA)	• <u>Oral</u> – *Augmentin* 875 mg PO bid **OR** IV/IM 3rd Cp[4]
	• <u>IV mild-moderate</u>– *Unasyn* 3 g IV q6h **OR** *Fortaz* 2g IV q8h **OR** cefoperazone 2 g IV q6h **OR** cefepime 2g IV q12: (See cefepime caution page 88) <u>IV severe disease</u> - imipenem 0.5-1 g IV q 6-8 h **OR** meropenem 1 g IV q8h.
	• See <u>methicillin resistant</u> *S. aureus* if MRSA possible
	• See <u>diabetic foot infection</u> – see page 93
Cellulitis – lake/sea H₂0 *(IV regimen differs if salt or fresh water etiology)*	• <u>Oral</u>: *Septra* 1 DS PO bid x 10 d **OR** FQ[2] x 10 d
	• <u>If salt water</u> – aminoglycoside (page 113) **AND** doxycycline 200 mg IV X 1, + 50-100 mg IV q 12h
	• <u>If fresh water</u> – ciprofloxacin 400 mg IV q 12 **OR** (ceftazidime 2 g IV q 8h **AND** gentamicin)
Cervicitis	• Treat as per urethritis
Chancroid	• azithromycin (*Zithromax*) 1g PO X 1 **OR** ceftriaxone 250 mg IM X 1 **OR** *Cipro* 500 mg PO bid X 3 days **OR** erythromycin 500 mg PO tid X 7 days.

Chicken pox	• See varicella
Chlamydia trachomatis urethritis, or cervicitis Also treat for gonorrhea	• azithromycin 1 g PO X 1 **OR** doxycycline 100 mg PO bid **OR** erythromycin base 500 mg qid x 7 d **OR** *Floxin* 300 mg PO bid X 7 d **OR** *Levaquin* 500 mg PO daily X 7 d (also treat gonorrhea) • IF PID, see <u>pelvic inflammatory disease page 103</u> • If LGV – see <u>lymphogranuloma venerum</u>
Chlamydia trachomatis In pregnancy	• azithromycin *(Zithromax)* 1 g PO X 1 **OR** amoxicillin 500 mg PO tid X 7 d **OR** erythromycin base 500 mg PO qid X 7 d **OR** erythromycin base 250 mg PO qid X 14 d
Cholecystitis/cholangitis	• See abdominal infection choices page 88
Chorioamnionitis	• *(Mefoxin* 2g IV q6-8h **OR** *Unasyn* 3.0 g IV q6h **OR** *Zosyn* 3.375-4.5 g IV q8h) **AND** doxycycline 100 mg IV OVER 1-4h bid, switch to 100 mg PO bid when stable • **OR** *Cleocin* 600-900 mg IV q8h **AND** [ceftriaxone 1 g IV q12h or gentamicin (1.7 mg/kg IV q8h or 5 mg/kg/24h]
Clostridium difficile diarrhea	• metronidazole *(Flagyl)* 500 mg PO tid X 10-14 d **OR** vancomycin 125 mg PO qid X 10-14 days • If cannot take PO: *Flagyl* 500 mg IV q6h ± vancomycin 1-3 ml/min of 500 mg/L saline solution per small bowel catheter or cecal catheter to maximum of 2g per day
Conjunctivitis	• moxifloxacin *(Vigamox)* 1 gtt tid X 7 days **OR** gatifloxacin *(Zymar)*1-2 gtts q 2h up to 8X/day while awake on days 1 & 2, then qid X 5 days **OR** ofloxacin *(Ocuflox)* 2 gtts q2-4h X 2d, then 2 gtts qid X 5d **OR** ciprofloxacin *(Ciloxan)* 1-2 gtts q2h (while awake) X 2d, then q4h X 5 days **OR** *(Garamycin* or *Tobrex)* 1-2 gtts q2-4h or ointment applied bid-tid **OR** *Polysporin* applied q 3-4 h **OR** *Ilotycin* applied q3-4h. Note: there is ↑gram positive resistance to 2nd/3rd generation quinolones *(Ciloxan/Ocuflox)* • Antimicrobials effective against Pseudomonas are required for contact lens wearers. • If *N. gonorrhea* suspected/proven (e.g. gram negative intracellular diplococci), ceftriaxone IV and frequent saline irrigation required.
Corneal ulcer	• See bacterial *keratitis* recommendations. • Do not patch eye if Pseudomonas is a concern (e.g. contact lenses). Also, consult ophthalmology & ensure Pseudomonas coverage if contact lens wearer.

Coxiella burnetii	• (Q fever evaluation & treatment) See page 12.
Cryptosporidiosis	• nitazoxanide (*Alinia*) 500 mg PO bid X 3 days • Immunocompromised/HIV – nitazoxanide (*Alinia*)) 1 g PO bid X 2 weeks. (Less effective if CD4 < 50.) Ensure compliance with protease inhibitors as they have anticryptosporidiosis activity. • Alternatives – paromomycin (*Humatin*) and macrolides (azithromycin/*Zithromax*, clarithromycin/*Biaxin*) have activity vs. this parasite, but not as effective as *Alinia*.
Cutaneous larval migrans *(creeping eruption)*	• albendazole (*Albenza*) 200 mg PO bid X 3 days OR ivermectin (*Stromectol*) 200 mcg PO X 1 dose OR thiabendazole 222 mg/kg up to 1500 mg PO bid X 2 days OR thiabendazole cream (15%) or suspension (500/5 ml) applied topically bid X 2 weeks
Cyclospora	• *Septra* DS 1 PO bid X 10 days (use qid dosing if immunocompromised/HIV) OR *Cipro* 500 mg PO bid X 10 days
Dental infection	• Oral therapy – amoxicillin-clavulanate (*Augmentin*) 875 mg PO bid OR clindamycin 300-450 mg PO qid OR penicillin (↑resistance) 500 mg PO qid OR erythromycin 250-500 mg PO qid x 10 days • IV therapy – *Cleocin* 600 mg IV q6h OR *Unasyn* 1.5-3g IV q6h OR cefotetan 2g IV q12h
Diabetic foot infection *Depth Classification* 0 at risk, no ulcer 1 superficial, no infection 2 expose tendon or joint 3 extensive ulcer/abscess *Ischemia Classification* A not ischemic B ischemia, no gangrene C forefoot gangrene D complete foot gangrene 2,3 need debridement, antibiotics (3) amputation C,D (±B) vascular consult D amputation	• Oral agents – (IDSA recommendations) *Septra* DS or *Bactrim* 1 PO bid OR linezolid (*Zyvox*) 600 mg PO bid OR clindamycin 150-450 mg PO qid OR if not methicillin resistant - levofloxacin (*Levaquin*) , dicloxacillin, amoxicillin/clavulanate • IV agents – ceftobiprole 500 mg IV q 8-12 h (not approved in US yet) OR (IDSA recommendations) vancomycin 1 g IV q12h + ceftazidime 1 g IV q 12h OR linezolid (*Zyvox*) ± aztreonam (*Azactam*) OR daptomycin (*Cubicin*) ± aztreonam (*Azactam*) OR clindamycin + [levofloxacin or ciprofloxacin] OR imipenem-cilastatin (*Primaxin*) OR ertapenem (*Invanz*) OR ticarcillin/clavulanate (*Timentin*) OR piperacillin/tazobactam (*Zosyn*) • IDSA – Infectious Disease Society of America

See further antibiotic categories, detail, & caveats page 113.

Diarrhea ...(*Salmonella, Shigella,* ...*Campylobacter, E.coli* or *Traveler's diarrhea*) Only treat Salmonella if older, septic, immune - compromised, or ill enough to be hospitalized	• azithromycin (*Zithromax*) 1g PO X 1 dose, or 500 mg PO X 3 days **OR** Cipro 500 mg PO bid X 3 days **OR** *Levaquin* 500 mg PO daily 1-3 days **OR** rifaximin (*Xifaxan*) 200 mg PO tid X 3 days *(for severe symptoms – fever, bloody diarrhea)* • <u>Traveler's diarrhea prophylaxis</u> – 1 of following daily until 1-2 days after return from travel: Bismuth subsalicylate 2 tabs (262 mg tablet) or 30 mL qid **OR** rifaximin (*Xifaxan*) 200 mg PO daily **OR** Cipro 500 mg PO daily **OR** *Levaquin* 500 mg PO daily
Diarrhea *(Vibrio cholera)*	• azithromycin (*Zithromax*) 1 g PO X 1 dose **OR** Cipro 1 g PO X 1 **OR** doxycycline 300 mg PO X 1 **OR** Septra DS 1 PO bid X 3 days.
Diverticulitis – outpatient	• (*Septra* DS 1 PO bid *OR* Cipro 500 mg PO bid **OR** *Levaquin* 750 mg daily) **AND** metronidazole 500 mg PO qid at least 7-10 days • **OR** *Augmentin* 500 mg PO tid X 7-10 days
Diverticulitis – inpatient	• See Infect Dis Soc America guidelines (page 88)
Ehrlichiosis	• doxycycline 100 mg PO bid X 7-14 days
Encephalitis	• See herpes encephalitis page 97,
Endocarditis *IV drug use* *(Staph. aureus most* *common) Tigecycline,* *linezolid, Synercid kill* *MRSA, but are not well* *studied in endocarditis* *(may require 2nd additional* *agent for best coverage)*	• vancomycin 1 g IV q 12 h **OR** daptomycin (*Cubicin*) 6 mg/kg IV q 24 h **OR** tigecycline (*Tygacil*) 100 mg IV 1st dose + 50 mg IV q 12h **OR** linezolid (*Zyvox*) 600 mg IV q 12h **OR** quinupristin/dalfopristin (*Synercid*) 7.5 mg/kg IV q12h • <u>If known methicillin sensitive</u> (nafcillin 2 g IV q4h ± gentamicin 1 mg/kg IV q8h)
Endocarditis *native valve –* *empiric treatment*	• (penicillin G 20 mill units IV q 24h [continuous or divided q4h] **OR** Ampicillin 2g IV q4h) **AND** Nafcillin 2g IV q4h **AND** gentamicin 1mg/kg IV q8h • <u>Penicillin allergic</u> – vancomycin 15 mg/kg IV q12h **AND** gentamicin 1 mg/kg IV q8h
Endocarditis *Prosthetic valve empiric Rx*	• vancomycin 15 mg/kg IV q12h (max 2 g/day) **AND** gentamicin 1 mg/kg IV q8h **AND** Rifampin 300 mg PO/IV q 8h **ADD** cefepime 2 g IV q 8h if ≤ 2 months from valve surgery (see cefepime caution page 88)
Endocarditis *Prophylaxis* See page 83– disorders/procedures requiring prophylaxis	• Administer 1 of following 30-60 min pre-procedure: amoxicillin 2 g PO **OR** cephalexin 2 g PO **OR** clindamycin 600 mg **OR** azithromycin 500 mg **OR** clarithromycin 500 mg **OR** ampicillin 2 g IM/IV **OR** ceftriaxone 1 g IVIM **OR** clindamycin 600 mg IV/IM

Entamoeba histolytica	• Asymptomatic carrier –paromomycin (*Humatin*) 30 mg/kg/d (divided tid) X 7 days **OR** metronidazole 750 mg PO tid X 10 days **OR** diloxanide (*Furamide*) 500 mg PO tid X 10 days • Rectocolitis – [metronidazole 750 mg PO tid X 7 d **OR** tinidazole (*Tindamax*) 2 g PO daily X 3 days] **AND THEN** paromomycin, iodoquinol or diloxanide (see asymptomatic dosing) • Liver abscess or severe disease – [metronidazole 750 mg IV/PO X 7-10 d **OR** tinidazole (*Tindamax*) 2 g PO daily X 5 days] **THEN** paromomycin, iodoquinol or diloxanide (see asymptomatic dosing)
Enterobius vermicularis pinworms	• albendazole (*Albenza*) 400 mg PO **OR** mebendazole 100 mg PO **OR** pyrantel pamoate 11 mg/kg (max 1 gram) - *give selected drug X 1 dose with repeat single dose in 2 weeks.*
Enterococcus faecalis & *Enterococcus faecium*	• Vancomycin sensitive – *ORAL agents:* (mild infection) amoxicillin 1 g PO qid **OR** ampicillin 500 mg PO qid **OR** nitrofurantoin 100 mg PO qid **OR** *Macrobid* 100 mg PO bid **OR** doxycycline 100 mg PO bid: *IV agents:* ampicillin 1-2 g IV q 4-6 h **OR** ampicillin/sulbactam (*Unasyn*) 1.5-3 g IV q 6 h **OR** vancomycin 1 g IV q 12 h • Vancomycin resistant – *ORAL agents (mild infection):* doxycycline 100 mg PO bid **OR** nitrofurantoin 100 mg PO qid **OR** nitrofurantoin sustained release (*Macrobid*) 100 mg PO bid **OR** linezolid (*Zyvox*) 600 mg PO bid **OR** (UTI only fosfomycin [*Monurol*] 3 g PO). *IV agents:* daptomycin (*Cubicin*) 4-6 mg/kg IV q 24h **OR** linezolid (*Zyvox*) 600 mg IV/PO q 12h **OR** quinupristin + dalfopristin (*Synercid*) 7.5 mg/kg IV q 8h **OR** tigecycline (*Tygacil*) 100 mg IV X 1, then 50 mg IV q 12h **OR** (*agents not available* in US: streptomycin 7.5 mg/kg IV q 12h **OR** teicoplanin [*Targocid*] 400 mg IV day 1,+ 200-400 mg IV q 24h) • **ADD** gentamicin (or streptomycin) if endocarditis (SBE) or serious infection. If SBE + high level resistance to aminoglycosides: ampicillin 2 g IV q 4h **AND** ceftriaxone 2 g IV q 12 h

See further antibiotic categories, detail, & caveats page 113.

Epididymitis	• ceftriaxone (*Rocephin*) 250 mg IV/IM **AND** doxycycline 100 mg PO bid X 14 days. **If enteric organisms** are likely (e.g. age > 35 years) or negative gonococcal testing consider: ofloxacin 300 mg PO bid **OR** levofloxacin 500 mg PO qd X 10 d
Epiglottitis – *steroid use is unproven*	• ceftriaxone (*Rocephin*) 2 g IV q24h **OR** cefuroxime (*Zinacef*) 0.75-1.5 g IV q8h **OR** Unasyn 3 g IV q6h
Erysipelas (upper dermis, painful, fever, nodes, <u>distinct</u> elevated borders)	• <u>Oral agents</u> – penicillin 250-500 mg PO qid **OR** dicloxacillin 250-500 mg PO qid **OR** cephalexin 250-500 mg PO qid **OR** cefadroxil 1-2 g PO daily. • <u>IV agents</u> – see cellulitis
Fasciitis	• See Necrotizing Fasciitis
Folliculitis	• <u>Topical</u> – mupirocin (*Bactroban*) apply tid **OR** clindamycin 1% gel/lotion (*Cleocin T, Evoclin*) apply bid **OR** erythromycin 1.5% solution/2% gel (*Eryderm, Erygel, Erycette*) apply bid. • <u>Systemic</u> – see cellulitis and MRSA • <u>Hot tub/swimming pool folliculitis</u>– Pseudomonas is cause and antibiotics are usually not required. Consider acetic acid 5% compress bid. Administer antibiotics if immunocompromised, persistent infection, mastitis: *Cipro* 500-750 mg PO bid.
Francisella tularensis	• (tularemia exposure & treatment) See page 14.
Gangrene-see page 88	• *Gas gangrene, Fournier's, Necrotizing fasciitis*
Gardnerella	• *Gardnerella vaginalis* – see vaginitis (bacterial)
Genital ulcer-See specific disease	• Do not rely on exam. Test for syphilis, herpes, and chancroid. See page 114 for differentiation.
Giardia lamblia	• metronidazole (*Flagyl*) 250 mg PO tid X 5 days **OR** tinidazole (*Tindamax*) 2 g PO X 1 **OR** nitazoxanide (*Alinia*) 500 mg PO bid X 3 d
Gingivitis – acute necrotizing, ulcerative	• penicillin 250-500 mg PO qid **OR** tetracycline 250 mg PO qid **OR** doxycycline 100 mg PO bid X 10 d
Gonorrhea – *cervicitis, urethritis, pharyngitis, proctitis - Not PID*	• ceftriaxone 125 mg IM (primary option for pharyngeal) X 1 **OR** cefixime or cefpodoxime (*Vantin*) 400 mg PO **OR** cefuroxime (*Ceftin*) 1 g PO **OR** spectinomycin 2 g IM (not available in US) **OR** (*Cipro* 500 mg PO or *Floxin* 400 mg PO X 1) – there is high resistance to quinolones, so only use these agents if culture shows sensitivity to these drugs. • See next page

Gonorrhea – *cervicitis, urethritis, pharyngitis, proctitis - Not PID* *See fluoroquinolone caution and dosing page 96* *Also treat Chlamydia – see page 92*	• If severe cephalosporin allergy consider cephalosporin desensitization **OR** azithromycin 2 g PO **OR** fluoroquinolone **AND** repeat culture. • <u>Disseminated disease:</u> ceftriaxone 1 g IM/IV q 24h **OR** cefotaxime 1 g IV q 8h **OR** ceftizoxime 1 g IV q 8h **OR** spectinomycin 2 g IM q 12h. • <u>Meningitis or endocarditis:</u> ceftriaxone 1-2g IV q12h • <u>PID:</u> see pelvic inflammatory disease, page 103.
Granuloma Inguinale	• 3 weeks of 1 of following: doxycycline 100 mg PO bid **OR** azithromycin 1 g q week **OR** Cipro 750 mg PO bid **OR** *Septra* DS 1 PO bid
Helicobacter pylori	• (1) *Prevpac* as directed **OR** • (2) amoxicillin 1g and *Biaxin* 500 mg and omeprazole 20 mg PO bid X 14 d **OR** • (3) lansoprazole 30 mg PO bid +*Pepto Bismol* 2 PO qid + metronidazole 500 mg PO tid + tetracycline 500 mg PO qid X 14 days
Herpes - encephalitis	• acyclovir 10 mg/kg IV over 1 hour q8h X 2-3 weeks
Herpes – simplex *Consult Ophthalmology for keratitis*	• <u>Genital-primary</u> - acyclovir (*Zovirax*) 400 mg PO tid x 7-10 d **OR** famciclovir (*Famvir*) 250 mg tid X 7-10 d **OR** valacyclovir (*Valtrex*) 1 g PO bid x 7-10 d • <u>Genital-recurrence</u> – acyclovir (400 mg PO tid X 5 days or 800 mg PO bid X 5 days or 800 mg PO tid X 2 days) **OR** famciclovir (125 mg PO bid X 5 days or 1 g PO bid X 1 day) **OR** valacyclovir (500 mg PO bid X 3 days or 1 g PO daily X 5 days) • <u>HIV positive episodic genital infection</u> – acyclovir 400 mg PO tid X 5-10 d **OR** famciclovir 500 mg PO bid X 5-10 d **OR** valacyclovir 1 g PO bid X 5-10 d • <u>HIV positive prophylaxis</u> – see prophylaxis below • <u>Keratitis</u> – trifluridine (*Viroptic*) 1 gtt q 2h up to 9X/day, after re-epithelization decrease to 1 gtt q 4-6h X 7-14 days **OR** vidarabine (*Vira-A*) 3% ointment apply 5X/day **OR** (available in Europe) acyclovir 3% ophthalmic ointment 5X/day. Acyclovir 400 mg PO 5X/day X 14-21 days may be effective for corneal disease if topical agent toxicity. • See next page for further recommendations (labialis, gingivostomatitis, prophylaxis, severe disease, [pneumonitis])

Herpes – simplex *continued*	• <u>Labialis/gingivostomatitis – primary</u> – acyclovir 200 mg 5X/day or 400 mg PO 3X/day **OR** famciclovir 250 mg PO bid **OR** valacyclovir 1 g PO bid X 7-10 d
	• <u>Labialis/gingivostomatitis - recurrent</u> – famciclovir (start during prodrome) (1.5 g PO X 1 dose or 750 mg PO bid X 1 day) **OR** valacyclovir 500 mg PO bid X 3 days **OR** penciclovir (*Denavir*) apply topically q2h while awake for 4 days OR doconasol (*Abreva*)
	• <u>Prophylaxis</u> - acyclovir 400 mg PO bid **OR** famciclovir 250 mg PO bid **OR** valacyclovir 500-1000 mg PO daily
	• <u>Prophylaxis, HIV positive</u> – acyclovir 400-800 mg PO bid-tid **OR** famciclovir 500 mg PO bid **OR** valacyclovir 500 mg PO bid
	• <u>Severe (disseminated, pneumonitis,- see</u> <u>*encephalitis* above</u>): acyclovir 5-10 mg/kg IV q 8 h X 2-7 followed by PO therapy for total of 10 days therapy
Herpes – zoster (including keratitis) *if immunocompromised or ill consider IV therapy*	• acyclovir 800 mg PO 5 x per day x 5-7 days **OR** famciclovir 500 mg PO tid x 7 days **OR** valacyclovir 1 g PO tid x 7 days (± steroids - efficacy in reducing post herpetic neuralgia is controversial)
HIV exposure	• See page 80-81
Hookworms	• albendazole (*Albenza*) 400 mg PO x 1 **OR** mebendazole 500 mg PO x 1 **OR** mebendazole 100 mg PO bid X 3 d) **OR** pyrantel pamoate 11 mg/kg (max 1 g) PO daily X 3 days.
Impetigo	• mupirocin (*Bactroban*) topical tid OR retapamulin (*Altabax*) apply bid X 5 days
	• ± see cellulitis page 91.
Influenza treatment *(start ≤48 hours of onset)*	• <u>Influenza A or B</u>: Oseltamivir (*Tamiflu*) 75 mg PO bid X 5 d **OR** zanamivir (*Relenza*) 10 mg (2 puffs) bid X 5 d
Influenza prophylaxis	• <u>Influenza A or B</u>: Oseltamivir (*Tamiflu*) 75 mg PO daily X at least 7 d **OR** zanamivir (*Relenza*) 10 mg (2 puffs) qd X 10 days if household contact or 28 days if community outbreak
Isospora belli	• *Septra* DS 1 PO bid X 10 days (qid X 10 days if HIV) **OR** *Cipro* 500 mg PO bid X 1 week

IV catheter line infection	• vancomycin 1g IV q12h **OR** linezolid (*Zyvox*) 600 mg IV q 12h **OR** daptomycin (*Cubicin*) 6 mg/kg IV q 24 h **OR** tigecycline (*Tygacil*) 100 mg IV 1st dose + 50 mg IV q 12 h • **ADD** rifampin to increase eradication of MRSA. *Antimicrob Agents Chemother.* 2007 May; 51: 1656 • If sepsis, immunocompromised or ill see Sepsis-Wound/Vascular catheter page 88
Keratitis *Coordinate care with ophthalmologists for most cases.*	• <u>Bacterial</u> – Bacteria cause 65-90% of all keratitis cases. Consider Nocardia and Mycobacterium after refractive surgery (LASIK). *Treatment*: (1) Fortified tobramycin (14 mg/ml) **AND** [fortified cefazolin (50 mg/ml) or fortified vancomycin (15-50 mg/ml)] **OR** (2) Fortified cefazolin + 3rd/4th generation fluoroquinolone topically **OR** (3) gatifloxacin (*Zymar*) or moxifloxacin (*Vigamox*) *Dosing*: One drop is applied every 5-15 minutes X 1st hour. Then, antibiotic is applied every 30 minutes, but alternated so that a drop is instilled every 15 minutes, for 6–12 hours. Then, administer one gtt of each q hour while awake X 24-72 hours, then slowly reduce to q 6-8 hours X 10-14 days. Reserve single agent therapy for mild cases. • <u>Viral</u> - See herpes simplex and herpes zoster • <u>Parasitic/amebic</u> – Acanthamoeba can cause infection in contact lens wearers (esp. if wear overnight). Propamidine isethionate (*Brolene*) [may not be available in United States] + neomycin/polymycin B/gramicidin solution q hour while awake X 1week, then taper.
Lice	• See *Pediculus Humanis*
Ludwig's angina	• See submandibular abscess
Lyme disease	• See page 115.
Lymphogranuloma venereum (LGV)	• doxycycline 100 mg PO bid x 21 days • **OR** erythromycin 500 mg PO qid x 21 days
Mastitis (also see breast abscess page 90)	• Treat as MRSA cellulitis – see methicillin resistant Staphylococcus aureus
Mastoiditis	• cefotaxime 1g IV q4h **OR** ceftriaxone 1-2g IV q24h

See further antibiotic categories, detail, & caveats page 113.

Measles exposure	• Prophylactic vaccine if *susceptible* & exposed. *Susceptible* = all persons unless they had documented measles, born < 1957, lab evidence immunity, or completed appropriate live-virus vaccination. **DO NOT** give if neomycin allergy, TB, immunosuppressed, steroid use, hematological cancer, pregnant, ≤ 3 months from blood or immunoglobulin use. Use of live vaccine ≤ 72 hours after exposure prevents disease. Use monovalent vaccine if 6-12 months old. • Use immune globulin (IG) if immunosuppressed, < 1 yo or pregnant:(1) 0.25 ml/kg (max 15 ml) IM within 6 days exposure.(2) Double (max 15 ml) if immune-compromised. (3) Give vaccine ≥ 5 mo after IG.
Meningitis - bacterial < 50 years and healthy	• cefotaxime 2g IV q4-6h **OR** ceftriaxone 2g IV q12h • **AND** vancomycin 15 mg/kg IV q12h • **AND** dexamethasone 0.15 mg/kg IV concurrent or 15 min pre-antibiotic administration and 0.15 mg/kg IV q6h X 4 days. This therapy is primarily indicated if *Strep. pneumoniae* or *H. influenzae* is suspected.
Meningitis – bacterial > 50 years or unhealthy See dexamethaxone comments above	• < 50 year old regimen above + ampicillin 2 g IV q4h • *Severe Penicillin allergy –Septra* 15-20 mg/kg/day (divided q 6-8 h) **AND** *Vancocin* 500-750 mg IV q6h
Meningitis exposure *(Neisseria meningitidis and Haemophilus influenzae)*	• *N. meningitidis* exposure –Rifampin 600 mg PO bid X 2 days **OR** ceftriaxone X 1 dose 250 mg IM **OR** ciprofloxacin 500 mg PO X 1 in adults. Treat household, day care, nursery contacts within 24h of case, older children/adults if kissed, shared food or drink or medical personnel exposed to secretions. • *H. influenzae* exposure - Rifampin 600 mg PO bid 2 days (Max dose 600 mg) if household contact if (1) household has unimmunized child < 4 years or immunocompromised child regardless of vaccine status (2) nursery or child care contacts if ≥ 2 cases of Hib invasive disease in prior 60 days
Meningitis/ventriculitis ...CSF shunt or trauma	• Shunt - vancomycin 15 mg/kg IV q 8-12h **AND** (ceftazidime [*Fortaz*] 2 g IV q 8h or meropenem [*Merrem*] 2 g IV q 8h or cefepime [*Maxipime*] 2 g IV q 8h [see cefepime caution page 88]).
Meningococcemia	• See *Neisseria meningitidis*

See further antibiotic categories, detail, & caveats page 113.

Methicillin resistant *Staphylococcus aureus* (MRSA)	• <u>Oral agents</u> –*Bactrim* or *Septra DS* 1 PO bid **OR** clindamycin 150-450 mg PO qid [5-10% resistance, which is inducible with macrolide resistance] **OR** linezolid (*Zyvox*) 600 mg PO bid **OR** doxycycline 100 mg PO bid [10-15% resistance] **ADD** consider adding rifampin 300-600 mg PO bid to other oral drugs (do not use as sole agent) • <u>IV agents</u> – vancomycin 1 g IV q 12h **OR** linezolid (*Zyvox*) 600 mg IV q 12h **OR** tigecycline (*Tygacil*) 100 mg IV 1st dose + 50 mg IV q 12h **OR** daptomycin (*Cubicin*) 4-6 mg/kg IV q 24h **OR** quinupristin/dalfopristin (*Synercid*) 7.5 mg/kg IV q12h **OR** not yet available in US: [teicoplanin (*Targocid*) 400 mg IV day 1,+ 200-400 mg IV q 24h **OR** ceftobiprole 500 mg IV q 8-12 h]
Necrotizing fasciitis	• See Sepsis due to necrotizing fasciitis page 88.
Neisseria gonorrhea	• See gonorrhea OR pelvic inflammatory disease
Neisseria meningitidis	• <u>Disease</u> – Penicillin G 4 million units IV q 4h **OR** ceftriaxone 2 g IV q 12h • <u>Exposure</u> – See *Meningitis* exposure
Neutropenic fever	• See neutropenic fever guidelines page 83, 84.
Onychomycosis	• See tinea unguium
Osteomyelitis	• <u>MRSA possible</u> - vancomycin 1 g IV q 12h **OR** linezolid (*Zyvox*) 600 mg IV q 12h **OR** tigecycline (*Tygacil*) 100 mg IV 1st dose, then 50 mg IV q 12h **OR** daptomycin (*Cubicin*) 4-6 mg/kg IV q 24h **OR** quinupristin/dalfopristin (*Synercid*) 7.5 mg/kg IV q 12h • **ADD** ciprofloxacin 400 mg IV q 12 h or ceftazidime 2 g IV q 8 h or cefepime 2 g IV q 12h or ceftobiprole 500 mg IV q 8-12 h (pending FDA approval) if immunocompromised, punctured rubber sole, dialysis, IV drug use. (See cefepime caution pg 88) • (if known methicillin sensitive) nafcillin **OR** oxacillin 2g IV q4h **OR** cefazolin 2g IV q8h
Osteomyelitis – *if IV drug user, or dialysis, or immunocompromised*	• ciprofloxacin (*Cipro*) 200-400 mg IV q 12h • **AND** [(Nafcillin or oxacillin 2 g IV q4h or cefazolin 2 g IV q 8h) **OR** vancomycin 1g IV q12h] • See <u>Methicillin Resistant Staphylococcus aureus</u> • If diabetic + foot, see <u>Diabetic Foot</u>

Otitis externa	• _Cortisporin otic_ 4 gtts qid **OR** _Cipro HC otic_ 3 gtt bid X 7d **OR** _Floxin otic_ 10 gtt bidX10d • If severe – dicloxacillin **OR** cephalexin (_Keflex_) 500 mg PO qid **OR** diabetic regimen below. • If diabetes (Pseudomonas) – imipenem (_Primaxin_) 0.5-1.0 g IV q6h **OR** meropenem (_Merrem_) 1 g IV q 8h **OR** ciprofloxacin (_Cipro_) 400 mg IV q12h **OR** ceftazidime 2 g IV q8h **OR** [anti-pseudomonal penicillin + aminoglycoside (page 113)]
Otitis media	• [amoxicillin 250-500 mg PO tid or 500-875 mg PO bid (some experts recommend 1 g PO tid)] **OR** [_Augmentin_ 500 mg PO tid or 875 mg PO bid (some experts _Augmentin XR_ 2g/125 PO bid)] **OR** cefdinir (_Omnicef_) 600 mg PO daily **OR** cefpodoxime (_Vantin_) 200 mg PO bid **OR** cefuroxime (_Ceftin_) 250 mg PO bid X 10 days • See otitis externa diabetic if suspect _Pseudomonas_
Papillomavirus	• See warts
Parapharyngeal abscess	• See submandibular abscess page 109
Parotitis – infectious	• nafcillin or oxacillin 2 g IV q4 **OR** cefazolin (_Ancef_) 1 g IV q8h (ineffective if HIV, mumps, CMV, DM, mycobacteria, cirrhosis, malnutrition, or medication induced parotitis)
Pediculus humanus capitis (pediculosis or lice)	• permethrin 1% (_Nix_) applied to hair/scalp X 10 min, may repeat in 1-2 weeks **OR** permethrin 5% cream (_Elimite_) applied overnight **OR** malathion (_Ovide_) 0.5% shampoo X 10 min, reapply in 1 week • Resistance or treatment failure: Septra DS or _Bactrim_ 1 PO bid X 3 days repeat in 1 week, (most effective if combined with permethrin) **OR** ivermectin (_Stromectol_) 200 mcg/kg PO X 1 – may repeat in 1 week [3, 6 mg tabs] **OR** lindane 1% shampoo applied for 4 minutes, then rinse **OR** lindane 1% lotion apply > 8 hours, repeat in 1 week [avoid lindane if pregnancy or seizures]

See further antibiotic categories, detail, & caveats page 113.

Pelvic inflammatory disease (PID) – *inpatient (cdc) treatment* Choose Regimen, A, B, or C	• <u>Regimen A:</u> [cefoxitin (*Mefoxin*) 2g IV q 6 h **OR** cefotetan 2g IV q12h] **AND** doxycycline 100 mg PO or IV q 12h x 14 d • <u>Regimen B:</u> clindamycin 900 mg IV q 8h **AND** gentamicin (see dosing page 113) • <u>Regimen C:</u> ampicillin/sulbactam (*Unasyn*) 3 g IV q 6h **AND** doxycycline 100 mg IV q 12h • See <u>PID-outpatient</u> for fluoroquinolone discussion • <u>Switch</u> to oral outpatient medications below once clinically improved for 24 hours.
PID – *outpatient (cdc) treatment*	• (ceftriaxone 250 mg IM or cefoxitin 2 g IM with probenicid 1 g PO) **AND** doxycycline 100 mg PO bid x 14 days ± **ADD** metronidazole (*Flagyl*) 500 mg PO bid x 14 days • **Alternate Regimen** – if parenteral cephalosporins are not feasible & the community prevalence and individual risk of resistant gonorrhea is low, may attempt to use fluoroquinolone regimen: [ofloxacin (*Floxin*) 400 mg PO bid x 14 days **OR** levofloxacin (*Levaquin*) 500 mg PO daily X 14 days] **AND** metronidazole (*Flagyl*) 500 mg PO bid X 14 days
Peritonitis – *bowel perf.*	• See abdominal infection recommendations page 88
Peritonitis - *spontaneous*	• cefotaxime 2 g IV q8h **OR** Unasyn 3 g IV q6h **OR** Timentin 3.1 g IV q6h **OR** Zosyn 4.5 g IV q 8h • <u>Resistant E.coli/Klebsiella (ESBL+[extended spectrum β lactamase +)</u> ciprofloxacin (*Cipro*) 400 mg IV q12h or imipenem (*Primaxin*) 0.5 g IV q 6-8h or -1 g IV q 8h
Peritonsillar abscess	• See *Submandibular* abscess
Pharyngitis *If group A strep. likely*	• benzathine penicillin (*Bicillin LA*) 1.2 million units IM X 1 **OR** penicillin VK 500 mg PO bid **OR** cephalexin 250-500 mg PO qid x 10 days **OR** cefadroxil 0.5-1g PO daily x 10 days **OR** azithromycin 500 mg PO day 1, then 250 mg PO X 4 days **OR** clarithromycin 250 mg PO bid X 10 days
Plague	• (Exposure and disease treatment) See page 12.
Pneumonia – *aspiration or lung abscess*	• (clindamycin 600-900 mg IV q8h **OR** cefoxitin 2g IV q 8h **OR** ticarcillin-clavulanate (*Timentin*) 3.1g IV q6h **OR** piperacillin-tazobactam (*Zosyn*) 4.5g IV q 8h) **AND** consider MRSA coverage – see page 101

Community Acquired Pneumonia (CAP)[1] – Infect Dis Soc Am 2007	
Pneumonia – CAP **Healthy,** and no use of antibiotics in past 3 months	• azithromycin (*Zithromax*) 500 mg PO X 1, then 250 mg PO daily X 4 days (inpatient dosing – 500 mg IV q 24 h X 1-2 days, then 500 mg PO X 7-10 days) **OR** clarithromycin (*Biaxin*) 250 mg PO bid X 7-14 days **OR** Biaxin XL 1 g PO daily X 7 days **OR** doxycycline 100 mg PO/IV bid
Pneumonia – CAP **Outpatient** therapy if **Comorbidity present** *(heart, lung, liver, renal disease, or diabetes, alcoholism, asplenia, immunosuppression, cancer, or antibiotic use in prior 3 months)* Also see Pneumonia – CAP: Pseudomonas & MRSA	• See page 151, 152 for admission recommendations • gemifloxacin (*Factive*) 320 mg PO daily X 7d **OR** levofloxacin (*Levaquin*) 750 mg PO/IV daily X 5d **OR** moxifloxacin (*Avelox*) 400 mg PO/IV daily X 7-14 d • **OR** (azithromycin or clarithromycin–see pneumonia /**healthy** dose) **PLUS** β lactam (amoxicillin 1 g PO tid or Augmentin 2 g PO bid or cefpodoxime 200 mg PO bid or cefuroxime 250 mg PO bid • If > 25% macrolide resistant (MIC ≥ 16 mcg/ml) *Strep. pneumonia* choose option without macrolide.
Pneumonia – CAP **Inpatient** (non-ICU) therapy	• gemifloxacin (*Factive*) 320 mg PO daily X 7 d **OR** levofloxacin (*Levaquin*) 750 mg PO/IV daily X 5 d **OR** moxifloxacin (*Avelox*) 400 mg PO/IV daily X 7-14 d • **OR** (azithromycin/*Zithromax* or clarithromycin /*Biaxin*– see pneumonia/**healthy** dose) **PLUS** (ceftriaxone 1-2 g IV q 24h or cefotaxime 1 g IV q 12h or ampicillin 1-2 g IV q 4-6 hours) • **OR** doxycycline 100 mg PO/IV bid **PLUS** ertapenem (*Invanz*) 1 g IV q24 hours
Pneumonia – CAP **ICU admit** ICU Admit criteria: (1) septic shock, vasopressor use or (2) respiratory failure/intubation, or (3) *any 3 of following:* RR ≥ 30, PaO2/FiO2 ≤ 250, multilobar, confusion, uremia (BUN ≥ 20), WBC < 4,000, platelets < 100,000, temperature < 36°C,↓ BP requiring aggressive fluids	• See ICU admission criteria to left. • (ceftriaxone/*Rocephin* 1-2 g IV q 24 hours or cefotaxime/*Claforan* 1 g IV q 12 hours or ampicillin-sulbactam/*Unasyn* 1.5 – 3 g IV q 6hours) **PLUS** (azithromycin/*Zithromax* or clarithromycin/*Biaxin* or gemifloxacin/*Factive* or levofloxacin/*Levaquin* or moxifloxacin/*Avelox*) – use dosing listed above for <u>Pneumonia healthy with outpatient comorbidity present.</u> • Penicillin allergy: (levofloxacin (*Levaquin*) 750 mg IV daily **OR** moxifloxacin (*Avelox*) 400 mg IV daily **PLUS** aztreonam (*Azactam*) 1-2 g IV q 8-12h

[1] See page 151, 152 for use of scoring system (CURB-65, PORT/PSI - Pneumonia severity index) to determine need for inpatient or outpatient treatment of CAP

Community Acquired Pneumonia (CAP) – continued	
Pneumonia – CAP **MRSA** methicillin resistant *S. aureus* possible (see hospital acquired pneumonia)	• If MRSA is a concern (e.g. recent skin infection, prior MRSA, recent admission/ED visit, post-influenza, lung abscess or lung effusion, intubation/ventilator use, tracheostomy) **ADD** one of following to the inpatient regimen above (1) linezolid (*Zyvox*) 600 mg IV q 12 hours **OR** (2) vancomycin 1 g IV q 12 hours to above inpatient or ICU regimens
Pneumonia – CAP **Pseudomonas** possible (see hospital acquired pneumonia)	• If Pseudomonas is a concern (e.g. COPD, aspiration, alcoholism, chronic steroid use, structural lung disease such as bronchiectasis, tracheostomy, ventilator use, frequent antibiotic use) consider one of following regimens:
	• [Piperacillin-tazobactam (*Zosyn*) 3.375-4.5 g IV q 6 hours or cefepime (*Maxipime*) 1-2 g IV q 12 hours (See cefepime caution page 88) or imipenem (*Primaxin*) 1 g IV q 6-8 hours or meropenem (*Merrem*) 1 g IV q 8 hours] **AND** (2) ciprofloxacin (*Cipro*) 400 mg IV q 8-12 hours or levofloxacin (*Levaquin*) 750 mg IV q 24 hours
	• **OR** [Piperacillin-tazobactam (*Zosyn*) 3.375-4.5 g IV q 6 hours or cefepime (*Maxipime*) 1-2 g IV q 12 hours [See cefepime caution page 88] or imipenem (*Primaxin*) 1 g IV q 6-8 hours or meropenem (*Merrem*) 1 g IV q 8 hours] **PLUS** (gentamicin or tobramycin – see dosing on page 113) **PLUS** azithromycin (*Zithromax*) 500 mg IV q 24 h X 1-2 days, then 500 mg PO X 7-10 days
	• **OR** [Piperacillin-tazobactam (*Zosyn*) 3.375-4.5 g IV q 6 hours or cefepime (*Maxipime*) 1-2 g IV q 12 hours [See cefepime caution page 88] or imipenem (*Primaxin*) 1 g IV q 6-8 hours or meropenem (*Merrem*) 1 g IV q 8 hours] **PLUS** (gentamicin or tobramycin – see dosing on page 113) **PLUS** ciprofloxacin (*Cipro*) or levofloxacin (*Levaquin*)
	• Penicillin allergy – substitute aztreonam (*Azactam*) 1-2 g IV q 8-12h for (1) above

[1] See page 151, 152 for use of scoring system (CURB-65, PORT/PSI - Pneumonia severity index) to determine need for inpatient or outpatient treatment of Community acquired pneumonia (CAP)

Hospital Acquired Pneumonia (HAP), Ventilator Associated (VAP) and Healthcare Associated Pneumonia (HCAP) – Infect Dis Soc Am 2007	
HCAP definition	Anyone hospitalized ≥ 2 days in an acute care hospital within 90 days of pneumonia, or lives in nursing home or long term care facility OR within past 30 days received recent IV antibiotics, chemotherapy, wound care, or attended a hospital or hemodialysis clinic.
HAP definition	Pneumonia occurring ≥ 48 hours after admission
VAP definition	Pneumonia arising > 48-72 hours after intubation
Early onset Pneumonia (≤ 4 days of admission) with NO Multi-Drug Resistant Risk Factors (see late onset) HAP/VAP (not HCAP)	• ceftriaxone (*Rocephin*) 1-2 g IV q 24h **OR** levofloxacin (*Levaquin*) 750 mg IV q 24h **OR** moxifloxacin (*Avelox*) 400 mg IV q 24h **OR** ampicillin-sulbactam (*Unasyn*) 1.5 – 3 g IV q 6h **OR** ertapenem (*Invanz*) 1 g IV q 24h
Late Onset Pneumonia ≥ 5 days from admit OR **Multi-Drug Resistant** Risk Factors present HAP/VAP/ (all HCAP cases) *Recommendations are for initial empiric therapy. Streamline therapy based upon cultures and clinical response to treatment.*	• <u>Multi-Drug Resistant Risk Factors:</u> All patients defined as HCAP above or who have a family member with a multidrug-resistant pathogen, high frequency of antibiotic resistance in the community or the admission hospital unit, or immunosuppression (disease or therapy) • **Choose one of following:** (cefepime [*Maxipime*] 1-2 g IV q 8-12h [See cefepime caution page 88] or ceftazidime (*Fortaz*) 2 g IV q 8 h or imipenem (*Primaxin*) 1 g IV q 8h or meropenem (*Merrem*) 1 g IV q 8 h) • **PLUS choose 2nd agent** – (piperacillin-tazobactam (*Zosyn*) 4.5 g IV q 6h or Cipro 400 mg IV q 8h or Levaquin 750 mg IV q 24h or gentamicin 7 mg/kg/24h or tobramycin 7 mg/kg q 24h or amikacin 20 mg/kg q 24h [√ aminoglycoside trough levels]) • <u>IF MRSA</u> risk factors are present or high local incidence **ADD** linezolid (*Zyvox*) 600 mg IV q 12h or vancomycin 15 mg/kg (max 1 g) IV q 12h. • If ESBL+ (extended spectrum β lactamase +) organism suspected, use (1) carbepenem (imipenem or meropenem) or β-lactam/ β -lactamase inhibitor (*Zosyn*) **AND** (2) ciprofloxacin or levofloxacin or aminoglycoside • If Legionella possible, **ADD** macrolide or respiratory quinolone.

Pneumonia – *Pneumocystis jiroveci (formerly carinii)*	• *Septra* DS 2 PO q 8h **OR** IV *Septra* - 15 mg/kg of TMP if ill q8h X 21 days **OR** [(clindamycin 600 mg IV q8h or 300-450 mg PO qid) and primaquine 15- 30 mg of base PO daily X 21 d] • **OR** pentamidine (*Pentam*) 4 mg/kg IV q24h X 21 d • **OR** dapsone 100 mg PO daily and trimethoprim (*Primsol*) 5 mg/kg PO tid X 21 days • **OR** atovaquone 750 mg PO bid X 21 days • **ADD** prednisone X 2-3 weeks if pO$_2$ < 70 mm Hg
Proctitis - infectious	• Ceftriaxone 125 mg IM **AND** doxycycline 100 mg PO bid X 7 days.
Prostatitis ≤ 35 years	• see PID - outpatient treatment
Prostatitis > 35 years	• ciprofloxacin 500 mg PO bid X 14d **OR** *Septra* 1DS PO bid x 14d **OR** see epididymitis-all ages • <u>Chronic prostatitis</u> – may require 4 weeks of treatment
Pseudomemb. colitis	• See *Clostridium difficile*
Pyelonephritis – *Healthy, Not pregnant* Septra/Bactrim resistance is increasing. Clinicians should be aware of local resistance patterns while culturing urine of all pyelonephritis patients to ensure adequacy of treatment regimen.	• <u>One of following oral X 7 days</u>: ciprofloxacin (*Cipro*) 500 mg bid, *Cipro XR* 1g daily, levofloxacin (*Levaquin*) 250-500 mg daily, ofloxacin (*Floxin*) 200-400 mg bid, lomefloxacin (*Maxaquin*) 400 mg daily • **OR** *Septra* DS mg PO bid, or oral cephalosporin (see UTI pregnancy dose) each for 14 days • <u>IV</u> (ampicillin 2 g IV q4h **AND** gentamicin [pg 113]) **OR** *Cipro/Levaquin* (upper PO dose IV) **OR** cefotaxime 1g IV q12h **OR** ceftriaxone 1g IV q24h **OR** ticarcillin-clavulanate (*Timentin*) 3.1g IV q6h, **OR** piperacillin-tazobactam (*Zosyn*) 3.375-4.5mg IV q6-8h • If pregnant - IV cefotaxime or ceftriaxone as above
Pyelonephritis – *nursing home or Foley catheter*	• ampicillin 2 g IV q4h **AND** gentamicin [page 113] • **OR** IV fluoroquinolone-healthy pyelonephritis dose above **OR** *Timentin* 3.1 g IV q8h **OR** *Zosyn* 4.5 g IV q 8h **OR** imipenem **OR** meropenem
Q fever	• (Exposure and disease treatment) See page 12
Rabies	• See page 82
Retropharyngeal abscess	• See submandibular abscess page 109
Rocky Mtn. Spot. Fever	• See page 115

See further antibiotic categories, detail, & caveats page 113.

Salmonella diarrhea Treatment not indicated for mild disease.	• Consider treatment if > 50 years, severe atherosclerosis, immunosuppressed state, cardiovascular abnormalities or prostheses • azithromycin 1 go PO X 1, then 500 mg PO daily X 6 days **OR** ciprofloxacin 500 mg PO bid X 7 days. • Severe disease or bacteremia: ceftriaxone 2 g IV q 24h **OR** ciprofloxacin 400 mg IV q 12h.
Scabies	• permethrin 5% cream (*Elimite*) or 1% *Nix* to entire body overnight then wash off **OR** crotamiton (*Eurax*) apply chin to feet, repeat in 24 h, wash off in 48 h **OR** ivermectin (*Stromectol*) 200 mcg/kg PO [3, 6 mg tabs] **OR** 6% sulfur in petroleum cream applied overnight **OR** lindane 1% lotion to body overnight then wash off [avoid if pregnancy or seizures]
Sepsis – *Xigris has multiple side effects & primarily reserved for ICU patients and not used in the ED.*	*See page 88 for suspected source and antibiotics* • drotrecogin alfa/recombinant human activated protein C (*Xigris*) 24 mcg/kg/h X 96h if evidence sepsis induced organ dysfunction > 24 h**AND** high risk of death (APACHE II ≥ 25)
Septic arthritis (no trauma or operation) *Consult Orthopedics*	• (nafcillin **OR** oxacillin 2 g IV q4h) **AND** (antipseudo-monal cephalosporin - see page 88 or ciprofloxacin (*Cipro*) 400 mg IV bid) • If suspect gonorrhea: 3rd generation cephalosporin • If suspect MRSA, see Osteomyelitis (MRSA possible) recommendations.
Septic arthritis (post trauma/surgery or prosthetic joint) *Consult Orthopedics*	• vancomycin 1 g IV q 12h **AND** [ciprofloxacin 400 mg IV q12h or gentamicin 1.7 mg/kg IV q8h or aztreonam (*Azactam*) 1 g IV q8h or antipseudomonal cephalosporin IV] • See Osteomyelitis - Methicillin resistant *Staph. aureus* for alternatives to vancomycin
Septic bursitis	• IV therapy: nafcillin or oxacillin 2 g IV q4h **OR** cefazolin 2 g IV q8h **OR** vancomycin 1g IV q12h • PO therapy: dicloxacillin 500 mg PO qid **OR** cipro-floxacin 750 mg PO bid + rifampin 300 mg PO bid • MRSA possible, see Methicillin resistant *S. aureus*.
Sexual assault prophylaxis See HIV post exposure prophylaxis - page 80	• Hepatitis B vaccine series if no prior vaccine (not HBIG) **AND** ceftriaxone 125 mg IM **AND** metronidazole 2 g PO X 1 **AND** (azithromycin 1 g PO X 1 or doxycycline 100 mg PO bid X 7 days)

Shigella diarrhea	• azithromycin (*Zithromax*) 500 g PO X1, then 250 mg PO X 4 days **OR** ciprofloxacin 500 mg PO bid X 3 days **OR** levofloxacin 500 mg PO daily X 3 days **OR** Septra DS 1 PO bid X 3 days
Shunt infection	• <u>Vascular shunt</u> – see IV catheter infection, page 99 • <u>CNS shunt</u> – see Meningitis/ventriculitis, page 100
Sinusitis	• Debate exists as to whether antibiotics are superior to placebo in treating simple, uncomplicated sinusitis. Watching and waiting may be most appropriate initial course. *JAMA* 2007; 298; 2487. • <u>Mild disease</u>: treat as Otitis Media (page 102) • <u>Severe disease</u> (if stable for outpatient treatment): moxifloxacin (*Avelox*) 400 mg PO daily X 10 d, **OR** levofloxacin (*Levaquin*) 500 mg PO daily X 10-14 d • <u>Severe disease (inpatient)</u> cefotaxime 1g IV q4h **OR** ceftriaxone 1-2g IV q24h **OR** *Avelox* 400 mg IV daily X 10 d **OR** *Levaquin* 500 mg IV daily X 10-14 days
Smallpox	• See page 13.
Sporotrichosis	Source – soil/thorny plants (e.g. roses, hay, straw) Typical incubation is 7-30 days (max 3 months) • <u>Lymphocutaneous</u>– itraconazole (*Sporonox*) – 100-200 mg PO given q24h or divided bid [max 200 mg/day] X 3-6 months OR fluconazole (*Diflucan*) 400 mg PO daily X 6 months
Staphylococcus aureus	• See - Methicillin resistant *Staphylococcus aureus*
Submandibular abscess (surgery usually required)	• clindamycin (*Cleocin*) 600-900 mg IV q8h **OR** cefoxitin (*Mefoxin*) 2 g IV q8h **OR** *Unasyn* 1.5-3.0 g IV q8h **OR** *Timentin* 3.1 g IV q4-6h **OR** *Zosyn* 3.375-4.5 g IV q6h.
Syphilis – *primary or secondary < 1 year*	• benzathine penicillin (*Bicillin LA*) 2.4 million Units IM X 1 **OR** doxycycline 100 mg PO bid x 14 days • <u>HIV + *Bicillin LA*</u> (above dose) q wk X 3 wk.
Syphilis – *secondary >1 year or tertiary*	• benzathine penicillin (*Bicillin LA)* 2.4 million Units IM q week X 3 **OR** doxycycline 100 mg PO bid x 28 d • <u>Neurosyphilis or ocular disease</u> – aqueous penicillin 3-4 million units IV q 4 h X 10-14 days **OR** (if no prior anaphylaxis/urticaria) consider ceftriaxone 2 g IM/IV X 10-14 d **OR** desensitization to penicillin if positive allergy skin testing.
Tick bite-Lyme endemic	• Doxycycline 200 mg PO X 1 (Lyme endemic areas)

Tinea - capitis & barbae (scalp & beard)	• terbinafine (*Lamisil*) 250 mg PO daily X 4-8 weeks **OR** griseofulvin (*Grifulvin V*) 500 mg PO daily X 6 weeks **OR** itraconazole (*Sporanox*) 3-5 mg/kg/d PO daily X 6 weeks **OR** fluconazole (*Diflucan*) 8 mg/kg q week X 8-12 weeks [max 150 mg/week] (**non-FDA** recommendations *J Am Acad Derm* 1999;40:S27) • **ADD** ketoconazole 2% or selenium sulfide shampoo
Tinea - corporis, cruris, pedis (skin, inguinal, feet) *Am Fam Physician* 1998; 58: 163 & *J Am Acad Derm* 1999; 40: S31-34. (not all oral agents are FDA approved for these indications)	• <u>Topical options</u>- ciclopirox (*Loprox*) bid, clotrimazole (*Lotrimin*) bid, econazole/*Spectazole* daily, miconazole (*Micatin*) bid, naftine (*Naftil*) bid, oxiconazole daily, terbinafine (*Lamisil*) bid, tolnaftate bid • <u>Unresponsive to topicals</u>–fluconazole (*Diflucan*) 150 mg/week X 2-4 weeks **OR** terbinafine (*Lamisil*) 250 mg PO dailyX 2 weeks (longer regimen for tinea pedis) **OR** ketoconazole (*Nizoral*) 200 mg PO daily X 4 weeks **OR** griseofulvin 500 mg PO daily X 4-6 weeks
Tinea unguium – nails & onychomycosis (not all orals are FDA approved for this indication) *J Am Acad Derm* 1999; 40: S21	• terbinafine (*Lamisil*) 250 mg PO daily X 6 weeks or 500 mg PO daily X 1 week on/3 weeks off X 2 mo (use longer regimen for toes, shorter for fingers) **OR** fluconazole (*Diflucan*) 150-300 mg/week X ≥ 3 mo **OR** itraconazole (*Sporanox*) 200 mg PO daily X 3 mo or 200 mg PO bid X 1 wk on/3 wks off X 2-3 mo
Tinea versicolor	• <u>Topical options</u>– ciclopirox (*Loprox*) bid, clotrimazole (*Lotrimin*) bid, econazole (*Spectazole*) daily, ketoconazole (*Nizoral*) daily, miconazole (*Micatin*) bid, terbinafine (*Lamisil*) bid • <u>Orals</u> – ketoconazole (*Nizoral*) 400 mg PO X 1 or 200 mg/d X 7 d **OR** fluconazole 400 mg PO X 1
Toxic shock syndrome	• See page 116
Traveler's diarrhea	• See diarrhea, page 94
Trichomonas	• metronidazole 2 g PO X 1 **OR** 500 mg PO bid x 7 d. See vaginosis for pregnancy recommendation
Tularemia	• (Exposure and disease treatment) See page 14
Urethritis *Also treat for gonorrhea page 96*	• Treatment for Chlamydia + *Ureaplasma urealyticum Mycoplasma genitalium* [azithromycin (*Zithromax*) 1 g PO X 1 **OR** doxycycline 100 mg PO bid X 7 days **OR** erythromycin base 500 mg PO qid X 7 days **OR** ofloxacin (*Floxin*) 300 mg PO bid X 7 days **OR** levofloxacin (*Levaquin*) 500 mg PO daily X 7 days] • Other causes -Trichomonas, HSV, adenovirus

See further antibiotic categories, detail, & caveats page 113.

Urinary tract infection *Healthy, young, females,* *Non-pregnant, non-* *recurrent.* *If pyelonephritis,* *see page 107*	• <u>Simple UTI</u> 3 days PO of any of following (if complicated outpatient, use for 10-14 days): - *Septra* 1 DS bid, ciprofloxacin 250-500 mg bid, *Cipro XR* 500 mg daily, levofloxacin 250 mg daily, lomefloxacin 400 mg daily, norfloxacin 400 mg bid, ofloxacin 200-300 mg bid
Urinary tract infection *Pregnant &* *Uncomplicated without* *pyelonephritis* *OR* *Pregnant asymptomatic* *bacturia*	• Treat 7-10 days for simple infection **OR** 3 days for asymptomatic bacturia - choose one of following: • nitrofurantoin (*Macrodantin*) 50-100 mg PO qid **OR** *Macrobid* 100 mg PO bid **OR** cefadroxil (*Duricef*) 1 g PO bid **OR** cephalexin (*Keflex*) 500 mg PO bid **OR** cefuroxime (*Ceftin*) 125-250 mg PO bid **OR** cefixime 400 mg PO daily **OR** cefpodoxime (*Vantin*) 100 mg PO bid
Vaginosis/Vaginitis	• <u>Bacterial (BV)</u> – (1) <u>Oral</u> - metronidazole (*Flagyl*) 500 mg PO bid or clindamycin 300 mg PO bid x 7 d **OR** (2) <u>Intravaginal</u> - metronidazole gel 5g (1 applicator) 1-2X/d x 5 d or clindamycin vaginal cream 2% qhs X 7 d • <u>Candida</u> – butoconazole 2% sustained release cream (*Gynazol*) 5 g X 1 application **OR** miconazole cream or suppository daily-bid X 1 week **OR** fluconazole (*Diflucan*) 150 mg PO X 1 dose **OR** itraconazole(*Sporonox*) 200 mg PO bid X 1 day • <u>Trichomonas</u> – metronidazole (*Flagyl*) 2 g PO x 1 pill **OR** 500 mg PO bid x 7 days **OR** tinidazole (*Tindamax*) 2 g PO X 1 dose (250, 500 mg tabs) • <u>Pregnancy</u> – Per the American College of Obstetrics & Gyndecology, "there is no evidence that supports the screening and antibiotic treatment of BV in pregnant women in the 2nd or 3rd trimester, either in the general population or in high-risk women, to prevent preterm birth. However, studies are needed to see if this applies to screening and treatment of women in the first trimester of pregnancy. There is also no evidence that supports the treatment of *trichomonas* in pregnancy, and there is some evidence that it may actually be harmful." www.acog.org. In contrast, the cdc recommends treatment if prior premature delivery or low birth weight baby. www.cdc.gov

Varicella	• <u>Exposure</u> – prophylaxis with VariZIG is indicated if immunocompromised, pregnant, or at risk neonate and premature infant (see www.cdc.gov). <u>Dose</u> VariZIG – 125 units/10kg IV/IM up to 625 units maximum. Availability is limited – call 800-843-7477 if needed. Institute antivirals if disease occurs after vaccine. Varicella vaccine is recommended postexposure (within 96-120 hours) for other persons without varicella immunity who have no contraindications to vaccination. • <u>Disease</u> - acyclovir 800 mg PO qid x 5 days **OR** valacyclovir (*Valtrex*) 1 g PO tid X 7 days **OR** (use IV acyclovir dosing if immunocompromised, pneumonia or 3rd trimester pregnancy)
Vascular infection	• see IV catheter page 112 or endocarditis page 94
Ventriculitis	• See Meningitis/ventriculitis
Vibrio	• <u>Diarrhea</u> – see diarrhea, page 94. • Soft tissue infection – see cellulitis, sea water pg 91
Viral encephalitis	• See herpes encephalitis, page 97, or see viral encephalidites page 14
Viral hemorrhagic fever	• (Marburg, Yellow fever, Ebola) See page 14
Warts	• <u>Anal/Cervical/Vaginal</u> warts – require specialist • <u>Genital</u> – imiquimod (*Aldara*) apply 3X/week qhs until clear (max 16 weeks) – wash off in 6-10 hours **OR** podofilox 0.5% solution or gel (*Condylox*) apply bid for 3 consecutive days/week, continue X 4 weeks (only apply 3 days/week and Max of 0.5 ml/day) **OR** physician applied podophyllin 25% applied to wart for 30 min 1st treatment, then minimum time for desired result (1-4h) q week **OR** <u>Other therapy</u> by physician: cryo-therapy, laser, trichloroacetic acid, bleomycin, surgery • <u>Cutaneous</u> – (1) topical salicylic acid (*Dr. Scholl's/Duo-Film/Clear Away wart remover*) bid or q48h if plaster or pad application X 4-12 weeks (over the counter) (2) tretinoin gel (*Retin A*) 0.025-0.1% topically qhs for verruca plana (flat warts) or (3) <u>Other therapy</u> above for anogenital warts.
Yellow fever	• See page 14 (viral hemorrhagic fever)
Yersinia pestis	• (Plague exposure/ treatment) See page 12

Antibiotic Selection

- The decision to use IV or PO regimens is complex. Listed medications are only recommendations. Consult textbooks, recent literature, and experts if uncertain about proper treatment options. Certain disease (e.g. fasciitis, gangrene, septic arthritis, osteomyelitis) may require surgical treatment. Drug doses may need to be changed or selections altered depending on cultures, renal function, underlying disease &new published data.
- FQ – fluoroquinolone oral dosing: ciprofloxacin [*Cipro*] 250-500 mg PO bid or 1 g extended release (*Cipro XR*) 1 g daily, gatifloxacin [*Tequin – caution may cause high or low blood sugars*] 400 mg PO daily, levofloxacin [*Levaquin*] 250-750 mg PO daily, moxifloxacin [*Avelox*] 400 mg PO daily, ofloxacin [*Floxin*] 200-400 PO bid)
- Macrolides – azithromycin (*Zithromax*) 500 mg PO X1, then 250-500 mg PO daily (or 1 g PO X 1 for Chlamydia); clarithromycin (*Biaxin*) 250-500 mg PO bid or extended release (*Biaxin XL*) 1 g daily, erythromycin 250-500 mg PO qid X 7-10 days
- 3rd Cp – 3rd generation cephalosporins (e.g. cefotaxime, ceftizoxime, ceftriaxone)
- Gas gangrene, necrotizing fasciitis, Fournier's gangrene, and Meleney's synergistic gangrene require similar antibiotics and surgical debridement. Consider hyperbaric O_2.
- AG – aminoglycoside - amikacin - least *Pseudomonas* resistance, tobramycin most intrinsic activity, & gentamicin - most *Pseudomonas* resistance.

Aminoglycoside Dosing with Normal Renal Function[1,2]

amikacin (*Amikin*)	15 mg/kg/d IV divide q8-12h, max dose 1500 mg/d.
gentamicin (*Garamycin*)	1.7 mg/kg IV/IM q8h, or 5-7 mg/kg/d
tobramycin (*Nebcin*)	1.7 mg/kg IV/IM q 8h,

[1] Gentamicin and tobramycin can be given once/day at 5-7 mg/kg IV q 24 h or amikacin can be given at 15 mg/kg q 24h. Administer over 60 min to avoid neuromuscular blockade. Draw level 8-12 h after starting infusion. Level is plotted on once daily algorithm & interval (not dose) is adjusted for subsequent doses. Endotoxin reactions have been reported with this regimen.

[2] Adjust aminoglycoside dosing regimen so that peak serum levels (drawn 60 minutes after the start of a 30-60 minute infusion or 60 minutes after an IM injection) are sufficiently high to be bactericidal. See peak and trough levels on chart below with trough levels on chart drawn 30 minutes prior to next dose.

Peak and Trough Aminoglycoside Levels

Drug	Peak	Trough
amikacin	15-30 mcg/ml	< 5-10 mcg/ml
gentamicin	6-12 mcg/ml	< 2 mcg/ml
tobramycin	6-12 mcg/ml	< 2 mcg/ml

Aminoglycoside Dosing in Renal Failure

Loading dose – Administer the same loading dose regardless of renal function.

Calculate creatinine clearance

Calculation of Creatinine Clearance (CLcr)	
	• Male CLcr = $\dfrac{[140 - \text{age (years)}] \times \text{weight (kg)}}{\text{serum creatinine (mg/dl)} \times 72}$
	• For women, multiply above result by 0.85.
	• Normal creatinine clearance is ~ 100 ml/min

Maintenance dose for Traditional Dosing based on Creatinine Clearance

Creatinine clearance	Dose to administer OR interval alteration
> 50 ml/minute	• Administer 60-90% of traditional dose q 8-12 hours **OR** • Increase interval alone to q 12-24 hours
10-50 ml/min	• Administer 30-70% of traditional dose q 12 hours **OR** • Increase interval alone to q 24-48 hours
< 10 ml/min	• Administer 20-30% of traditional dose q 24-48 hours **OR** • Increase interval alone to q 48-72 hours

Maintenance dose for once daily aminoglycosides, alter 1st maintenance dose timing

Creatinine clearance	Timing of maintenance dose (gentamicin example given)
> 60 ml/min	Normal time for recommended interval (q 24h for gentamicin)
40-59 ml/min	At 1.5 X recommended dosing interval (q 36h for gentamicin)
20-39 ml/min	At 2.0 X recommended dosing interval (q 48h for gentamicin)

Check 12 h level with this regimen. For **subsequent** doses, if 12 h gentamicin or tobramycin level is ≤ 3 mcg/ml widen the dosing interval to q 24 h, if 3-5 mcg/ml administer q 36h if, 5-7 mcg/ml administer q 48 h

Differentiation Between Genital Ulcers[1] (see specific disease for treatment)

Disease	Ulcer Description	Incubation	Painful	Inguinal Nodes
Syphilis	Indurated, nonclean base, heals on own	≥ 2 weeks	No	Firm, rubbery, tender nodes (painless ulcer)
Herpes simplex	Multiple, small grouped vesicles or ulcers with scalloped borders	2-7 d	Yes	Tender, bilateral lymph nodes
Chancroid	Irregular purulent, undermined edges, no induration, occasionally multiple	2-12 days	Yes	Very painful, fluctuant, craters may form, unilocular
Lympho-granuloma venereum	Usually not observed, small and shallow, often heal spontaneously	5-21 days	No	Matted clusters of nodes, unilateral or bi-lateral, multiloculated.
	May be above and below inguinal ligament forming "groove sign"			

[1]25% of cases of genital ulcers the agent never identified. There is a large overlap in appearance of genital ulcers.

Tick Borne Disease

Lyme Disease

Most common tick borne disease. Usually coast Northeast, Midwest, & West although reported in 43 states. Less than 1/3 recall a tick bite. Bites usually in spring/ summer. *Diagnosis* – Erythema migrans (EM) is diagnostic if endemic area. Labs are nonspecific with ↑ Sed rate, ↓Hb, normal WBC count (↓lymphocytes) ELISA is positive beyond 2 weeks. IgM peaks 2-6 weeks, and IgG peaks 12 mo into illness (onset ≥ 4 weeks). False ⊕ if syphilis, mono., RMSF, autoimmune disease.	*Clinical Stages: Early local* EM- single lesion ~ 7-10 d after tick bite. Expands centrifugal, clears centrally. Ave 15 cm. See in 75-90% *Early disseminated* (1) many EM lesions 20-50% (2) neuro – lymphocytic meningitis, 7th nerve palsy (↑bilat), radiculoneuritis (3) AV block, myopericarditis (4) ↑spleen, nodes (5) GI – ↑LFTs (6) keratoconjunctivitis, iritis *Late disseminated* – mono-or polyarthritis (esp. large joints), acrodermatitis, retinal vasculitis/optic atrophy, fatigue, dementia, multiple sclerosis like syndrome.
CDC Criteria for Diagnosis	**Treatment**
Endemic area [within 2 counties with one definite case or with tick vector] (1) Erythema migrans (EM) with exposure ≤ 30 days from onset OR (2) Laboratory confirmation and > one organ system involved [cardiac, neurologic, arthritis] *Nonendemic area* (1) EM and > 2 organ systems (2) EM and lab confirmation.	*Early Lyme or mild cardiac disease*– (1) doxycycline 100 mg PO bid X 10-21 d or (2) amoxicillin 500 mg PO tid X 10-21 d or (3) cefuroxime 500 mg PO bid X 10-21 d or (4) erythromycin 250 mg PO qid X 10-21 d *Isolated 7th nerve* – above drugs X 30 days *Meningitis, severe cardiac or arthritis* – Rocephin 2 g IV daily X 14-21 d or penicillin G 20 million U q24h divided doses X 10-21d *Clin Infect Dis* 2000; 31: 533.

Rocky Mountain Spotted Fever

Most common sites South/South Atlantic (OK, NC #1/#2). Typical rash onset 2-3 days after illness (esp. May to Sept), 1st 1-4 mm macules, later petechiae. 1st ankles+ wrists then trunks, palm/soles. Can cause: encephalitis, pulmonary edema, arrhythmia, GI bleed, skin necrosis, DIC, neuro deficits. Death in 8-15 days (≤ 5 d if G6PD deficient) due to hemolysis Labs: Normal WBC, ↓ (platelets, Na, Hb), ↑ (AST, bilirubin, CK, CSF WBC [monocytes] while serological tests are often negative until convalescence.	**Clinical Features**	
	Fever (88-90% > 102°F)	88-100%
	Headache/myalgias (each)	83-93%
	Rash anywhere	74-90%
	Rash palms/soles	49-82%
	Tick bite	54-66%
	Triad (fever, headache, rash)	45-67%
	Nausea, vomiting	56-60%
	Other (cough, ↑liver/spleen, abd pain, diarrhea, anorexia, nodes, edema, ataxia, meningismus, stupor, conjunctivitis)	each present in > 10% of patients
Diagnosis	**Treatment**	
(1) Treat based on clinical criteria (e.g. fever, headache, myalgias, with or without rash during summer in endemic areas (2) if rash, direct immunofluoresce stain of skin. (3) Anti-bodies [immune fluorescent antibody] are detected at 7-10 days [altered by treatment] (4) PCR ↓sensitivity (5) Weil-Felix should not be used	(1) doxycycline 100 mg PO or IV bid X 7 days or at least until afebrile for 2 days. (2) chloramphenicol – 500 mg PO or IV qid X 7 days or afebrile X 2 days (worse outcome compared to doxycycline). (3) fluoroquinolones may have utility if contraindication or allergy to above. *Clin Infect Dis* 1998; 27: 1353.	

Procedure for Tick Removal

- Apply gloves.
- Consider injecting small wheal of lidocaine + epinephrine directly beneath tick.
- Application of petroleum jelly, isopropyl alcohol, fingernail polish or a hot match to the underside of the tick may actually cause regurgitation (of spirochete & other organisms) and **should be avoided**.
- Using blunt tweezers, grasp the tick as close as possible to the skin.
- Pull slowly in a firm perpendicular direction away from the skin.
- Do not squeeze the tick and do not rotate as pulling away from skin.
- Cleanse area thoroughly after procedure with disinfectant.
- Person performing procedure should thoroughly wash hands afterwards.
- Place tick into alcohol or flush down toilet.
- See tick bite prophylaxis (if endemic region), page 109.

Toxic Shock Syndrome

Toxic shock syndrome is due to toxin (TSST-1) produced by *S. aureus*. TSST-1 sources include tampons (50% of cases), nasal packing, wounds, post partum vaginal colonization and many other sites.

Criteria for Diagnosis - Must have each (•) of following

- Temperature > 38.9 C (102F)
- Systolic BP < 90, orthostatic decrease of Systolic BP 15 mm Hg **or** syncope.
- Rash - diffuse, macular erythroderma, with subsequent desquamation.
- Involvement of *3 of the following* organ systems either clinically **or** by labs.

GI - vomiting, or profuse diarrhea	Muscular - myalgias or ↑ CPK X 2
Renal - ↑ BUN + Cr X 2, sterile pyuria	Heme - platelets < 100,000/mm3
Liver – AST, ALT ↑ X 2	Mucosa - vaginal, conjunctiva, or
CNS - disoriented, nonfocal exam	pharyngeal hyperemia

- Negative serology for Rocky Mountain spotted fever, leptospirosis, measles, hepatitis B, antinuclear antibody, VDRL, monospot, blood, urine, throat cultures.

Management

- Restore intravascular volume with NS. Pressors may be needed. Admit to ICU.
- Follow sepsis protocol, page 87 if shock.
- Obtain blood for CBC, platelets, coagulation studies, electrolytes, liver function tests, culture urine, blood ± CSF. Obtain CXR, arterial blood gas, and ECG.
- Search for focus of infection and remove source (e.g. tampon).
- If bleeding, treat coagulopathy with platelets, fresh frozen plasma or transfuse. Nafcillin or oxacillin 1-2 g IV q 4 h until clinically improved then oral anti-staphy-lococcal agents (dicloxacillin, or 1st generation cephalosporin) for 10-14 days. Consider vancomycin if suspect methicillin resistant *S. aureus*. <u>Note</u>: antibiotics only reduce recurrence of toxic shock and do not treat actual disease.

Diagnostic Tests

High Yield Criteria for Non-Trauma Cranial CT in ED Patients

Clinical Feature	Utility (95% Confidence Intervals)[1]	
• Age 60 years or greater	Sensitivity	100% (94-100)
• Headache with vomiting	Specificity	31% (28-33)
• Focal neurologic deficit	Positive predictive value	11% (8-13)
• Altered mental status	Negative predictive value	100% (98-100)

[1] Wide confidence intervals and low incidence of serious disease (e.g. subarachnoid hemorrhage) means that these criteria should NOT be used alone for clinical decision making.   *J Accid Emerg Med* 2000; 17:15; *Acad Emerg Med* 1997; 3: 654.

Dizziness & Vertigo

Dizziness is a vague symptom that manifests as (1) a definite rotational sensation (2) a sensation of impending faint or loss of consciousness (3) dysequilibrium or (4) an ill defined lightheadedness other than vertigo, syncope, or dysequilibrium

Most Common Final Cause of "Dizziness" in ED Patients[1]

Peripheral vestibular disorder	43%	Hyperventilation	6%
Cardiovascular including vaso-		Endocrine	5%
vagal, HTN, CNS disease	21%	Infectious	4%
Medication	10%	Seizure or Anemia (each 2%)	2%
Post-traumatic	7%	Ménière's syndrome	1%
Other	6%	Multiple sensory deficit	1%
Psychogenic	6%	Unknown	10%

Age > 69, focal neuro exam, & absent vertigo identified 86% of patients with a serious cause for "dizziness".   *Ann Emerg Med* 1989; 18: 664.

Vertigo – the illusion of motion

Differentiation of Central (brain stem/cerebellar) from Peripheral Vertigo	
Central Vertigo	*Peripheral Vertigo*
Gradual onset, less intense	Acute onset, intense spinning, swaying
Mild peripheral symptoms	Nausea, vomiting, diaphoresis
Nonfatigable, multidirection nystagmus	Aggravated by change in position
Nystagmus uninhibited by eye fixation	Fatigable, unidirectional nystagmus
Vertical Nystagmus (always central)	Nystagmus inhibited by fixing on object
Focal cerebellar or brain stem findings	Otic symptoms (pain,tinnitus, ↓ hearing).
	No central focal examination findings.

Nylen Barany (Hallpike-Dix) Maneuver

Maneuver – With patient sitting and the physician supporting the head, the patient rapidly assumes the supine position with head hanging 45 degrees off bed, 1st with head straight, then head turned 45 degrees to left, then 45 degrees to right.

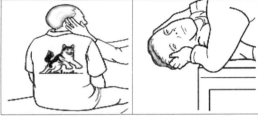

Peripheral vertigo – The above maneuver elicits vertigo and nystagmus with a latency of several seconds and duration of < 1 minute. Nystagmus is unidirectional and nystagmus/vertigo are fatigable.

Central Vertigo – The above maneuver may elicit nystagmus with no latency, nonfatigable, multidirectional & generally lasts > 1 minute.

Benign Paroxysmal Positional Vertigo (BPPV) Repositioning Maneuvers

BPPV is one of most common causes of vertigo and "dizziness" in ED patients (esp. > 50 years old). Free floating debris within the semicircular canals are felt to be responsible for symptoms. The canalith-repositioning procedures outlined below have been found effective for relieving symptoms of BPPV of the posterior semicircular canal & may not be effective if horizontal canal involvement.

Maneuver	Description (Diagram next page)
Epley Maneuver	• <u>Seat patient</u> & have patient turn head 45 degrees toward **affected** ear (*holding physician's arm for support*) • <u>Lower patient to supine position</u> with head still at 45 degrees toward the affected ear and head hanging off the end of the bed • Hold the patient in this position until nystagmus/vertigo abate (*some recommend holding position for 4 minutes*) • Then, turn head 90 degrees toward alternate ear. • With head still turned, roll the patient onto the side of the unaffected ear (patient is now looking at the floor) • This may precipitate more nystagmus/vertigo (maintain X 3-4 min.) • <u>Return patient to seated position</u> • Tilt head 30 degrees down toward chest (maintain X 3-4 minutes) • Remain upright, avoid bending over, or driving for 1-2 days

Epley Maneuver

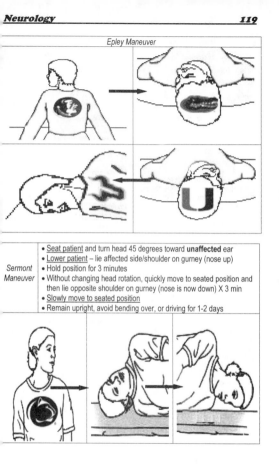

Sermont Maneuver	• <u>Seat patient</u> and turn head 45 degrees toward **unaffected** ear • <u>Lower patient</u> – lie affected side/shoulder on gurney (nose up) • Hold position for 3 minutes • Without changing head rotation, quickly move to seated position and then lie opposite shoulder on gurney (nose is now down) X 3 min • <u>Slowly move to seated position</u> • Remain upright, avoid bending over, or driving for 1-2 days

---

Headache – see page 123-128 for Subarachnoid & Stroke

Most Frequent Cause of Headaches in 485 Adult ED Patients

medical Illness	33%	subarachnoid hemorrhage[1]	0.8%
muscle contraction – tension	32%	meningitis	0.8%
migraine	22%	neuritis	0.6%
unidentified	7%	temporal arteritis	0.4%
central nervous system tumor	3%	subdural hematoma	0.2%

[1] Subarachnoid bleed is present in up to 17% of ED patients with worst headache ever.
Ann Emerg Med 1980; 9: 404; *Acad Emerg Med* 1998; 32: 297.

Weakness

Acute Weakness (Upper vs. Lower Motor Neuron)

Upper motor neuron (UMN) lesions cause damage to cortex (e.g. stroke), brain stem, or spinal cord. Lower motor neuron (LMN) lesions damage the anterior horn cells, peripheral nerve, and the neuromuscular junction.

	Category	UMN disease	LMN disease
Differentiation of	Muscular deficit	Muscle groups	Individual muscles
upper motor neuron	Reflexes	↑ (± acutely ↓)	Decreased/absent
from lower motor	Tone	↑ (± acutely ↓)	Decreased
neuron disease	Fasciculations	Absent	Present
	Atrophy	Absent/minimal	Present (late)

Assessment of Acute Muscle Weakness

Assess ventilation: FVC should be ≥ 15ml/kg and max. inspiratory force > 15cmH$_2$0

Spinal Cord	Peripheral Neuropathy	Myoneural Junction	Muscle disease
Lower limbs weak	Weak distal>proximal	Cranial nerves	Generally weak
Absent lower DTR[1]	General areflexia	Generally weak	Weak proximally
Sharp sensory level	Stocking/glove	Fasciculations	Muscles tender
Bladder/bowel	Sensory loss	No sensory loss	No sensory loss
(B/B) incontinence	OK B/B	OK B/B	OK B/B
↓ examples[2]	↓ examples[2]	↓ examples[2]	↓ examples[2]
transverse myelitis	Guillain Barre	Myasthenia gravis	polymyositis
cord tumor/bleed,	porphyria, arsenic	organophosphates	alcohol/endocrin
abscess or disc	toxic neuropathy	botulism	myopathy
herniation	tick paralysis		electrolyte abnl[3]

[1] DTR - deep tendon reflexes, [2] - lists are not comprehensive, [3] - abnormality (K, Na, Ca)

Bell's Palsy

A peripheral 7th cranial nerve palsy. Etiology is usually viral (e.g. herpes), but should consider Lyme disease, middle ear infection/lesion, CNS mass, or vascular disease. If forehead not unilaterally weak or suspect mastoiditis obtain neuroimaging study.

Clinical Features		Management
Unilateral forehead weakness	100%	• Exclude CNS and otic disease
Maximum deficit in 96 h	>95%	• Administer *Lacrilube* to eye & use eye patch qhs to prevent corneal abrasion.
Maximum deficit in 48 h	50%	
↑ tearing	68%	• Prednisone 60 mg PO daily X 5 days, then 40 mg/day X 5 days
Mastoid pain	61%	
Abnormal taste	57%	• Antiviral (1) valacyclovir 1 g PO daily X 5 days (started within 7 days onset) OR (2) conflicting studies indicate acyclovir may be ineffective – if used administer 400 mg PO 5 times/day for 10 days (esp. if onset < 3 days)
Hyperacusis	29%	
↓ tearing	16%	
Numbness (may signify 5th cranial nerve involvement)	<50%	
		• Follow up - neurologist or primary care

N Engl J Med 2007; 357: 1598; *Otol Neurotol* 2007; 28: 408 & 2003; 24: 948.

Guillain-Barre

Guillain-Barre is post-infectious autoimmune destruction of peripheral nerves. 85-95% have full recovery (weeks to months after weakness progression stops).

Clinical Features	Diagnosis
• Recent viral illness in 50-67%	• CSF – protein normal or > 400 mg/L
• Weakness begins symmetrically in legs and ascends to arms and trunk. Reflexes are absent or hypoactive.	• CSF –WBC normal or monocytosis
	• Nerve conductions study (slowing)
	• MRI shows nerve root enhancement
• Paresthesias in distal extremities	**Management**
• Weak onset rapid ↓ or absent DTRs	• Assess ventilation: forced vital capacity should be ≥ 15-20 ml/kg and Maximum Inspiratory Force should be > 15-30 cm H_2O
• Face involvement in 25-50%	
• Hypesthesias or paresthesias in 33%, with loss of vibration, proprioception, touch distally.	
	• Plasmapheresis
• Autonomic dysfunction: arrhythmias, hypotension, urine/stool retention.	• IV immune globulin 0.4 g/kg IV X 5d
	• Both plasmapheresis and IVIG can shorten recovery time.
• Miller-Fischer variant – weakness begins in face and descends with ophthalmoplegia and ataxia	• Steroid use is controversial

Myasthenia Gravis

An autoimmune disease where antibodies destroy acetylcholine receptor at myoneural junction. Thymus abnormalities (thymoma in 10-25%) are often present.

Clinical Features	
• Ptosis, diplopia, blurring (common)	• Either truncal or extremity weakness
• Dysarthria, dysphagia, jaw muscle weakness, head drooping	• Weakness worsens with repetition
• Asymmetric weakness	• Heat worsens & cold improves weakness (cold pack improves ptosis)

Myasthenia crisis	Crisis Management
• Due to worsening disease with weakness, difficulty swallowing and respiratory insufficiency.	• Tensilon test: edrophonium (*Tensilon*) 1-2 mg IV while on cardiac monitor. If no adverse response, give 8 mg IV. Improvement = myasthenic crisis. Worsening = cholinergic crisis.
• Precipitants – infection, antibiotics Aminoglycosides, tetracycline, clindamycin), CNS depressants, β blockers, quinidine, procainamide, lidocaine, metabolic (↑K,↑Mg, ↓K,↓Ca)	• Assess ventilation – Forced Vital Capacity should be $\geq$ 15 ml/kg and Maximum inspiratory force should be > 15 cm H_2O

Cholinergic crisis	
• Overdose of anticholinesterase meds.	• Look for and treat precipitants.
• Weakness occurs with SLUDGE (salivation, lacrimation, urination, defecation, GI upset, and emesis)	• Admit all patients with either a myasthenic crisis or with a cholinergic crisis.

Stroke, TIA, and Subarachnoid Hemorrhage

ABCD-2 Score for Predicting Risk of Stroke after Transient Ischemic Attack[1]

Risk Factor (points)	Total # Points	7 Day Stroke Risk
Age > 60 years (1)	0	0%
BP - Systolic $\geq$ 140 or Diastolic $\geq$ 90 (1)	1	0%
Clinical features	2	0-1%
- Unilateral weakness (2)	3	1-4%
- Speech disturbed, not weak (1)	4	3-11%
Duration of symptoms, $\geq$ 60 minutes (2)	5	6-13%
- or 10-59 minutes (1)	6	7-25%
Diabetes (1)	7	8-50%

[1] Some experts recommend mandatory admit & evaluation for all moderate (3 or 4 to 5) and high risk ABCD-2 scores (6 or 7). ABCD score does not include diabetes. ABCD(2) does.
[2] A CT finding of *leukoaraiosis* (decreased vascular density or scattered loss of deep white matter) or ischemia (new or old) also increases risk and the ABCDI (ABCD with Imaging) score adds 1 point for these findings to ABCD score. MRI diffusion weighted imaging findings also predict high risk of early stroke (esp. within 90 days).

Lancet 2007; 36:283; *Stroke* 2008; 39: 297; *Lancet Neurol* 2006; 6: 323.

Subarachnoid Hemorrhage (SAH)

Saccular (berry) aneurysms are most common cause (> AV malformations, anticoagulation or vasculitis). *Risks:* personal or family history, pre-eclampsia, polycystic kidney disease, atherosclerosis, hypertension, alcohol, cigarettes, aspirin, cocaine. Mean age at rupture is 40-60 y. 56% occur at rest, 25% while working, 10% while sleeping.

Clinical features	
Any headache (H/A)	70%
Warning (sentinel) H/A	55%
Neck pain or stiffness	78%
Altered mental status	53%
3rd cranial nerve deficit	9%
Seizure	3-25%
Focal deficit	19%
No H/A, deficit, or nuchal rigidity	11%

Cooperative Aneurysm Study *Neurology* 1983; 33: 981.

Grade	Hunt and Hess Classification of SAH	Normal CT
I	Asymptomatic, minimal headache (H/A) and mild nuchal rigidity	15%
II	Moderate-severe H/A, nuchal rigidity, cranial nerve deficits only	7%
III	Drowsy, confused or mild focal deficit	4%
IV	Stupor, mild/mod hemiparesis, early decerebrate or vegetative Δ	1%
V	Deep coma, decerebrate rigidity, moribund appearance	0%

SAH Diagnosis	SAH Treatment
• CT abnormal > 95% if onset < 12 h • CT abnormal 77% if onset > 12 h • CSF > 100,000 RBCs/ mm³ (mean) although any # RBC's can be found • Xanthochromia (traumatic spinal taps do not cause acute xanthochromia) • ECG – peaked, deep or inverted T waves, ↑ QT, or large U waves	• ↓systolic BP to ≤ 160 mm Hg or MAP to ≤ 110 mm Hg • Nimodipine (*Nimotop*) 60 mg PO q6h to decrease vasospasm • Consider seizure prophylaxis • Neurosurgical consult • Early angiography & surgical intervention per neurosurgeon

CT angiography can detect up to 99% of aneurysms that are ≥ 3 mm and is superior to conventional CT at diagnosing SAH. While MRI is equivalent to CT at detecting acute hemorrhage, it is superior at detecting subacute and chronic hemorrhage (> 4 days). 5th gen. multidetector CT may be more sensitive than older CT. *Am J Neuroradiol* 2008; 29: 134; *Acad Emerg Med* 2006; 486. *JAMA* 2004;292: 1823.

Stroke

Ischemic strokes (85%) are (1) thrombotic (2) embolic or (3) hypoperfusion. Hemorrhagic strokes (15%) are intracerebral or subarachnoid (see below).

Major stroke syndromes

- *Anterior cerebral artery:* paralysis of contralateral leg > arm. Sensory deficits parallel weakness, with altered mentation, gait apraxia, and incontinence.
- *Middle cerebral artery:* paralysis contralateral arm, face > leg. Sensory deficits parallel paralysis, blind (½ visual field), dysphasia, & agnosia.
- *Posterior cerebral artery* (occipital, parietal lobes): Blind in half of visual field, 3rd nerve paralysis, visual agnosia, altered mental status and cortical blindness.
- *Vertebrobasilar artery:* vertigo, nystagmus, dysphagia, facial numbness, dysarthria, contralateral loss of pain, temperature, diplopia, syncope.

Management: See page 124-128

**American Heart Association Recommended Studies
in Suspected Acute Ischemic Stroke**

All patients		If clinically suspected alternate disease	
CT (or MRI)	Renal function	Liver function	Oxygen saturation
ECG	CBC/platelets	Toxicology screen	CXR
Glucose	PT/INR	Blood alcohol	Lumbar puncture
Electrolytes	PTT	Pregnancy test	EEG

American Heart Association (AHA) Suspected Stroke Algorithm

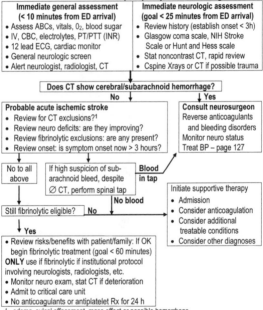

Immediate general assessment (< 10 minutes from ED arrival)	Immediate neurologic assessment (goal < 25 minutes from ED arrival)
• Assess ABCs, vitals, O_2, blood sugar • IV, CBC, electrolytes, PT/PTT (INR) • 12 lead ECG, cardiac monitor • General neurologic screen • Alert neurologist, radiologist, CT	• Review history (establish onset < 3h) • Glasgow coma scale, NIH Stroke Scale or Hunt and Hess scale • Stat noncontrast CT, rapid review • Cspine Xrays or CT if possible trauma

Does CT show cerebral/subarachnoid hemorrhage?

No → **Probable acute ischemic stroke**
• Review for CT exclusions?[1]
• Review neuro deficits: are they improving?
• Review fibrinolysis exclusions: are any present?
• Review onset: is symptom onset now > 3 hours?

Yes → **Consult neurosurgeon**
Reverse anticoagulants and bleeding disorders
Monitor neuro status
Treat BP – page 127

No to all above

If high suspicion of sub-arachnoid bleed, despite ∅ CT, perform spinal tap

Blood in tap

Still fibrinolytic eligible?   No

No blood

Initiate supportive therapy
• Admission
• Consider anticoagulation
• Consider additional treatable conditions
• Consider other diagnoses

↓ Yes

• Review risks/benefits with patient/family: If OK begin fibrinolytic treatment (goal < 60 minutes)
ONLY use if fibrinolytic if institutional protocol involving neurologists, radiologists, etc.
• Monitor neuro exam, stat CT if deterioration
• Admit to critical care unit
• No anticoagulants or antiplatelet Rx for 24 h

[1] - edema, sulcal effacement, mass effect or possible hemorrhage
AHA/ACC. *Circulation* 2000; 102 (suppl I): I-204-I-216. *Stroke* 2005; 36: 916; 2003:1056.

Thrombolytic (rTPA) use in Acute Ischemic Stroke

Indications for rTPA[1] use in Acute Ischemic Stroke[2, 3]	Age 18-80 years
	Onset of symptoms ≤ 3 hours before treatment initiated
	No CT evidence of bleeding or major early infarct (below)
	Acute focal neurologic deficits excluding contraindications

[1] rTPA - tissue plasminogen activator. (Streptokinase is NOT used for acute stroke)
[2] Facilities administering rTPA should have ability to manage intracranial bleeding (may involve in house neurosurgeon or rapid transfer protocol).
[3] Some published studies on fibrinolytic therapy in stroke treated at community hospitals show worse outcome than traditional therapy. Fibrinolytic therapy for stroke should only be performed in the context of a well established hospital protocol.
  Stroke 2005; 36: 916; 2003:1056. JAMA 2000; 283: 1151 Neurology 1996; 47: 835. Stroke 2003; 34: 1056, 1106. (www.strokeaha.org)

Contraindications to rTPA (alteplase) Use in Acute Ischemic Stroke

Onset symptoms > 3 hours from rTPA	Active bleed or trauma (e.g. fracture)
Any known or suspected CNS bleed (current or prior history)	CT with major early infarct signs[1]
Noncompressible artery puncture in prior 7 days (or spinal tap)	Use caution if mild or rapidly improving deficit (e.g. NIH stroke scale ≤ 5)
	Pregnancy or lactating females
Myocardial infarction in past 3 months	*Known bleeding diathesis including:*
Blood glucose < 50 or > 400 mg/dl	● INR > 1.7
Uncontrolled HTN[2] (BP ≥ 185/110)	● Platelets < 100,000/mm³
Seizure with residual postictal neurological deficit	● heparin use ≤ 48 hours or high PTT
	Isolated mild neurologic deficit below
CNS neoplasm, or aneurysm	● isolated ataxia or dysarthria
GI or GU bleeding in prior 21 days	● isolated sensory deficit
Non-CNS major surgery in prior 14 days	● mild weakness

[1] Edema, sulcal effacement, mass effect, bleed, multilobard infarct (> 1/3 hemisphere)
[2] HTN - hypertension (after treatment), [3] See page 128 for NIH stroke scale.
  Neurology 1996; 47: 835. Stroke 2005; 36: 916; 2003:1056. (www.strokeaha.org)

Protocol for rTPA Administration

- Administer rtPA 0.9 mg/kg (max dose of 90 mg) with 10% given as IV bolus followed by infusion of remaining drug over 60 minutes.
- Monitor arterial blood pressure during ensuing 24 hours
  - (1) Monitor q 15 min X 1st 2 hours
  - (2) Then q 30 min for next 6 hours
  - (3) Then q 60 min for next 16 hours
  - (4) Treat blood pressure (see below)
- Do not administer aspirin, heparin, warfarin, ticlopidine or other antiplatelet or antithrombotic agents within 24 hours of rtPA treatment.
- Do not place central venous line or perform arterial punctures in first 24 hours.
- Do not place bladder catheter for 30 min or NG tube for 24 hours after infusion.

Management of Blood Pressure in Acute Ischemic Stroke

Not Eligible for Thrombolytics

Blood Pressure [1,2]	Management
Systolic BP ≤ 220 OR Diastolic BP ≤ 120	• Only treat if end organ damage (e.g. aortic dissection, MI, pulmonary edema, hypertensive encephalopathy). • Treat symptoms (e.g. headache, nausea, vomiting, pain or agitation) as needed. • Treat complications (e.g. hypoxia, ↑ICP, seizures prn)
Systolic BP > 220 OR Diastolic BP 121-140	• Labetalol 10-20 mg IV over 1-2 minutes, may repeat or double q 10 minutes to max. total dose 300 mg **OR** • Nicardipine 5 mg/hour IV infusion initially, titrate to desired effect by increasing 2.5 mg/hour q 5 minutes to maximum of 15 mg/hour • GOAL: 10-15% reduction of blood pressure
Diastolic BP > 140	• Nitroprusside 0.5 micrograms/kg/min IV as initial dose with continuous BP monitoring • GOAL: 10-15% reduction of blood pressure

Eligible for Thrombolytic Therapy - Pretreatment

Systolic BP > 185 OR Diastolic BP > 110	• Labetalol 10-20 mg IV over 1-2 minutes, may repeat X 1 OR Nitropaste 1-2 inches • If BP is not reduced and maintained with SBP < 185 AND Diastolic BP < 110 do not give thrombolytics

Thrombolytic Therapy – During Posttreatment

Check BP q 15 min X 2 hours, then q 30 min X 6 hours, then q hour X 16 hours	
Diastolic BP > 140	• Nitroprusside 0.5 mcg/kg/min as initial dose and titrate to desired blood pressure
Systolic BP > 230 OR Diastolic BP > 121-140	• Labetalol 10 mg IV over 1-2 minutes, may repeat or double q 10 minutes to maximum total dose 300 mg OR give initial bolus, then drip at 2-8 mg/min OR • Nicardipine 5 mg/hour IV infusion initially, titrate to desired effect by increasing 2.5 mg/hour q 5 minutes to maximum of 15 mg/hour. • If BP not controlled by above consider nitroprusside
Systolic BP 180-230 OR Diastolic BP 105-120	• Labetalol 10 mg IV over 1-2 minutes, may repeat or double q 10 minutes to maximum total dose 300 mg OR give initial bolus and then start drip at 2-8 mg/min

[1] BP – blood pressure in mm Hg   *Stroke* 2007; 38: 1655.
[2] Preliminary data from the Control of Hypertension /Hypotension Immediately Post Stroke (CHHIPS) study found a reduced 3 month mortality if BP treated acutely (if > 1 hour of stroke symptoms, ≤ 36 h onset, & SBP > 160 mm Hg) by reducing SBP to 145-155 mm Hg with oral 5 mg lisinopril or 50 mg labetalol. At 4 & 8 hours, if SBP had not dropped to 145-155 mm Hg or ↓15%, the same doses were repeated. If dysphagic, SL lisinopril (not FDA approved) or IV labetalol was used initially. Exclusions: undergoing thrombolysis, impaired consciousness, HTN encephalopathy, prestroke dependency (modified Rankin score > 3), coexisting cardiac or vascular emergencies, contraindications to medications, or primary bleed with SBP > 200 mm Hg or diastolic BP > 120 mm Hg. Until final study published reviewed, repeated and validated in multiple settings, this strategy is **NOT recommended.** (See www.strokeaha.org for future changes in treatment recommendations).
www.le.ac.uk/cv/research/CHHIPS/HomePage.html

Acute Intracranial/Intraventricular Hemorrhage (ICH/IVH) Recommendations

	Imaging – Either CT or MRI are first choice imaging options.
Class I	Cardiopulmonary, neurological monitoring should take place in an ICU.
	• Administer antiepileptics for **seizures** (page 158). (see Class IIb)
	• If fever, treat with antipyretics and exclude infection.
	• Use protamine sulfate (page 42) to reverse heparin associated ICH.
	• If **warfarin** associated ICH, administer IV vitamin K and replace clotting factors (e.g. fresh frozen plasma, See Class IIb recommendations).
	• If **cerebellar ICH** > 3 cm with neurologic deterioration, brain stem compression, or hydrocephalus – stat neurosurgical consult for consideration of early evacuation.
	• If hemiplegia/hemiparesis, apply intermittent pneumatic compression.
Class IIa	• Elevate the head of the bed 30° and avoid/limit head turning.
	• In select cases, aggressive therapy to decrease high intracranial pressure (ICP) including osmotic diuretics (mannitol, hypertonic saline), CSF drainage, neuromuscular blockade, and hyperventilation requires monitoring of ICP and BP to maintain cerebral perfusion pressure (CPP) > 70 mm Hg. [CPP = mean arterial pressure (MAP) − ICP]
	• Keep blood **glucose** ≤ 185 mg/dl (& possibly ≤ 140 mg/dl) with insulin.
Class IIb	• There is incomplete evidence for how to manage **blood pressure.** Agents to consider include labetalol, nicardipine, esmolol, enalapril, hydralazine, *Nipride*, and nitroglycerin (see page 79, 222 for dosing).
	▪ If Systolic BP > 200 mm Hg or MAP > 150 mm Hg: Consider continuous IV infusion with BP monitoring q 5 min.
	▪ If Systolic BP > 180 mm Hg or MAP > 130 mm Hg: AND there is evidence/suspicion of elevated ICP, consider ICP monitor and reduce BP using IV medications to keep CPP > 60 to 80 mm Hg
	▪ If Systolic BP > 180 mm Hg or MAP > 130 mm Hg: AND there is NO evidence or suspicion of elevated ICP consider modest reduction of BP (MAP = 110 mm Hg or target BP of 160/90 mm Hg)
	• If lobar clot within 1 cm of surface, consider **craniotomy** within 12 h.
	• Recombinant factor VII is not recommended outside of clinical trials.
	• A brief period of **prophylactic antiepileptic** therapy soon after ICH onset may reduce the risk of early seizures if lobar hemorrhage.
	• Prothrombin complex conc., factor IX complex, and recombinant FVIIa normalize INR rapidly with lower volumes than FFP but more emboli. FFP is associated with greater volumes & longer infusion.
	• Treatment of ICH due to thrombolytics includes empirical replacement of clotting factors and platelets.
	• If acute proximal venous thrombosis (esp. if pulmonary emboli), consider acute placement of vena cava filter.
	• Consider cause of hemorrhage, arterial thrombotic risk, and health & mobility of patient when deciding to add long term antithrombotics.
Class III	• Routine evacuation of supratentorial ICH within 96 hours of onset is not recommended unless lobar clot within 1 cm of surface.

[1] More detailed recommendations are detailed within text.   *Stroke* 2007; 38: 2001.

National Institute of Health Stroke Scale

1a. Level of consciousness (LOC)	Alert	0	6. Best motor leg [2]	No drift in 5 sec.	0
	Arouses to obey respond, answers	1		Drift without hitting bed/support– 5 sec.	1
	Responds to pain	2		Drifts completely down in 5 sec.	2
	Autonomic reflexes or no response	3		No effort - limb falls immediately	3
				No movement	4
1b. LOC questions *(ask age & current month)*	Both correct	0	(6a. left leg, 6b. right leg)		
	One correct	1	7. Limb ataxia[3]	Absent	0
	Incorrect	2		Present in one limb	1
1c. LOC commands *(make fist, close eyes)*	Obeys both	0		Present in two limbs	2
	Obeys one	1	*Absent (0) if can't understand or paralysis*		
	Incorrect	2	8. Sensory	Normal	0
2. Best gaze	Normal	0		Partial loss– less sharp pinprick	1
	Partial palsy	1		Not aware of being touched	2
Forced deviation or total gaze paresis not overcome by oculocephalic reflex		2	9. Best language[4]	No aphasia	0
3. Best visual	No loss	0	*Mild/moderate aphasia –* loss of fluency or comprehension. Can identify material or content of pictures		1
	Partial hemianopsia	1			
	Complete hemianopsia	2	*Severe aphasia –* fragmented expression Cant ID material from patient response		2
	Bilateral hemianopsia	3			
4. Facial palsy	None	0		Mute, aphasia – no comprehension	3
	Minor asymmetry with smile	1	10. Dysarthria[5]	Normal	0
	Partial (near total paralysis low face)	2		Mild-moderate – understand slurring	1
	Complete	3		Severe – unintelligible	2
5. Best motor arm[1]	No drift in 10 sec.	0	11.Extinction/Inattention (Neglect) None		0
	Drift without hitting bed/support– 10 sec.	1	Visual, tactile, auditory, spatial, personal inattention or extinction to bilateral stimulation in one of senses tested		1
	Drifts completely down in 10 sec.	2			
	No effort - limb falls immediately	3			
	No movement	4	Profound hemi-inattention or extinction to > 1 mode (does not recognize hand or orients to only one side of space)		2
www.ninds.nih.gov/doctorsNIH Stroke Scale (version 10-03).					

1 Arm drift – 1 arm pronates from 90 degree or 45 degree elevation (10 second test)

2 Leg drift - While supine, 1 leg falls to bed from 30 degree elevation (5 second test)

3 Test finger-nose, heel to shin both sides. Ataxia only if out of proportion to weakness.

4 Aphasia – disturbance in processing language. Patient often uses inappropriate words or nonfluent sentences. Test *receptive aphasia* by having patient follow simple commands and test *expressive aphasia* by identifying objects.

5 Dysarthria – slurring from paralysis or incoordination of muscles for speech

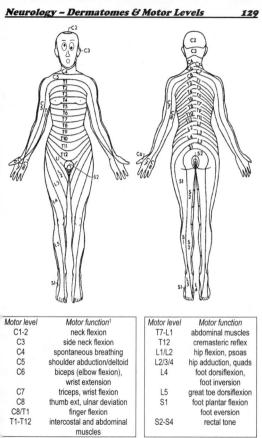

Motor level	Motor function[1]	Motor level	Motor function
C1-2	neck flexion	T7-L1	abdominal muscles
C3	side neck flexion	T12	cremasteric reflex
C4	spontaneous breathing	L1/L2	hip flexion, psoas
C5	shoulder abduction/deltoid	L2/3/4	hip adduction, quads
C6	biceps (elbow flexion), wrist extension	L4	foot dorsiflexion, foot inversion
C7	triceps, wrist flexion	L5	great toe dorsiflexion
C8	thumb ext, ulnar deviation	S1	foot plantar flexion foot eversion
C8/T1	finger flexion	S2-S4	rectal tone
T1-T12	intercostal and abdominal muscles		

[1] Do not test neck flexion (C-1), side flexion (C3) if neck trauma suspected.

Diagnosis of Ectopic Pregnancy in Clinically Stable Patients

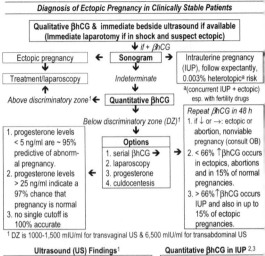

Qualitative βhCG & immediate bedside ultrasound if available
(Immediate laparotomy if in shock and suspect ectopic)

↓ *if + βhCG*

| Ectopic pregnancy | ← | **Sonogram** | → | Intrauterine pregnancy (IUP), follow expectantly, 0.003% heterotopic[a] risk |

↓   ↓   [a](concurrent IUP + ectopic) esp. with fertility drugs

Treatment/laparoscopy   *Indeterminate*

↑   ↓

Above discriminatory zone[1] ←   **Quantitative βhCG**

↓

Below discriminatory zone (DZ)[1]

Repeat βhCG in 48 h
1. if ↓ or →: ectopic or abortion, nonviable pregnancy (consult OB)
2. < 66% ↑βhCG occurs in ectopics, abortions and in 15% of normal pregnancies.
3. > 66% ↑βhCG occurs IUP and also in up to 15% of ectopic pregnancies.

	Options	→

1. progesterone levels < 5 ng/ml are ~ 95% predictive of abnormal pregnancy.
2. progesterone levels > 25 ng/ml indicate a 97% chance that pregnancy is normal
3. no single cutoff is 100% accurate

Options
1. serial βhCG →
2. laparoscopy
3. progesterone
4. culdocentesis

[1] DZ is 1000-1,500 mIU/ml for transvaginal US & 6,500 mIU/ml for transabdominal US

Ultrasound (US) Findings[1]
Intrauterine pregnancy (IUP)

1. Decidual reaction
2. Gestational sac seen at 4.5 wk with βhCG > 1000-1400 via transvaginal US or 6 wk with βhCG > 6,500 via transabdominal US
3. Yolk sac - see at 5.5 weeks (βhCG > 7200)
4. Fetal pole/heart beat are seen at 5.5 to to 7 weeks (βhCG > 10,800-17,200)

Ectopic pregnancy (% with finding)
1. Empty uterus, decidual reaction, or pseudosac (10-20%)
2. Cul-de-sac fluid (24-63%):echogenic=blood
3. Adnexal mass (60-90%)
4. Echogenic halo around tube (26-68%)
5. Fetal heart activity (8-23%)

Quantitative βhCG in IUP [2,3]	
Time	**mIU/ml**
< 1 week	< 5 - 50
1 - 2 weeks	40 - 300
2 - 3 weeks	100 - 1,000
3 - 4 weeks	500 - 6,000
1 - 2 months	5,000 - 200,000
2 - 3 months	10,000 - 100,000
2nd trimester	3,000 - 50,000
3rd trimester	1,000 - 50,000

[1] Transvaginal sonography unless otherwise noted.
[2] Time from conception
[3] Median time for βhCG to turn negative after spontaneous abortion is 16 days (30 days for elective)

See page 146 - detailed ultrasound review with examples

Difficult Deliveries (Breech and Shoulder Dystocia)

Techniques described are for instances when obstetrical expertise is unavailable and ED delivery is required. Call for OB back-up immediately for these occasions.

Breech Delivery	Mauriceau maneuver
• Grasp both feet index finger between ankles & pull feet through vulva. Wrap feet in towel, perform episiotomy. • Apply downward traction until hips delivered, with thumbs over sacrum & fingers over hip, continue down traction. • As scapula emerges rotate back laterally • Attempt shoulder delivery only after low scapula & axilla visible. • 1st deliver anterior shoulder & arm, then rotate and deliver posterior arm. • If unable, deliver posterior shoulder 1st – pull feet up above Mom's groin, ± guide 2 fingers along humerus + gently sweep fetal arm down. Ant arm may be delivered by depression of body alone or with finger sweep as per posterior shoulder. • Rotate occiput anteriorly as in diagram.	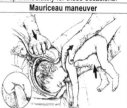 Used with permission Williams Obstetrics 20th ed, McGraw Hill, 1997 • Next, extract head using _Mauriceau-Smellie-Veit_ maneuver. Apply suprapubic pressure, gently flex head by pressing on maxilla (see picture insert).

Maneuvers for Managing Shoulder Dystocia

• 1st McRoberts maneuver (hyperflex Moms hips–rotates hips cephalad & flattens lumbar lordosis) + assistant applies suprapubic pressure. Assistant's pressure may be applied as an anterior to posterior (Mazzanti) or lateral to medial maneuver. (79% success)
• Gaskin maneuver – hand/knee position –allows post. shoulder descent (83% success)
• Wood's screw (**A below**) – push & rotate the posterior shoulder anteriorly 180° in clockwise direction & deliver this shoulder
• Rubin (**B below**) – adduct either shoulder 15-30° across the fetal chest to decrease the bisacromial diameter (distance between shoulders).
• Clavicle fracture – pull upward, anteriorly on distal clavicle to ↓ bisacromial diameter.

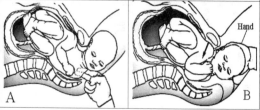

Gestational Hypertension - Preeclampsia - Eclampsia

Gestational Hypertension	
• BP ≥ 140/90 mm Hg **Or**	Measure BP on 2 occasions ≥ 6 hours apart (not practical in the ED)
• BP ↑of ≥ 30/15 above prior BP	

Pre-eclampsia	Severe pre-eclampsia
• Hypertension with general edema or proteinuria > 20 weeks gestation	• BP ≥ 160/110 mm Hg
• Weight gain > 2 lb./week, 6lbs/month	• Proteinuria ≥ 2+
• Proteinuria occurs late: > 300 mg protein/24h (300 mg/d = 1+ dipstick) or > 1 g/L on 2 urines > 6h apart	• Creatinine > 1.2 mg/dl (new onset)
	• Oliguria (urine output ≤ 500 ml/24h)
	• Elevated AST/ALT
• Serum uric acid > 5 mg/dl	• Platelets < 100,000 cells/mcL
• Urine protein/creatinine > 0.19, 90% sensitive, 70% specific	• Headache, visual Δ, abdominal pain, pulmonary edema, hyperreflexia

HELLP syndrome	ECLAMPSIA
• **H**emolytic anemia, **E**levated **L**iver function tests, **L**ow **P**latelets	• Seizures due to pre-eclampsia in 3rd trimester or ≤ 7 days of delivery (occasionally occurs later)
• Variant of pre-eclampsia with upper abdominal pain and/or vomiting	• This is the most common cause of death in Gestational Hypertension
• Minimal hypertension	

Treatment of Pre-eclampsia/Eclampsia

- *Seizure prophylaxis* - Load 4-6 g MgSO$_4$ IV in 100 ml NS over 30 min. <u>Maintenance</u>: Add 20 g MgSO$_4$ to 500 ml NS infuse at 50 ml/h (2g/h). <u>Side effects</u>: flushing, headache, dizziness, ↓reflexes, respiratory/cardiac arrest. Monitor patellar reflexes, respirations and keep urine output ≥ 25 ml/h. Reverse with calcium gluconate (10%) 10-20 ml slow IV push. <u>Caution</u>: MgSO$_4$ use in myasthenia gravis, maternal cardiovascular or renal disease, or use with nifedipine, β agonists may cause cardiorespiratory depresson.

- *Seizure treatment* - 1st MgSO$_4$ (see above) then barbiturates or benzo-diazepines (short-acting, e.g. midazolam) - both cause fetal depression. (see page 158)

- *Antihypertensives* - <u>Indications</u> – Systolic BP ≥ 160 or diastolic BP ≥ 105 mmHg. <u>Goal</u> - ↓diastolic BP to 90-95 mmHg & systolic 140-155 mm Hg.
  1. Hydralazine - 5 mg IV over 1-2 min. Repeat 5-10 mg IV q 20-30 min prn. If a total of 20 mg given without effect, try 2nd drug.
  2. Labetalol - 10 mg IV. Double q 10 min until BP goal or max. 300 mg (total).
  3. Nicardipine IV – limited studies suggest that this may be useful 2nd line agent (see page 79, 222 for dosing)

Third Trimester Vaginal Bleeding and Post Partum Hemorrhage

Placental Abruption (Separation of Normal Placenta prior to Birth)

Risk factors		Management (Discuss with Consultant)
• Hypertension, maternal age > 35 y		• Avoid pelvic examination until placenta previa excluded.
• Smoking, cocaine use, trauma		• Ultrasound is not sensitive.
• Causes 30% of 3rd trimester bleeds		• Administer O_2, and IV NS.
Clinical Features		• Obtain type & crossmatch, PT/PTT, CBC fibrinogen, platelets, fibrin degradation products.
• Vaginal bleeding (dark)	78%	
• Abdominal pain	66%	
• Uterine contractions	17%	• Administer blood, FFP, platelets prn
• Fetal death	15%	• OB consult, immediate delivery
• Maternal DIC[1]	-	

[1] bedside DIC screen: place 5 ml maternal venous blood in red top tube, DIC if no clots by 6 min

Placenta Previa

Defined	Management (Discuss with Consultant)
• Implanted placenta over cervical os	• If pre-term – consider tocolysis with (1) $MgSO_4$ 4-6 g IV (slow) + 2g/h IV
Clinical Features/Diagnosis	
• 20-30% of 3rd trimester bleeding	OR
• Sudden profuse bright red vaginal bleeding	(2) terbutaline 0.25 mg SC q 30 min up to 1 mg in 4 hours
• Absence of abdominal pain	OR
• Soft non-tender uterus	(3) terbutaline 2.5-5 mg PO q4-6h
• **AVOID** pelvic examination	If viable pregnancy (near term) – delivery via cesarean section
• Ultrasound is 95-100% sensitive	

Postpartum Hemorrhage

Definition	Most common causes
Postpartum hemorrhage is the loss of > 500 ml of blood in 1st 24 h after delivery	• Uterine atony
	• Cervical and uterine lacerations

Management
• IV NS, blood prn, oxygen, and fundal massage, deliver placenta, remove products of conception from cervical os, evaluate for lacerations/local trauma.
• Obstetrical consultation.
• oxytocin (*Pitocin*) 10 U IM or 10-40 U in 1L NS at 100-200 ml/h after placental delivery - may↓BP. If oxytocin ineffective administer methylergonovine tartrate (*Methergine*) 0.2 mg IM - may cause ↑or↓BP, seizures, headaches
• <u>Other Options</u>: (1)15-methyl $PGF_{2\alpha}$ (*Carboprost*) 0.25 mg IM q 15-90 min to maximum dose of 2 mg. May↓BP - monitor O_2. Use caution if ↑BP, cardiac, hepatic, renal, lung disease, seizure, ↓Hb or diabetes. **OR** (2) misoprostol (*Cytotec*) 0.6-1 mg PR **OR** (3) prostaglandin E_2 (*Dinoprostone*) 20 mg PR
• Uterine packing, surgery, or uterine embolization may be needed if severe

Rh Isoimmunization

Kleihauer Betke test estimates blood transfused into maternal circulation. (fetal cells/maternal cells X maternal blood volume [L] = fetomaternal hemorrhage [ml]).
(1) RhIG (Rh Immune globulin/*RhoGAM*) - 1 vial IM is indicated if fetal RBC's possibly entered circulation of Rh negative mother. 1 RhIG vial contains ~ 300 mcg of immune globulin and protects against transfusion of 15 ml of Rh$^+$ packed RBC's.
(2) RhIG (*MICRhoGAM, MiniGamulin Rh, HypRho-D Mini Dose*) - 1/6 dose neutralizes 2.5 ml RBC's. Indications - pregnancy termination, or ectopic ≤12weeks.[1]

Indications for RhIG therapy

Rh negative mother and one of the following	
• Delivery of Rh positive infant	• Threatened abortion (*controversial*) [1]
• Abortion or ectopic pregnancy	• Following amniocentesis, chorionic
• Following trauma (even if minor)	villi or umbilical blood sampling
• Any transfusion of Rh positive blood	• At 28 weeks

[1] Use of Rhogam is controversial in spontaneous or elective abortion < 12 weeks. Some authors recommend its use (Society of Obstetricians and Gynaecologists of Canada, *J Obstet Gynaecol Can* 2003; 765) while others do not (*Am J Emerg Med* 2006; 24: 48; *J Reprod Med* 2002; 47; 909)

Dysfunctional Uterine Bleeding - DUB

Exogenous steroids (birth control pills) and anovulatory cycles are most common cause. During evaluation, exclude pregnancy, treatable disorders: infection, trauma, bleeding disorder (20% admitted adolescents with DUB - esp. Von Willebrand's disease or platelet disorder); endocrine disorders, tumors, fibroids, and cysts.

Class	Hemoglobin	Management [1]
Mild	> 11 g/dl	(1)Iron supplementation, gynecology follow up
Moderate **NOTE:** Hormone therapy may cause vomiting (add anti-emetic)	9-11 g/dl without signs of volume depletion	(1)4 BCP[2] pills (estrogen/progestin) PO daily until bleeding stops, then taper over 1 week to 1 PO daily **OR** (2) (2)Medroxyprogesterone (*Provera*)[3] 30-40 mg PO daily X 1 week decreasing by 10 mg daily until 10 mg/day, then continue X 3-4 weeks. If bleeding does not stop by 1 week,↑ to 40-50 mg PO daily, then taper. This will NOT protect against pregnancy. use other birth control. (3)nonsteroidals (e.g. ibuprofen) lower prostaglandin E$_2$, + decrease bleeding + Iron and gynecology follow-up
Severe **Consult Obstetrics**	< 9 or hypovolemia (e.g.↓BP or ↑heart rate)	(1)GYN consult, fluid, blood,dilation & curettage as needed (2)Premarin 25 mg IV or PO q 6-12 h until bleeding stops. (max 4 doses). Then norethindrone 5 mg PO bid alone or with oral estrogen monophasic BCP (below) X 4 weeks

[1] Use caution with administration of listed agents if ≥ 35 y or cardiopulmonary disease, as cardiac ischemia, and thromboembolic disease risk is increased with these medicines.
[2] BCP - Birth control pill – ethinyl estradiol 30-35 mcg + norethindrone 1 mg (or norgestrel 0.3 mg in *Lo/Ovral*) (e.g. *Neocon 1/35, Nortrel 1/35, Ortho-Novum 1/35, Lo/Ovral*)
[3] Alternate regimen - *Provera* 10 mg PO daily, increasing dose 10 mg/day until bleeding stops. Once bleeding controlled, this dose can be maintained for total of 3-4 weeks.
Obstet Gynecol Clin North Am 2003; 30: 321. & 2000; 27: 287

Visual Acuity Screen

96 20/800

873 20/400

2843   **OXX** 20/200

6 3 8 5 2   X O O 20/100

8 7 4 5 9   O X O 20/70

6 3 9 2 5   X O X 20/50

4 2 8 3 6 5   o x o 20/40

3 7 4 2 5 8   x x o 20/30

9 3 7 8 2 6   x o o 20/25

Hold card in good light 14 inches from eye. Record vision for each eye separately with and without glasses. Presbyopic patients should read through bifocal glasses. Myopic patients should wear glasses only.

Pupil Diameter (mm)

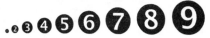

JG Rosenbaum. Pocket Vision Screen. Beachwood. Ohio

Common Causes of Red or Inflamed Eye

Feature	Conjunctivitis	Acute iritis	Acute glaucoma	Cornea trauma or infection
Discharge	moderate-high	none	none	watery,purulent
Vision	normal	sl. blurred	very blurred	usually blurred
Pain	none	moderate	severe	mod/severe
Photophobia	Minimal- none	severe	consensual[1]	Mild-moderate
Conjunctival injection	diffuse, esp. near fornices	mainly circumcorneal	diffuse or perilimbal	diffuse
Pupil	normal	small	mod dilate/fixed	normal
Light response	normal	poor	none	normal
IOP[2]	normal	normal or ↓, late ↑	elevated	normal
Slit lamp examination	clear anterior chamber	cell and flare reaction	corneal edema, appears steamy	positive fluorescein stain
Gram stain	± organisms	negative	negative	± organisms

[1] pain while shining light in unaffected eye, [2]IOP - Intraocular pressure normally is ≤ 20mmHg.

Conversion Chart for Schiotz Tonometer

Tonometer reading	Tonometer load in grams				Tonometer reading	Tonometer load in grams			
	5.5g	7.5g	10g	15g		5.5g	7.5g	10g	15g
	pressure in mmHg					pressure in mmHg			
0.0	42	59	82	128	7.0	12	18	27	47
0.5	38	54	75	118	7.5	11	17	25	43
1.0	35	50	69	109	8.0	10	16	23	40
1.5	32	46	64	101	8.5	9	14	21	38
2.0	29	42	59	94	9.0	8.5	13	20	35
2.5	27	39	55	88	9.5	8	12	18	32
3.0	24	36	51	81	10.0	7	11	17	30
3.5	22	33	47	76	10.5	7	10	15	27
4.0	21	30	43	71	11	6	9	14	25
4.5	19	28	41	67	12	5	7	12	21
5.0	17	26	37	62	13	4	6	10	20
5.5	16	24	34	58	14	3	5	8	15
6.0	15	22	32	54	15	-	4	6	13
6.5	13	20	29	50	17.5	-	-	4	8

Intraocular pressure (IOP) is falsely ↑ if sticky Schiotz plunger, blinking, accommodation, or looking toward nose. IOP is falsely ↓ with repeated measurements, myopia, anticholinesterase drugs, overhydration and scleral buckle operations.

Acute Narrow Angle Glaucoma

Clinical Features	Treatment (Consult Ophthalmology)
• More common Asians & female sex	• Pilocarpine (2-4%) – 2 drops q 15 min X 2 h or until pupilloconstriction
• Headache, vomiting, eye pain	• Pilocarpine 1 drop to unaffected eye
• Red eye, perilimbal injection	• Timolol (Timoptic) 0.1% 1 drop
• Conjunctival edema with "flare and cell" in anterior chamber	• Acetazolamide 500 mg IV, IM or PO
• Mid-dilated, poorly reactive pupil	• Mannitol 0.5 - 1g/kg IV
• Intraocular pressure often > 40 mm Hg	• Laser or surgical iridectomy

Central Retinal Artery Occlusion

Causes	Clinical Features
• Cardiac, carotid, vascular disease • Hyperviscosity, diabetes, sickle cell	• Sudden painless unilateral ↓ vision • Afferent pupil defect (no direct reaction to light, + reaction if light shine in contralateral eye) • Narrow retinal arterioles or "boxcars" from segmentation of arteriolar blood • Infarcted retina turns gray • Cherry red macula due to thin retina with clear view of underlying vessels
Treatment	
• Ophthalmology consult • Best to start within 2 h (try up to 48h) • Globe pressure/massage on 5 sec and off 5 sec for 5-30 minutes • ↑pCO₂ breath bag/95%O₂/5%CO₂ • Paracentesis by ophthalmologist	

Iritis

<u>Defined</u> – acute inflammation of anterior uvea. <u>Clinical features</u> - ↓ vision, perilimbal redness, photophobia (consensual), normal or ↓ IOP (late↑). Slit lamp cell & flare ant. chamber	<u>Treatment</u> – (1) Consult Ophthalmology (2) Homatropine 2% or 5% - 1 drop qid (3) Prednisolone 1% - 1 drop qid (4) Systemic nonsteroidal agents (4) IV antibiotics if infection

Temporal Arteritis

History		Examination	
• Mean age (years)	70	• ↓Temp. artery (TA) pulse	46%
• Polymyalgia rheumatica	39%	• Tender temporal artery (TA)	27%
• Headache	68%	• Indurated, red (TA)	23%
• Jaw claudication	45%	• Large artery with bruit	21%
• Unilateral vision loss	14%	• Afferent pupil, cranial nerve	-
• Claudication, eye pain, fever	<5%	palsies, pale, swollen disc	-

Diagnosis	Management
• ESR > 50 mm in most cases • Artery biopsy (not emergent)	• Ophthalmology consult • Prednisone 60-80 mg PO daily

Mydriatics/Cycloplegics

Drug *Trade Name*	Duration	Effect[1]	Indication	Comments
Atropine 0.5-3.0%	2-3 days	M, C	dilation	caution if narrow glaucoma
Cyclopentolate HCl *Cyclogyl* 0.5-2%	24 hours	M, C	dilation e.g. exam	same as atropine
Homatropine 2-5%	10-48hours	M, C	dilation	same as atropine
Phenylephrine HCl *Neosynephrine* 0.12-10%	2-3 hours	M	dilation, no cycloplegia	caution: cardiac disease, glaucoma or hypertension
Scopolamine HBr *Hyoscine* 0.25%	2-7 days	M, C	strong cycloplegia	same caution above with dizziness, disorientation
Tropicamide *Mydriacyl* 0.5-1%	6 hours	M, C	dilation, cycloplegia	same as atropine, only weak cycloplegia

[1] M - mydriatic (pupillodilation), C - cycloplegia. Usual dose of meds listed is 1 drop daily – tid. Higher doses may be used for specific diseases (e.g. acute angle glaucoma pg 136).

Note: Traumatic orthopedic injuries including cervical, thoracic, lumbosacral, pelvic, knee, ankle, shoulder and spinal cord injuries are described in the Trauma section of the text (pages 191-194)

Arthritis and Joint Fluid Analysis

Analysis of Joint Fluid

	Normal	Noninflammatory	Inflammatory	Septic
Clarity	Clear	Clear	Cloudy	Purulent/turbid
Color	Clear	Yellow or blood	Yellow	Yellow
WBC/ml	< 200	<200-2000	200-50,000	> 5000-50000
PMN (%)	< 25%	< 25%	> 75%	> 75%
Crystals	Absent	Absent	May be present	Absent
Glucose[1]	95-100%	95-100%	80-100%	< 50%
Culture	Negative	Negative	Negative	Positive > 50%
Disease	–	Osteoarthritis, trauma, rheumatic fever	Gout, pseudogout, spondyloarthropathy RA[2], Lyme, lupus	Nongonococcal and gonococcal septic arthritis

[1] Ratio of joint fluid to serum glucose X 100%, [2] Rheumatoid arthritis

Etiology of Arthritis Based on Number of Involved Joints

Monoarthritis (1 joint)	Trauma, Tumor Infection (septic arthritis) Gout or Pseudogout	Lyme disease Avascular necrosis Osteoarthritis (acutely)
Oligoarthritis[1] (2-3 joints)	Lyme disease Rheumatic fever Reiter's syndrome	Gonococcal arthritis Ankylosing spondilitis Polyarticular gout
Polyarthritis[1] (> 3 joints)	Rheumatoid arthritis Lupus	Viral (Rubella, hepatitis) Osteoarthritis (acute)

[1] Septic arthritis due to endocarditis may involve multiple joints.

Etiology of Migratory Arthritis

Gonococcal arthritis, viral arthritis, Rheumatic fever, Lyme disease Subacute bacterial endocarditis Pulmonary infection Mycoplasma, histoplasmosis, coccidiomycosis	Systemic lupus erythematous Drug hypersensitivity (esp. cefaclor) Septicemia (staphylococcus, streptococcus, meningococcus, & *Neisseria gonorrhea*) Henoch-Schonlein purpura

Conus Medullaris or Cauda Equina Syndromes

Etiology: loss of spinal space due to trauma, central disc herniation at L3-S1, ankylosing spondylitis, rheumatoid arthritis, epidural hematoma , cancer. _Conus medullaris syndrome_ has sudden onset with bilateral perineal & thigh pain. Motor loss is symmetric, mild fasciculations may be present, sensory loss is in saddle distribution, bladder/rectal/sexual function is severely impaired. _Cauda equina syndromes_ are gradual in onset, unilateral, with severe asymmetric pain in thighs, perineum, back & legs. Motor loss is asymmetric, severe and fasciculations are absent. Sensory loss in saddle area ± may be unilateral. Mild bladder-rectal-sexual function impairment. _Evaluate_ with CT myelogram or MRI & consult spine surgeon.

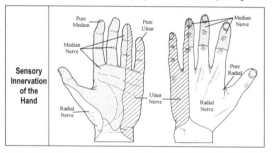

Sensory Innervation of the Hand

Nerve	Motor Tests for Nerve Injury
Median	lie dorsum of hand on flat surface, palmar abduct thumb vs. resistance while palpating radial border of the thenar eminence (abd. pollicis brevis)
Ulnar	abduct fingers or pinch paper between thumbs, + prox. index fingers as pull in opposite direction. Nerve injury if thumb IP bends (_Froment's_ sign)
Radial	extend fingers and wrist against resistance

Compartment Syndromes

Etiology: ↓ in compartment size (e.g. crush) or ↑ in contents (e.g. swelling, bleed). Most common in young males esp. with forearm, leg involvement.

Symptoms	Compartment Pressures (CP)	
• Pain (with passive muscle extension)	• Normal	< 10 mm Hg
• Paresthesias (lose vibratory sense 1st)	• Abnormal	10-30 mm Hg
• Pallor or Pulselessness (late signs)	• Compartment	> 30 mm Hg or MAP
• Paralysis	syndrome	minus CP < 40 mm

Psychiatry

Folstein Mini-Mental Status Exam

Score	Orientation, Registration, Attention, Recall, Language/praxis
5	What is the year, season, date, day, month?
5	Where are we (city, state, country, hospital, floor)?
3	Name 3 objects: one second to say each. Ask patient for all 3 after you have said them. 1 point for each correct answer.
5	Serial 7s backward from 100 (stop after 5X) or spell WORLD backwards
3	Ask 3 objects above to be repeated. 1 point for each correct answer
2	Show pencil & watch and ask subject to name them
1	Ask patient to repeat "no ifs, ands, or buts."
3	Obey:"Take this paper in your right hand, fold in ½, put it on floor"
1	Read & obey written command: "Close your eyes"
1	Write any sentence with a noun, verb (sentence must be sensible)
1	Copy design below: Copy must contain all angles and 2 must intersect

A score ≤ 23 is abnormal (organic brain syndrome)   *J Psychiat Res* 1975; 12: 189.

Differentiating Between Delirium, Dementia, and Acute Psychosis

Feature	Delirium	Dementia	Psychosis
Age of onset	Any	Usually older	13-40 years
Psychiatric history	Usually absent	Usually absent	Present
Emotion	Labile	Normal or labile	Flat or inappropriate
Vital signs	Abnormal	Normal	Normal
Onset	Rapid or sudden	Gradual	Sudden
24h course	Fluctuates	Stable	Stable
Consciousness	Hyper or ↓ alertness	Clear	Clear
Attention	Disordered	OK unless severe	Can be disordered
Cognition	Disordered	Impaired	Selective
Hallucinations	Visual or sensory	Rare	Auditory
Delusions	Fleeting	Rare	Sustained, grand
Orientation	Impaired	Often Impaired	Rarely impaired
Psychomotor	↑ or ↓ or Shifting	Normal	Variable
Speech	Incoherent	Perseveration, difficult find word	Normal, slow or rapid
Involuntary move	Asterixis or tremor	Often absent	Usually absent
Physical illness or drug toxicity	Drug toxicity or withdrawal	Either (esp. Alzheimer's)	Neither

Emerg Med Clin North Am 2000; 18: 243.

Final Diagnoses in ED Patients with NEW Psychiatric Complaints

Organic Disease		Functional/Psychiatric Disease	
Toxin ingestion/abuse	30%	Psychotic	17%
Dementia	7%	(not schizophrenia)	
Postictal	6%	Schizophrenia	13%
Metabolic (Ca, Na, glucose, O_2)	6%	Depressive disorders	3%
Infectious	5%	Other	4%
Other	9%		

Medical Evaluation of ED Patients with NEW Psychiatric Complaints[1,2]

Evaluation	Diagnostic	Evaluation	Diagnostic
• History	27%	Electrolytes with BUN,	
• Examination/O_2 sat.	6%	creatinine, glucose	10%
• Drug screen/alcohol	29%	CT scan	10%
• Complete blood count	5%	Lumbar puncture	8%

1. ACEP Clinical Policy – Level B recommendation: In adults with primary psychiatric complaints, diagnostic evaluation is based upon the history and physical examination. Routine laboratory testing of all patients is of low yield and testing (including drug screening) need NOT be performed routinely in the ED. *Ann Emerg Med* 2006; 47: 79.
2. Above evaluation should be considered for patients with new psychiatric complaints with abnormal vitals, or mental status, or abnormal history or physical: thyroid screen, CPK (to exclude rhabdomyolysis), CT, CXR & a more focused (limited or expanded) evaluation based on history & exam. Most patients in cited study with meningitis or a positive LP had no fever. *Ann Emerg Med* 1994; 24: 673.

"Modified SAD PERSONS" Scale[1]

Factor	Points[1]
Sex (male)	1
Age less than 19 years OR above 45 years	1
Depression or hopelessness (admits to depression or ↓ concentration, appetite, sleep, or libido)	2
Previous suicide attempts or previous psychiatric care (in or outpatient)	1
Excess alcohol or drug use	1
Rational thinking lost (organic brain syndrome or psychosis)	2
Separated, divorced, or widowed	1
Organized or serious suicide attempt	2
No social support (close family, friend, job, active religious affiliation)	1
Stated future intent to harm self	2

1. Before discharging a depressed patient from the ED, make sure patient is not actively suicidal, has a support system at home, and has no firearms.

0 – 5 total points – low probability (< 5%) of requiring psychiatric admission
6 – 8 total points – intermediate probability (~ 50%) of requiring admission
≥ 9 total points – high probability (≥ 75%) of requiring admission

Radiation Dose/Risk of Radiological Procedures and Patient Behaviors[1]

A 10 mSv (dose) increases lifetime risk of cancer 0.1% (and cancer death 0.05%)

	Dose[2]	↑ Cancer[3]		Dose[2]	↑ Cancer[3]
US baseline/year	3-3.6	0.03-0.036%	CT head	2	0.02%
Smoking X 1 year	2-20	0.02-0.2%	CT cervical spine	26	0.26%
Mammogram	0.6	0.006%	CT abd/pelvis	8-11	0.08-0.11%
PA/Lat CXR	0.08	0.0008%	CT angio PE study	3-5	0.03-0.05%
KUB Xray	1.7	0.017%	MDCT-Ca++ score	2-3.6	0.02-0.036%
Lumbar Xray	2.1	0.021%	MDCT angio	7-15	0.07-0.15%
Cervical Xray	4	0.04%	Coronary angio	3-5	0.03-0.05%
V/Q scan	3-6	0.03-0.06%	Triple rule out CT	25-50	0.25-0.5%

[1] PE – pulmonary embolism study, MDCT – multidetector CT (64 slice), angio – angiography, triple rule out – triple rule out aortic dissection, PE, coronary disease
[2] Dose in millisieverts (mSv) [3] Increased lifetime cancer risk (highest in children, women)
Clev Clin J Med 2006; 73: 583, Cardiol Clin 2003; 21: 515, J Trauma 2006; 61: 382.

Contrast Induced Nephropathy (CIN) – Risk Assessment

Risk factor	Score	Total Risk Score	Contrast Nephropathy (CIN) Risk **	Dialysis Risk
Hypotension	5	≤ 5	7.5%	0.04%
Intra-aortic balloon pump use	5	6-10	14%	0.12%
Congestive heart failure	5	11-16	26.1%	1.09%
Age > 75 years	4	≥ 16	57.3%	12.6%
Anemia	3			
Diabetes	3	*eGFR = estimated glomerular filtration rate (in		
1 point per 100 ml contrast	1 or >	ml/min/1.73 m²) = 186 X (creatinine)$^{-1.154}$ X		
Serum creatinine > 1.5 mg/dl or eGFR < 60 ml/min/1.73m²	2,4,6*	(Age)$^{-0.203}$ X (0.742 if female) X (1.21 if Af Am)		

* 2 points if GFR 40-60, 4 points if 20-40, and 6 points if < 20 ml/min/1.73 m²
** Intraarterial contrast poses higher risk than IV. Iso-osmolar contrast (iodixanol) poses least CIN risk, followed by lower then high osmolar agents. *Am J Cardiol 2006; 98; 27k.*

Contrast Nephropathy Prevention & Management

To reduce CIN risk, stop nephrotoxic drugs 24 hours pre-procedure if possible, hydrate (DO NOT use 0.45% saline) pre and post procedure, use iso-osmotic (iodixanol) more so than low osmotic contrast agents, administer the smallest amount of contrast, consider pre-, intra- and postprocedural drugs (below) and post procedural monitoring/intervention (e.g. hemofiltration) if needed.

- Sodium bicarbonate – Mix 154 ml of 1000mEq/L NaHCO$_3$ in 846 ml of D$_5$W. Administer 3 ml/kg/hour for 1 hour pre & 1 ml/kg/h X 6h hours post procedure.
- Ascorbic acid (vitamin C) 3 g PO 2 hours pre-procedure and 2 g PO X the night after and 2 g PO the morning after contrast administration (cuts CIN risk in half)
- N-acetylcysteine (Mucomyst) 600 mg PO bid pre + 600 mg PO bid post contrast OR 1 g 1h pre + 1 g PO 4 h post procedure (NAC efficacy is controversial)
- Theophylline, fenoldopam, dopamine, – use pre-contrast is undefined

Ann Emerg Med 2007;50:335; Am J Card 2006;59K; Crit Care Clin 2005;261; Am J Kid Dis 2004; 12.

Prevention of Contrast Induced Anaphylaxis/Anaphylactoid Reactions*

Definite risk factors: asthma/bronchospasm (10X risk), prior contrast reaction (5X risk), allergy/atopy (2-3Xrisk), cardiac disease, dehydration, sicke cell, thrombotic tendencies (e.g. polycythemia, multiple myeloma), renal disease, anxiety or apprehension, and use of ionic (vs. nonionic) contrast media.

Possible or unproven risk factors: β blockers, interleukin2, aspirin, and NSAIDs.

Pretreatment for adult contrast procedures if prior contrast reaction includes:

- If the patient requires an emergency radiographic procedure, administer
  1. hydrocortisone 200 mg IV immediately and q4 hours until contrast given
  2. diphenhydramine 50 mg intramuscularly (or IV) 1 hour pre-contrast
  3. *Optional* – ephedrine 25 mg PO 1 hour pre-contrast if no heart disease, hypertension, or hyperthyroidism
- If an elective procedure is planned, administer
  1. prednisone 50 mg PO at 13, 7, and 1 hour pre-procedure
  2. diphenhydramine 50 mg PO or IM one hour pre-procedure
- Consider using nonionic contrast agents
- H2 blockers are of marginal benefit in preventing reactions

*See page 7 for treatment of anaphylaxis/anaphylactoid reactions.
Task Force Allergy/Immunol. *J Allergy Clin Immunol* 2005; 115: S483; *BMJ* 2006; 333: 675;

Ultrasonography – Trauma

Abdomen Trauma (Transducer 3.5 MHz Abdomen/FAST exam)

FAST exam is comprised of subxiphoid (T-1), right upper quadrant (above T-2), left upper (above T-3), & suprapugic (T-4) views. Some authors add bilateral paracolic views (at T2/3) , and renal fossae for total of 8 views. A **scoring system** (chart below) assigns 1 point for each of 7 areas fluid is seen (bilateral upper quadrants, paracolic gutters , renal fossae and suprapubic view). The RUQ/hepatorenal space (Morison's pouch) is most common site for free fluid. Up to 500-600 ml fluid (~440 ml if Trendelenberg position) is needed for US to show fluid.
Cardiac views: C1 (subxiphoid), C2 (parasternal), C3 (apical 4 chamber view), C4 (suprasternal), C5 (supraclavicular)

Abdominal Trauma Fluid Score & Outcome

Total Score	% Abd. Injuries	% Surgical Cases	Mortality
0	1.4%	0.4%	0
1	59%	13%	2%
2	85%	36%	6%
3	83%	63%	10%
≥ 4	95%	81%	10%

0 points if *isolated* cul de sac fluid in female   *J Ultrasound Med* 2001; 20: 359.

Chest Trauma

A - lung (granular appearance) abuts adjacent parietal pleural to right (seashore sign). B – pneumothorax – horizontal pattern replaces normal granular lung (stratosphere sign)

- Transducer: 2.5-3.5 MHz for heart, 3.5-7.5 for lung views
- T-1/C-1 (subxiphoid/subcostal) & C2 (parasternal) views (prior page) are used to identify pericardial fluid and cardiac motion (arrest vs. low BP).
- Look for pneumothorax in supine patient by placing transducer in 3rd – 4th intercostal space, anterior clavicular line. Normally an echogenic line of visceral pleura, adheres to lung as it moves & slides during inspiration & expiration (sliding lung sign). Its absence = pneumothorax
- Look for hemothorax as anechoic area above diaphragm (T-2/3 prior page).

Head Trauma

- Transducer: Using 7.5 MHz transducer on uninjured closed eye, one small study found that an optic nerve diameter (see arrows) > 5 mm (measured 3 mm behind globe) was 100% sensitive in detecting increased intracranial pressure in trauma patients.
  Ann Emerg Med 2007; 49: 508.

Ultrasound – Non-Trauma

Abdominal Aortic Aneurysm (Transducer – 2.5-3 MHz)

Normal: aorta < 3 cm outer wall to outer wall infrarenal aorta, Aneurysm > 3 cm.

Appendix

Technically difficult exam with sensitivity of 60-90% (lower if perforation). The best sites have high volume and extensive experience with imaging the appendix.

Normal: ≤ 6 mm wall to wall diameter.

Diseased: > 6 mm wall to wall diameter during compression, or target sign

Cardiovascular *See Transducer Location, page 143.*

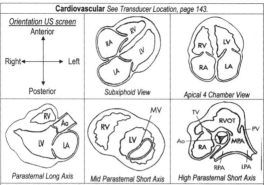

Orientation US screen

Anterior ↑ / Right ← → Left / Posterior ↓

Subxiphoid View

Apical 4 Chamber View

Parasternal Long Axis

Mid Parasternal Short Axis

High Parasternal Short Axis

Ao-Aorta, LA-left atrium, LPA-Left pulmonary artery, LV-Left ventricle, MPA-Main pulmonary artery, MV-Mitral valve, PV-Pulmonic valve, RA-Right atrium, RV-Right ventricle, OT-outflow tract. On page 143, see cardiac views: C1 (subxiphoid), C2 (parasternal-- improved if left lateral decubitus), C3 (apical 4 chamber view), C4 (suprasternal), C5 (supraclavicular) <u>Transducer</u>: Heart -2.5-3.5 MHz. Inferior vena cava/Int. Jugular Vein – 5-7.5 MHz. <u>Diseases</u>: <u>Cardiac standstill</u> and <u>pericardial effusions/tamponade</u> are best identified on subxiphoid and apical views. <u>Pulmonary embolism</u> causes a dilated RV in 75% (normal RV:LV ratio is 0.6:1), abnormal septal wall movement in ½, LV hyperkinesis, RV hypokinesis, left septal deviation, & tricuspid regurg. Central venous pressure (CVP) can be estimated by looking at inferior vena cava (IVC) & internal jugular vein (IJV). Normally, IVC narrows with inspiration & distends with expiration. With ↑CVP (e.g. <u>CHF</u>), IVC stays distended throughout inspiration/expiration. If IVC completely collapses with inspiration, low CVP (<u>Hypovolemia</u>) is present. If IJV is ≥ internal carotid diameter in semiupright position, CVP is > 10 cm H₂O. CVP can be estimated with patient at 45° by measuring IJV height above sternal notch and adding 5 cm.

Gallbladder /GB (Transducer 3.5-5 MHz)

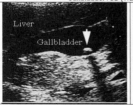

Liver

Gallbladder

<u>Normal</u>: 2-5 cm diameter, GB wall ≤ 3 mm, common bile duct (CBD) ≤ 6 mm, post operative CBD < 10 mm
<u>Diseased</u>: Gallstones (white arrow) with acoustic shadowing (black arrows), Murphy's sign, GB diameter < 2 cm (contracted), > 5 cm = distended, wall > 3 mm (mean cholecystitis wall = 9 mm), pericholecystic fluid, CBD > 6 mm (> 10 mm post operative)

Gynecologic (not pregnant)
Normal: phases of cycle – (1) endometrium thickness – *premenopausal*: 5-14 days after period/proliferative phase - 4-8 mm, after ovulation – 7-14 mm. *Post menopausal* – normal is < 5 mm (≤ 8 mm if on hormone replacement), (2) normal ovary size – 2.5-5 cm long X 1.4-3 cm wide X 0.6-1.5 cm thick, (3) cysts – normal follicular/corpus luteum cysts are ≤ 2.5 cm.   Abnormal: endometrium (see above), cyst > 2.5 cm (anechoic = blood), torsion (enlarged ovary, no Doppler flow, whirlpool sign – a twisted vascular pedicle), PID (tubal wall > 5 mm, incomplete septae in tube, fluid in cul-de-sac, cogwheel sign- a cogwheel appearance on the cross-section tubal view).

Obstetric (1st trimester)
Normal: TVUS - gestational sac at 4-5 weeks (βHCG 1000-2000), double decidual sac (earliest US sign of IUP). See timing of normal landmarks/milestones below.   Ectopic: findings include (1) empty uterus with quantitative BHCG ≥ 1000-1500. (2) cul de sac fluid in 24-63% (esp. if echogenic/blood), (3) empty sac, decidual reaction, or pseudosac (10-20%), (4) adnexal mass in up to 2/3, (5) echogenic halo around tube (26-68%), or (6) fetal heart activity in up to ¼.   Blighted ovum: gestational sac > 10 mm with no yolk sac or > 16 mm with no fetal pole (and no suspicion of ectopic pregnancy).

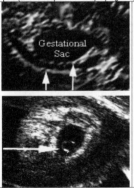

Timing of Landmarks/Milestones[1]

Double decidual sac	4-5 wks
double arrows top US	
Gestational sac (GS) (5 mm)	5 wks
Yolk sac[2] (YS) **single arrow**	5-5.5 wks
Embryo [3]	5.5-6 wks
Cardiac activity [4]	5.5-6 wks

[1] *See expected Quantitative HCG levels at different fetal ages, and when to suspect Ectopic Pregnancy, page 130.*
[2] *always see YS if GS > 20 mm on trans-abdominal or > 10 mm if transvaginal US*
[3] *always see embryo when GS is > 25 mm on transabdominal US, or > 18 mm on transvaginal US*
[4] *always see cardiac activity if embryo > 5 mm or GS > 18 mm*

Renal (Transducer 3.5-5 MHz)
Normal: Normal kidneys are 4-5 cm wide, 9-12 cm long, & within 2 cm in length compared to other side. Diseased: Renal colic – US will identify 2/3 of stones, & 85% with hydronephrosis (anechoic, blunted, enlarged, or rounded calices).

Upper Respiratory Infections

	Clinical Feature	Points	Total Score & (Strep. throat risk)
McIsaac modification of Centor score for Strep. pharyngitis	History of fever or temp >38°C	1	-1 or 0 (1%)
	Absence of cough	1	1 (10%)
	Tender anterior cervical nodes	1	2 (17%)
	Tonsillar swelling or exudates	1	3 (35%)
	Age < 15	1	4 (> 50%)
	Age ≥ 45	-1	5 (> 50%)

If total score ≤ 0, do not treat. If score 1-3, obtain rapid test. If score ≥ 4 , treat empirically.
See page 103 for antibiotics.   *JAMA* 2000; 284: 2912; *Ann Emerg Med* 2005; 87.

Diagnostic Tests

Alveolar-arterial Oxygen gradient (A-a gradient)

Formula:	(AP-47)xFiO$_2$ [150 room air at sea level] – (paO$_2$ + pCO$_2$/0.8)		
(AP) Atmospheric pressure – mm Hg	Altitude (feet)	Atmospheric pressure - mm Hg	Altitude (feet)
760	Sea level (0 feet)	609	6,000
707	2,000	564	8,000
656	4,000	523	10,000

Normal A-a gradient = (Patient's age)/4 +4,
FiO$_2$ = fraction inspired oxygen (21% on room air at sea level)

Dead Space

$\underline{VT}$ = tidal volume; $\underline{VDS_{aw}}$ = airway dead space volume
$\underline{VD_{phys}/VT}$ = (paCO$_2$ – pETCO$_2$)/paCO$_2$ [pETCO$_2$ = mean end-tidal CO$_2$]
Alveolar dead space fraction = $\underline{V_{ADS}/VT}$ = (VD$_{phys}$/VT- VDS$_{aw}$ /VT) X 100%
Modified dead space equation: = 100 X (PaCO$_2$ – PetCO$_2$)/PaCO$_2$
Normal alveolar dead space fraction < 20%

Acute Asthma & Chronic Obstructive Pulmonary Disease (COPD)

Predicted PEFR[1] in Adult Females								
Height (in)		58	60	62	64	66	68	70
Age (yr)	20	453	459	465	471	476	481	485
	25	464	471	477	482	488	493	498
	30	468	474	481	486	492	497	502
	35	468	474	480	485	491	496	501
	40	463	469	475	481	486	491	496
	50	446	452	458	463	469	474	478
	60	424	430	435	440	445	450	454

[1]PEFR = peak expiratory flow rate. (Liters/min)

Br Med J 1989 298: 1068-1070.

Predicted PEFR[1] in Adult Males							
Height (in)	**63**	**65**	**67**	**69**	**71**	**73**	**75**
Age (yr) 20	567	575	583	591	598	605	611
25	594	603	611	619	626	633	640
30	608	617	625	633	641	648	655
35	613	622	631	639	646	654	661
40	612	620	629	637	645	652	660
50	594	602	610	618	626	633	640
60	564	572	580	587	594	601	607

[1]PEFR = expiratory flow rate. (Liters/minute)

Br Med J 1989 298: 1068-1070.

Classifying Asthma Severity in the Emergency Department

	Signs & Symptoms	Initial PEFR[1] or FEV1	Clinical Course[2]
Mild	Dyspnea only with activity	PEFR ≥ 70% of predicted or best	Home care, quick relief with SABA, possible steroids
Moderate	Dyspnea interferes or limits activity	PEFR 40-69% of predicted or best	Relief with frequent SABA, oral steroids needed, symptoms may last > 1-2 day
Severe	Dyspnea at rest, limits conversation	PEFR < 40% of predicted or best	Often need admit, partial relief from frequent SABA, need oral steroids and adjunctive therapy
Life Threatening	Cannot speak, perspiring	PEFR < 25% of predicted or best	May need ICU, minimal or no relief with SABA, IV steroids needed, adjunctive therapy

[1] PEFR - Peak expiratory flow rate, FEV1 - Forced expiratory flow volume in one minute, [2] SABA – short acting β_2 agonists

EPR-3 National Heart Lung and Blood Institute 2007

Risk Factors for Death from Asthma

Asthma History	• Prior severe exacerbation (e.g. ICU admit, intubation)
	• 2 or more asthma hospitalization in past year
	• 3 or more ED visits for asthma in past year
	• Hospitalization or ED visit for asthma in prior month
	• Use of > 2 short acting B agonist canisters per month
	• Difficulty perceiving asthma symptoms or severity of exacerbations
	• Other risks: lack of written asthma action plan, sensitive to *Alternaria (fungus)*
Social History	• Low socioeconomic status or inner-city residence
	• Illicit drugs use or major psychosocial problems
Comorbidity	• Cardiovascular disease
	• Other chronic lung disease
	• Chronic psychiatric disease

EPR-3 National Heart Lung and Blood Institute 2007

Management Options for Acute Asthma in the Emergency Department

See Management algorithm page 150 (National Heart,Lung,Blood Inst NAEPP, NIH 2007)

General	Pulse oximetry, if severe or saturation < 91% administer O_2 and apply cardiac monitor, routine CXR is not indicated.	
Inhaled Short Acting β_2 Agonists (*preferred over systemic β agonists*)	Albuterol Nebulizer Solution (0.63, 1.25, or 2.5 mg/3 ml, OR 5 mg/ml)	2.5-5 mg every 20 min X 3 doses, then 2.5-10 mg every 1-4 h as needed, OR 10-15 mg/hour continuous
	Albuterol MDI (90 mcg/puff)	4-8 puffs q 20 min up to 4 hours, then every 1-4 hour as needed
	Levalbuterol/*Xopenex* (0.63 or 1.25 mg/3 ml OR 1.25 mg/0.5 ml)	1.25 mg-2.5 mg every 20 min X 3 doses, then 1.25-5 mg every 1-4 hours as needed
	Levalbuterol MDI 45 mcg/puff	4-8 puffs q 20 min up to 4 hours, then every 1-4 hour as needed
	Pirbuterol/*Maxair* MDI 200 mcg/puff	4-8 puffs q 20 min up to 4 hours, then every 1-4 hour as needed
Systemic β Agonists	Epinephrine 1:1000 (1 mg/ml)	0.3-0.5 mg SC every 20 minutes up to 3 doses
	Terbutaline (1 mg/ml)	0.25 mg SC every 20 minutes up to 3 doses
Anticholinergics	Ipratropium/*Atrovent* Nebulizer (0.25 mg/ml)	0.5 mg q 20 min X 3 doses, then as needed
	Ipratropium MDI (18 mcg/puff)	8 puffs every 20 min as needed up to 3 hours
Mixture	Ipratropium/albuterol (0.5 mg/2.5 mg /3ml)	3 ml q 20 min X 3 doses, then as needed
	MDI (18 mcg ipratropium+ 90 mcg albuterol per puff)	8 puffs every 20 min as needed up to 3 hours
Steroids	Systemic: Prednisone, prednisolone, Methylprednisolone	Mod./severe asthma & do not respond promptly or completely to short acting β_2 agonists, or if chronic steroid use. <u>Dose:</u> 40-80 mg/day (daily-bid) until PEF reaches 70% predicted or best; for outpatients add 40-60 mg/day (daily-bid) for 5-10 days total
	Inhaled steroids (*Aerobid, Azmacort, Beclovent, Flovent, Vanceril*)	After complete oral steroids or upon discharge from ED for all patients (especially if patient has severe asthma or uses oral steroids frequently)
Other options	Heliox	Consider heliox-albuterol neb. if life threatening exacerbation or severe asthma after 1 hour of standard treatment
	Magnesium sulfate	2 grams IV over 15 minutes if severe asthma and no renal failure.
	Montelukast – IV (not available in US)	Single study found 7 mg IV over 5 min effective.
	Noninvasive ventilation	See page 9
Unproven therapy	Antibiotics, IV β_2 agonists, hydration, methylxanthines, mucolytics	Antibiotics are NOT recommended unless pneumonia, sinusitis, or possibly fever with purulent sputum, IV β 2 agonists, mucolytics, and methylxantines are NOT recommended,

Guidelines for ED Management of Asthma NIH. Nat. Heart, Lung, Blood Institute 2007

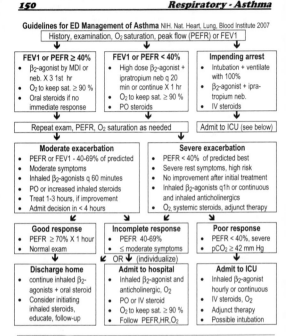

History, examination, O_2 saturation, peak flow (PEFR) or FEV1

FEV1 or PEFR ≥ 40%	FEV1 or PEFR < 40%	Impending arrest
• β_2-agonist by MDI or neb. X 3 1st hr • O_2 to keep sat. ≥ 90 % • Oral steroids if no immediate response	• High dose β_2-agonist + ipratropium neb q 20 min or continue X 1 hr • O_2 to keep sat. ≥ 90 % • PO steroids	• Intubation + ventilate with 100% • β_2-agonist + ipratropium neb. • IV steroids

Repeat exam, PEFR, O_2 saturation as needed | Admit to ICU (see below)

Moderate exacerbation	Severe exacerbation
• PEFR or FEV1 - 40-69% of predicted • Moderate symptoms • Inhaled β_2-agonists q 60 minutes • PO or increased inhaled steroids • Treat 1-3 hours, if improvement • Admit decision in < 4 hours	• PEFR < 40% of predicted best • Severe rest symptoms, high risk • No improvement after initial treatment • Inhaled β_2-agonists q1h or continuous and inhaled anticholinergics • O_2, systemic steroids, adjunct therapy

Good response	Incomplete response	Poor response
• PEFR ≥ 70% X 1 hour • Normal exam	• PEFR 40-69% • ≤ moderate symptoms	• PEFR < 40%, severe • pCO_2 ≥ 42 mm Hg

                       OR ↓ (individualize)

Discharge home	Admit to hospital	Admit to ICU
• continue inhaled β_2-agonists + oral steroid • Consider initiating inhaled steroids, educate, follow-up	• Inhaled β_2-agonist and anticholinergic, O_2 • PO or IV steroid • O_2 to keep sat. ≥ 90 % • Follow PEFR,HR,O_2	• Inhaled β_2-agonist hourly or continuous • IV steroids, O_2 • Adjunct therapy • Possible intubation

---

COPD– Global Initiative for Chronic Obstructive Lung Disease (GOLD)

Management of Severe/Non-Life-Threatening COPD	
• Assess severity, blood gas, CXR • O_2 to keep SaO_2 > 90%, PaO_2 > 60 • Bronchodilators (1) ↑dose and, or frequency (2) use spacers or air driven nebulizer (3)consider methylxanthines[1] • Oral or IV glucocorticosteroids	• Antibiotics if signs of bacterial infection • Consider noninvasive mechanical ventilation (see page 9, 151) • Monitor fluid balance, consider SQ heparin (if admitted), treat associated conditions (e.g. CHF, arrhythmias)

[1] American Thoracic Society states methylxanthines are not useful (2004)   GOLD 2007

COPD - Hospital Admission Criteria	COPD-ICU Admission Criteria
• Marked increased intensity symptoms • Severe underlying COPD (baseline FEV1 < 50% predicted or on home O_2) • New signs of cyanosis, edema • Failure to respond to initial treatment • Comorbidities, new arrhythmias • Frequent exacerbations • Diagnostic uncertainty • Insufficient home support	• Severe dyspnea that inadequately responds to initial ED therapy • Changes in mental status • Persistent or worsening hypoxia (PaO_2 < 40), hypercapnia ($PaCO_2$ > 60), or acidosis (pH < 7.25) despite treatment • Need mechanical ventilation • Hemodynamically unstable (i.e. on vasopressors)

Global Initiative for Chronic Obstructive Lung Disease 2007

Indications/Contraindications to Noninvasive Mechanical Ventilation in COPD

Inclusion Criteria	Moderate to severe dyspnea with use of accessory muscles/paradoxic abdominal movement, pH ≤ 7.35, paCO$_2$ > 45 mm Hg, Resp. rate > 25/min.
Exclusions	Respiratory arrest, cardiovascular instability, altered mentation /uncooperative high aspiration risk, viscous or copious secretions, recent face/GI-esophageal surgery, facial trauma, burns, extreme obesity, fixed nasopharyngeal abnormalities limiting use of equipment.

See page 9 for equipment parameters

Global Initiative for Chronic Obstructive Lung Disease 2007

Community Acquired Pneumonia – Outcome Prediction

CURB & CURB-65 Scores (both scores have been used in adults at any age)

CHARACTERISTIC	CURB-65 POINTS	CURB POINTS
Confusion (abbreviated mental test ≤ 8 or new disorientation to person, place or time)	1	1
Urea (BUN > 19 mg/dl or 7 mmol/L)	1	1
Respiratory rate ≥ 30/minute	1	1
Blood pressure/BP (systolic BP < 90 or diastolic BP ≤ 60 mm Hg)	1	1
Age ≥ **65** years	1	-

Mortality and Inpatient/Outpatient Treatment Recommendations[1,2]

	Points	30 day Mortality	Inpatient/Outpatient
CURB-65	0	0.6-0.7%	Outpatient
	1	2.1-3%	Outpatient
	2	6.1-9.2%	Inpatient[1]
	3	13-14.5%	Inpatient
	4	17-40%	Inpatient
	5	43-57%	Inpatient
CURB	0	0.3%	Outpatient
	1	2.5%	Inpatient[1]
	2	5.1%	Inpatient
	3	12%	Inpatient
	4	16%	Inpatient

[1] Patients with CURB-65 =2, or CURB = 1, should be considered for inpatient care OR intensive outpatient treatment. If hypoxia or hypotension, admit regardless of CURB or CURB-65.[2] See page 104-107 for antibiotic recommendations.

Am J Med 2005; 118: 384., *Clin Infect Dis* 2007; 44: S27.

Pneumonia Severity Index or Pneumonia Outcomes Research Team (PORT)

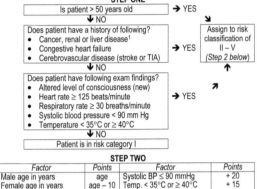

STEP ONE

| Is patient > 50 years old | → YES |

↓ NO

| Does patient have a history of following?
• Cancer, renal or liver disease[1]
• Congestive heart failure
• Cerebrovascular disease (stroke or TIA) | → YES |

Assign to risk classification of II – V *(Step 2 below)*

↓ NO

| Does patient have following exam findings?
• Altered level of consciousness (new)
• Heart rate ≥ 125 beats/minute
• Respiratory rate ≥ 30 breaths/minute
• Systolic blood pressure < 90 mm Hg
• Temperature < 35°C or ≥ 40°C | → YES |

↓ NO

| Patient is in risk category I |

STEP TWO

Factor	Points	Factor	Points
Male age in years	age	Systolic BP ≤ 90 mmHg	+ 20
Female age in years	age – 10	Temp. < 35°C or ≥ 40°C	+ 15
Live in nursing home	+ 10	Heart rate ≥ 125/minute	+ 10
Neoplastic disease[1]	+ 30	Arterial pH < 7.35	+ 30
Liver disease[1]	+ 20	BUN 30 > mg/dl	+ 20
Congestive heart failure[1]	+ 10	Sodium < 130 mEq/L	+ 20
Cerebrovascular disease[1]	+ 10	Glucose ≥ 250 mg/dl	+ 10
Renal disease[1]	+ 10	Hematocrit < 30 g/dl	+ 10
Altered mentation	+ 20	PaO2 < 60 mm Hg	+ 10
Respirations ≥ 30/min	+ 20	Pleural effusion	+ 10

Add Points from Step 2 Above to Determine Risk Category, Total Points, and 30 Day Mortality[2,3]	Risk Category	Total Points	30 Day Mortality
	Class I	-	0.1 – 0.4%
	Class II	≤ 70	0.6 – 0.9%
	Class III	71 – 90	0.9 – 2.8%
	Class IV	91 – 130	8.5 – 9.3%
	Class V	> 130	27.0 - 31.1%

1   Neoplastic – any non skin basal/squamous skin cancer active or diagnosed in past year; Liver – liver histology (biopsy) or clinical exam evidence chronic hepatitis or cirrhosis; Cerebrovascular – any prior stroke or TIA; Renal – abnormal BUN/creatinine, Congestive heart failure – systolic or diastolic ventricular dysfunction documented by history, exam, CXR, Echo, MUGA scan or ventriculogram.

2   Class I – III. outpatient treatment, Class IV – admit to floor, Class V –ICU admit.

3   Use scoring system in conjunction with physician judgment. If hypotension, vomiting, no support system, immune defect, or O$_2$ Sat < 91% may require admission despite low PORT score. (PORT). *N Engl J Med* 1997; 336: 243.; *Clin Infect Dis* 2000; 31: 347

Thromboembolism-Pulmonary Embolism (PE)-Deep Venous Thrombosis (DVT)

Pulmonary Emboli Risk Factors	Clinical Features	
• Immobility, Venous damage	Chest pain (pleuritic-75%)	80-90%
• Hypercoagulability (e.g. cancer, prior	Dyspnea	73-84%
clot, nephrotic syndrome, inflam-	Cough (wheeze – 9%)	37-53%
matory disease, recent pregnancy < 3	Hemoptysis	13-30%
months), estrogens, sepsis, lupus,	Respirations ≥ 16/min (≥ 20)	92(70%)
• No risk factors in 15% overall	Fever > 100° F/tachycardia	43/40%
• No risk factors in 28% < 40 years old	Calf swelling	30%

Diagnostic Studies	ECG Findings	
• CXR – abnormal in 60-84%	• Nonspecific ST-T changes	50%
• Art. blood gas – 92%↑A-a gradient[1]	• T wave inversion	42%
• Vent.-perfusion scan V/Q – pg 155	• New right bundle branch	15%
• D-Dimer- 85-95% sensitive	• S in 1,Q in 3, T in 3	12%
• Angiography- > 98% sensitive/specific	• Right axis deviation	7%
• Echo – detects 90% causing ↓BP	• Shift in transition to V5	7%
• CTA - > 95-99% sensitive for central PE	• Right ventricle hypertrophy	6%
• MRI – > 90-95% sensitive for PE	• P pulmonale	6%

A-a gradient: $150 - (paO_2 + pCO_2/0.8)$; Normal = age/4 +4.

Pulmonary Embolism Rule-Out (PERC) Criteria

Inclusion Criteria	• If all PERC **BREATHS** criteria absent, no D-dimer needed. • Suspicion of PE low enough that clinician would be confident enough to exclude if they had normal D-dimer (low risk group which comprises a population with ~8% PE risk) • Patients with dyspnea and PE was not felt to be the most likely diagnosis (very low risk group ~ 2% overall PE risk)
Exclusion Criteria	• DO NOT use this rule if PE suspicion high enough that you would not be confident in excluding PE with a normal D-dimer.

Kline's PERC (BREATHS) criteria	Operator Characteristics[1]	
• **B** - blood in sputum (hemoptysis)	Low Risk Group (see inclusion criteria)	
• **R** - room air sat < 95%	Sensitivity	96%
• **E** - estrogen or hormone use	Specificity	27%
• **A** – age ≥ 50 years	False negative rate	1.4%
• **T** - thrombosis in past (DVT, PE) or	Very Low Risk Group (inclusion criteria)	
. possible DVT/swollen calf.	Sensitivity	100%
• **H** – heart rate ≥ 100 beats/minute	Specificity	15%
• **S** - surgery in past 4 weeks	False negative rate	0%

[1] Operator Characteristics reflect sensitivity, specificity, false negative rate if NO BREATHS criteria above are present.

[2] More recent 7527 patient validation study found these criteria 96% sensitive for detecting PE. In the 1519 low risk patients, 0.9% with no PERC (BREATHS) criteria had PE, and 0 (0-0.2%) died.

Acad Emerg Med 2007;14:S7;J Thromb Haemost 2004;2:1247;Am J Emerg Med 2008;181

Pulmonary Embolus - *Wicki* (Geneva) Clinical Probability Score

PE Probability[1]		Total	PE Probability[2]	Predictor	Points
Low (10%)		0	~ 4%	Age 60-79 years	+1
		1	~ 8%	Age ≥ 80 years	+2
		2	~ 7%	Prior PE or DVT	+2
		3	~ 10%	Recent surgery[3]	+3
		4	~ 17%	Heart rate > 100	+1
Intermediate (38%)		5	~ 22%	$PaCO_2 < 36$ mm Hg	+2
		6	~ 42%	$PaCO_2 = 36 - 38.9$ mm Hg	+1
		7	~ 43%	$PaO_2 < 48.7$ mm Hg	+4
		8	~ 55%	$PaO_2 = 48.7 - 59.9$ mm Hg	+3
High (81%)		9	~ 77%	$PaO_2 = 60 - 71.1$ mm Hg	+2
		10	~ 77%	$PaO_2 = 71.1 - 82.3$ mm Hg	+1
		11	~ 85%	Plate-like atelectasis	+1
		12	100%	Elevated hemidiaphragm	+1

[1] Aggregate and [2] Individual probability of pulmonary embolism based on total points
[3] Recent surgery = orthopedic, hip, knee, pelvic or abdominal surgery during prior month
Arch Intern Med 2001; 161: 92-97.

Clinical Estimate of the Probability of DVT *(total points)*[1,2]

Active cancer (or treated past 6 mo)	1	Calf > 3 cm larger than other side[3]	1
Paralysis, paresis, recent leg cast	1	Pitting edema, greater in one leg	1
Entire leg swollen	1	Collateral superficial veins (nonvaricose)	1
Tender along deep venous system	1		
Recent bed-ridden for > 3 days or major surgery within 4 weeks	1	Alternative diagnosis as likely or greater than that of DVT	-2

[1] High probability (75% DVT prevalence) if score ≥ 3; Moderate probability (17% DVT) if score = 1 or 2; Low probability (3% DVT) if score ≤ 0. [2] Score is not useful if prior thromboembolism, suspect pulmonary embolus, pregnancy, or patient taking warfarin.
[3] Measure 10 cm below tibial tuberosity. *JAMA* 1998; 279: 1094.

Evaluating Suspected DVT Based on Pretest Probability (PTP)- (above score)

Low PTP - Doppler		Moderate PTP - Doppler		High PTP - Doppler	
Normal	Abnormal[1]	Normal	Abnormal	Normal	Abnormal
↓	↓	↓	↓	↓	↓
No DVT	venogram	Repeat US In 1 week	Treat DVT	venogram[2]	Treat DVT
	↙ ↓				↙ ↘
Abnormal	Normal			Normal	Abnormal
Treat DVT	No DVT			No DVT	Treat DVT
		Normal	Abnormal		
		No DVT	Treat DVT		

[1] most experts would treat instead of obtaining venogram
[2] most experts would repeat Doppler instead of venogram   *JAMA* 1998; 279: 1094.

American College of Emergency Physicians
Clinical Policy in Suspected Pulmonary Embolism (PE) www.acep.org

Level	Specific Recommendations
Level A	• No level A recommendations for D-dimer testing or CT chest alone • In patients with a low to moderate pretest probability of PE, a normal perfusion scan reliably excludes a clinically significant PE
Level B	• If low pretest probability of PE (1) a negative quantitative D-dimer (turbimetric or ELISA) or (2) a negative whole blood cell qualitative D-dimer assay & a Well's score < 2 excludes PE. Well's score can be found at (http://en.wikipedia.org/wiki/Pulmonary_embolism) • If low to moderate pretest probability of PE & an indeterminate V/Q, one of following can be used to exclude clinically significant PE: (1) a negative quantitative D-dimer (turbimetric or ELISA), (2) a negative whole blood cell qualitative D-dimer with a Well's score ≤ 4, (3) a negative single bilateral venous US scan for low probability patients, (4) a negative serial bilateral venous US for moderate probability patients. • Thin collimation spiral thoracic CT with 1-2 mm image reconstruction may be used as an alternative to V/Q scan for suspected PE.
Level C	• If low pretest probability of PE, a negative whole blood D-dimer assay alone or immunofiltration D dimer assay excludes PE. • If low to moderate pretest probability of PE and a nondiagnostic V/Q use a negative whole blood D-dimer assay to exclude PE. • Spiral CT of the thorax with delayed CT venography may be used for increased detection of significant PE.

Level A – generally accepted principles of management.
Level B – a range of strategies with moderate clinical certainty
Level C – strategies based on preliminary, inconclusive or conflicting evidence.

Diagnostic Imaging in Suspected Pulmonary Embolism
• CT angiography (CTA) with 1 mm slices is equivalent to pulmonary angiography in diagnosing pulmonary emboli (> 99% negative predictive value).
• If contrast allergy, elevated creatinine, or unable to obtain appropriate large IV access for CTA, V/Q scan is performed (see accuracy below)
• If unable to CT or V/Q, consider Doppler lower extremities, Echocardiography - findings include tricuspid regurgitation > 90%, pulmonary hypertension & dilated right ventricle (2/3 each), underfilled hyperdynamic left ventricle (1/2).
• If above imaging unavailable, consider risks/benefits of empiric therapy.

Ventilation-Perfusion Scan (V/Q) & Probability of Pulmonary Embolism/PE

Clinical Suspicion	Ventilation-Perfusion Scan Result		
	Low probability[1]	Intermediate	High probability
Low	4%	16%	56%
High	40%	66%	96%

[1]If low probability scan+comorbidity, mortality = 8%. If no comorbidity, mortality = 0.15%.

Initial Management Options in Pulmonary Embolism

ACCP 7th Conference on Antithrombotic Therapy Guidelines *Chest* 2004; 188 & 401S	• For confirmed nonmassive PE, short term (at least 5 days) SC LMWH or IV UFH is appropriate (for acute treatment, LMWH preferred). Treat before testing for PE if high clinical suspicion. • If renal failure, IV UFH is recommended over LMWH. • Routine anti-factor Xa levels are not suggested *unless* cannot achieve therapeutic aPTT and taking large daily doses of UFH. If renal failure or pregnancy Q on LMWH measure check anti-factor Xa levels. Obtain blood for level 4 hours after SC dose. • If IV UFH chosen, adjust dose to maintain aPTT equivalent to plasma heparin levels of 0.3-0.7 IU/ml anti-Xa activity. • Start oral vitamin K antagonists on the 1st day of treatment if no contraindications exist (e.g. pregnancy)

Weight Based Dosing Unfractionated Heparin (UFH) Option

Heparin 80 U/kg IV+ 18 U/kg/h (15U/kg/h if obese). √ PTT q6h. Adjust as follows:

Measured PTT	Heparin Adjustment
< 35 sec (1.2 X control)	• 80 U/kg bolus, then ↑rate by 4 U/kg/hour
35-45 sec (1.2 - 1.5 X control)	• 40 U/kg bolus, then ↑rate by 2 U/kg/hour
46-70 sec (1.5 - 2.3 X control)	• No change
71-90 sec (2.3 - 3 X control)	• ↓ rate by 2 U/kg/hour
> 90 sec (3 X control)	• stop infusion X 1 h, then ↓rate by 3 U/kg/h

Low Molecular Weight Heparin (LMWH) or Fondaparinux Option

• Enoxaparin (*Lovenox*) –1 mg/kg SC q 12h or 1.5 mg/kg SC q 24h
• Dalteparin (*Fragmin*) – 100-120 U/kg SC q 12h or 200 U/kg SC q 24h
• Tinzaparin (*Innohep*) – 175 U/kg SC q 24h
• Non-LMWH option: Fondaparinux (*Arixtra*) – 5 mg (< 50kg), 7.5 mg (50-100 kg), 10 mg (> 100 kg) SC q 24h
• Contraindications: major bleed risk, poor compliance/follow-up, renal failure.

Thrombolytics[1] *Only footnoted[2] regimens to right are FDA approved for this Indication*	• Indications (some are controversial): shock (BP < 90 mm Hg), significant respiratory distress, hypoxia or RV dysfunction.[1] • Dose: rtPA/alteplase 100 mg IV over 2 hours (or 0.6 mg/kg [max 50 mg] IV over 15 min) OR streptokinase 250,000 U IV over 30 min, then 100,000 U/hour X 24 hours (administer infusion over 72 hours if concurrent DVT)[2] OR r-PA/reteplase 10 units IV repeat 10 units IV in 30 min. OR TNKase/tenecteplase (see weight base bolus dosing page 35).
Vena Cava filter	• Indications: (1) strong contraindication to anticoagulation OR (2) clot develops while adequately anticoagulated
Embolectomy	• Indication: If not anticoagulation candidate & acutely unstable

[1] Other risk factors for adverse outcome include 1. bedside risk panel [troponin T > 0.1 ng/ml, pulmonary hypertension on ECG (Daniel score > 8)], 2. Echo - moderate or severe right ventricle (RV) hypokinesis with dilation or RV systolic pressure > 40 mm Hg, 3. CT angio. with > 49% occlusion or 4. elevated brain naturietic peptide [> 90 pg/ml associated with RV dysfunction] or D-dimer. No specific criteria for use of thrombolytics based on these risk factors can currently be recommended. The Pulmonary Embolism Severity Index may identify a subset who can be treated as outpatients (next page).*Crit Care Med* 2006; 2773.

Pulmonary Embolism Severity Index

Feature	Points	Feature	Points
Age in years	Age	Systolic BP < 100 mm Hg	+ 30
Male sex	+ 10	Respiratory rate ≥ 30/minute	+ 20
Cancer	+ 30	Temperature < 36°C (96.8°F)	+ 20
Heart failure	+ 10	Altered mentation (disoriented, lethargy, stupor, or coma)	+ 60
Chronic lung disease	+ 10		
Pulse ≥ 110 beats/minute	+ 20	O_2 saturation < 90%	+ 20

Total points (30 day mortality in %) – Class I – 65 (very low risk, 0-1.6%), Class II – 66-85 (low risk, 1.7-3.5%), Class III – 86-105 (intermediate, 3.2-6.5%), Class IV – 106-125 (high risk, 4-11.4%), Class V - > 125 (very high risk, 10-24.5%). *Am J Resp Med* 2005; 172: 1041. More recent study found 0.9% - 30 day mortality for ClassI/II. Currently, studies are analyzing whether a subset of Class I/II patients can safely undergo early hospital discharge or discharge from the ED with close follow up. *Chest* 2007; 132: 24.

Initial Management of Deep Venous Thrombosis

- Low molecular weight heparin (LMWH) is recommended over unfractionated heparin (UFH) in acute DVT
- If LMWH is used, routine anti-factor Xa levels are not recommended
- If renal failure, IV UFH is recommended over LMWH
- IV thrombolysis only recommended if massive ileofemoral DVT and at risk of limb gangrene due to venous occlusion
- See dosing of LMWH and UFH for PE previous page.

American College Chest Physicians. *Chest* 2004; 401S.

Management of Suspected Pulmonary Embolism in Pregnancy

There is minimal fetal risk from V/Q scan or CT angiography of chest. Keep Foley in to empty bladder and lessen fetal exposure during imaging (CT, V/Q scan).

(1) Doppler (Duplex) legs	• If abnormal, treat patient. False positive Doppler studies can occur after 20 weeks gestation due to vena cava compression.
(2) D-dimer	• 1st trimester D-dimer > 700 ng/ml, 2nd trimester D-dimer > 1,000, and 3rd trimester D-dimer > 1,420 are abnormal.
(3) Imaging Option 1 CT	• Many experts feel that CT may deliver less radiation to the fetus than V/Q scan and feel that CT is appropriate radiological study if Doppler of lower extremities is normal.
Imaging Option 2 V/Q scan	• If Doppler normal, perform reduced dose perfusion scan after IV NS & Foley placed to empty dye from bladder. Normal = no PE. • Perform ventilation scan if perfusion scan is abnormal.
Treatment	• The American College of Chest Physicians states that unfractionated heparin (UFH) and low molecular weight heparin (LMWH) are the anticoagulants of choice in pregnancy. See dosing previous page. Warfarin is contraindicated.

Radiology 2002; 487.; *Acad Emerg Med* 2004; 269.; *AJR* 2003; 1495.; *Chest* 2004; 627S.

Seizures and Status Epilepticus

Status epilepticus – Continuous seizure for ≥ 30 minutes or ≥ 2 seizures during same time period without full recovery of consciousness between seizures.

Most Common Causes of Status Epilepticus in Adults

Etiology	Percent[1]
• Anticonvulsant withdrawal or alcohol withdrawal (25% each)	50%
• CNS infection (12%), CNS tumor (8%), congenital CNS lesion (8%)	28%
• Cerebrovascular (stroke, anoxia, and hemorrhage)	22%
• Metabolic (encephalopathy due to low glucose, or infection)	22%
• Trauma	15%
• Drug toxicity (see page 162 for drugs that cause seizures)	15%
• Prior epilepsy	33%
• Idiopathic – no cause is found	30%

[1] Total adds up to > 100% due to multiple causes   *Neurol Clin North Am* 1998;16:257

Seizure Management

1. Protect airway, administer O_2, start IV, attach cardiac monitor and pulse oximeter, check glucose, electrolytes, drug levels, and prepare intubation equipment.
2. Administer D_{50} 1 amp IV if hypoglycemia, and thiamine 100 mg if malnourished.
3. Intravenous drug therapy as per table. If the first drug (A) is unsuccessful, try another agent (B, then C or D). If unsuccessful, consider general anesthesia.
4. Treat fever and correct sodium, calcium, or magnesium abnormalities.
5. Consider initiation of empiric antibiotics or antivirals.

Intravenous Drug Therapy for Status Epilepticus[1]

	Drug	Dose & route	Maximum rate	Special features
A	lorazepam	4 mg IV	2 mg/min	repeat X 1 in 5 min
	or diazepam	5-10 mg IV	5 mg/min	q10-15 min x 2
	or diazepam	20 mg PR	--	may repeat X 1
B	fosphenytoin[2]	20 mg/kg IV	< 150 mg/min	monitor closely
	phenytoin	20 mg/kg IV	< 50 mg/min	
C	phenobarbital	20 mg/kg IV	50-100 mg/min	monitor closely
C	midazolam	0.2 mg/kg IV (10 mg IM)	<1-2 mg/min	respiratory & blood
	drip	0.1-2 mg/kg/hour		pressure depression
D	valproic acid	30-40 mg/min	3 mg/kg/min	NOT for post-
	(Depakote)	may repeat 20 mg/kg		traumatic seizures
D	pentobarbital	5 mg/kg	slow IV	may repeat bolus X 1
	(coma)	0.5-10 mg/kg/h	(intubation/vasopressors required)	
D	propofol	1-2 mg/kg (load)	25-50 mg	respiratory & BP
	(Diprivan)	1-15 mg/kg/h	per bolus	depression

[1] If toxin induced status epilepticus, also manage as per specific toxin overdose.
[2] Dose in fosphenytoin PE (phenytoin equivalents) – administer at rate of < 150 mg/min.

Crit Care Clin 2007; 22: 637; *Lancet Neurol* 2006; 5: 246.

Surgical Abdominal Disorders

Diagnoses in ED patients > 65 y with Acute Abdominal Pain (≤ 1 week)

Physicians should have a low threshold for surgical consultation and admission/observation in elderly patients with undiagnosed abdominal pain.

Pain of unknown etiology	23%	Incarcerated hernia	4%
Biliary colic, cholecystitis	12%	Pancreatitis, UTI, volvulus, abscess	
Small bowel obstruction	12%	constipation, medications	Each 2%
Gastritis	8%	Aneurysm, ischemic bowel, hiatal	
Perforated viscus	7%	hernia, herpes zoster,	
Diverticulitis	6%	reducible hernia, myocardial	
Appendicitis	4%	infarction, pulmonary embolus	
Renal colic	4%	colon obstruction	Each < 1%

Ann Emerg Med 1990; 1383.

Appendicitis (MANTRELS diagnostic score)

Item	Score		Total	Action
Migration of pain to RLQ	1		≥ 7	Candidates for surgery
Anorexia or acetone in urine	1		4-6	Serial exams or further
Nausea with vomiting	1			testing is needed
Tenderness in right low quadrant	2			(e.g. CT or US)
Rebound tenderness	1		< 4	Extremely low probability
Elevated temperature > 100.4 F	1			of appendicitis, rare
Leukocytosis; WBC > 10,500	2			cases have score < 4
Shift of WBC's; >75% neutrophils	1			See US features pg 144

MANTRELS score is less accurate in women compared in men. Therefore, it may be appropriate to obtain a CT or US in women with high scores.

Biliary Tract Disease (Biliary Colic)

Clinical Features - Biliary Colic	Management of Biliary Colic
• Pain duration < 6-8 hours	• Treat pain
• Absence of fever	• Anticholinergics (e.g. dicyclomine
• WBC < 11,000 cells/mm³ in most	[Bentyl], atropine) are no more
• Normal liver function tests in 98%	effective than placebo for pain relief.
• US is > 98% sensitive for gallstones	• Surgery follow up

Acute Cholecystitis

Clinical Features - Acute Cholecystitis		Management of Acute Cholecystitis
Pain duration > 6-8 hours	> 90%	• Exclude complications by US or CT
Temperature ≥ 100.4° F	25%	(e.g. choledocholithiasis, acute
Murphy's sign	> 95%	pancreatitis in 15%, gallstone ileus)
WBC > 11,000 cells/mm³	65%	• Treat pain
Elevated liver function tests	55%	• Administer antibiotics (page 88)
Ultrasound sensitivity (see page 145 for imaging details)	85%	• IV NS and take nothing by mouth

Mesenteric (Arterial) Ischemia

Causes: arterial embolus in 25-50% (esp. to superior mesenteric artery), arterial thrombosis 12-25%,

Risk factors: age, vascular/valvular disease, dysrhythmias (esp. atrial fibrillation), congestive heart failure, recent MI, hypovolemia, diuretics, β blocker use, splanchnic vasoconstrictors (e.g. digoxin).

Clinical Features		Diagnostic Studies	
• Abdominal pain	80-90%	• Elevated lactate	70-90%
• Sudden onset pain	60%	• WBC > 15,000 cells/mm^3	60-75%
• Vomiting	75%	• Elevated LDH	70%
• Diarrhea (often heme +)	40%	• Elevated CK	63%
• Gross GI bleeding	25%	• Elevated phosphate	30-65%
• *Early*: Excess pain with minimal abdomen exam findings or tenderness	variable	• Elevated D-dimer	> 50%
		• Plain Xray – obstruction	30%
		• Plain Xray–thumb printing portal gas or free air	< 20%
• *Late*: shock, fever confusion, abdominal distension, rebound rigidity	variable	• CT, US sensitivity	<50-70%
		• CT angio. sensitivity	$\geq$ 95%
		• Angiography sensitivity	> 95%

Management
• Fluid and blood resuscitation, broad spectrum antibiotics (page 88)
• Surgical consult for possible emergency laparotomy (esp. if bowel necrosis or perforation is suspected)
• Mesenteric arteriography will demonstrate thrombosis, emboli, and mesenteric vasoconstriction and allow for selective papaverine administration until symptoms gone or surgery performed.
• Avoid digoxin & vasopressors (if possible) due to vasoconstriction.

Emerg Med Clin North Am 2004; 909. , *Radiol Clin North Am* 2007; 461.

Mesenteric Venous Thrombi – Risk factors – hypercoaguable state (prior PE/DVT, malignancy, sepsis, liver disease, pregnancy). Less acute symptoms than arterial occlusion. Anticoagulation may be needed.

Nonocclusive Mesenteric Ischemia - Risk factors – low flow states including hypovolemia, congestive heart failure, sepsis, post operatively (esp. hemodialysis patients), drugs (digoxin, ergots, cocaine use). 25% have no pain or GI bleeding. Surgery needed for bowel infarction. If stable, papaverine via angiographic catheter may be needed.

Chronic Mesenteric Ischemia – Intestinal angina occurring 1-2 hours after eating causing weight loss and food avoidance. Risk factors - coronary and peripheral artery disease, hypertension, diabetes, and cigarette use. Treatment consists of surgical revascularization.

Pancreatitis

Causes: gallstones, alcohols, drugs (table), infections (e.g. viral, Mycoplasma, Legionella, Ascaris, Salmonella), trauma, ↑ calcium, high triglycerides and certain metabolic disorders.

Clinical features – Epigastric pain radiating to back ± vomiting. Abdomen may be only mildly tender as pancreas is a retroperitoneal organ.

Complications: ↓Ca⁺², ↑glucose, ARDS, renal failure, bowel perforation, sepsis, pseudocyst or abscess formation, bleeding and death.

Select Drugs Causing Pancreatitis	
Definite	Probable
azathioprine	acetaminophen
cisplatin, ddl	cimetidine
furosemide	diphenoxylate
l-asparginase	estrogen
tetracycline	indomethacin
thiazides	mefenamic acid
sulfonamides	opiates
pentamidine	valproic acid

Diagnostics - Serum amylase is ↑ in 90-95% with acute pancreatitis. Many diseases cause hyperamylasemia (e.g. salivary gland & add disorders, pregnancy renal failure, burns, alcoholism, DKA, pneumonia). If amylase ≥ 2-3 X normal, specificity is > 95%. ↑ lipase is more specific than ↑ amylase for pancreatitis.

Ranson's Prognostic Signs in Pancreatitis[1]	
On admission[1]	In 48 hours[1]
Age > 55 y _(70 y)_	hematocrit fall > 10%
WBC > 16,000 _(18k)_	BUN rise > 5 mg/dl _(>2)_
glu > 200 mg/dl _(220)_	calcium < 8 mg/dl
LDH ≥ 350 IU/L _(400)_	PaO₂ < 60 mm Hg
AST ≥ 250 U/L	base deficit > 4mEq/L _(>5)_
	fluid sequestration > 6L_(>4)_

Mortality: < 1% if < 3, 25% if 3-4, 40% if 5-6, and 100% if > 6 prognostic signs listed above.

[1]Criteria for gallstone pancreatitis in parentheses

Diagnostic Studies	Management
• Suspect abscess, hemorrhage, or pseudocyst if fever, persistently ↑ amylase, mass, ↑ bilirubin, ↑ WBC	• ICU admit if Ranson > 3, sepsis, CT with necrosis, C-reactive protein > 130 mg/L
• US - 60-80% sensitive, 95% specific	• IV fluids and narcotics prn
• CT - 90% sensitive, 100% specific	• NG tube if persistent vomiting/ileus
• Obtain CT or US if suspect pseudocyst, abscess, necrosis, gallstones, cholecystitis, trauma, unknown cause	• If do not improve after 1 week, rule out abscess, pseudocyst, or ascites.
• MRI – equal to CT for severe disease	• Surgery if gallstones, bleeding, abscess, pseudocyst > 4 cm, deteriorate despite supportive care
• MRCP (magnetic resonance cholangiopancreatography) 81-100% sensitive (for common bile duct stone)	• Antibiotics (page 88) are indicated if necrosis, abscess, cholecystitis, cholangitis
• ERCP (endoscopic retrograde cholangiopancreaticography) may be required to diagnose and treat gallstone pancreatitis	• ERCP may be required for cholangitis or biliary obstruction

N Engl J Med 1994; 1198; _Gastroenterol Clin_ 2004; 855: _Surg Clin North Am_ 2007; 1341.

Toxins that Affect Vitals Signs and Physical Examination

Hypotension			Hypertension
Antihypertensive	Antidepressants	Nitroprusside	Amphetamines
α & β antagonists	Disulfiram	Opioids	Anticholinergics
Anticholinergics	Ethanol, methanol	Organophosphates	Cocaine, Lead
Arsenic (acutely)	Iron, Isopropanol	Phenothiazines	MAO inhibitors
Ca^{+2} channel block	Mercury, GHB	Sedatives	Phencyclidine
Clonidine, cyanide	Nitrates	Theophylline	Sympathomimetics

Tachycardia		Bradycardia
Amphetamines	Ethylene glycol, iron	Antidysrhythmics
Anticholinergics	Organophosphates	α agonists, β antagonists
Arsenic (acutely)	Sympathomimetics	Ca^{+2} channel blockers
Antidepressants	PCP, Phenothiazines	Digitalis, opioids, GHB
Digitalis, disulfiram	Theophylline	Organophosphates

Tachypnea		Bradypnea	
Ethylene glycol	Salicylates	Barbiturates	Isopropanol
Methanol	Sympathomimetics	Botulism	Opioids
Nicotine	(cocaine)	Clonidine	Organophosphates
Organophosphates	Theophylline	Ethanol	Sedatives

Hyperthermia		Hypothermia
Amphetamines	Phencyclidine	Carbon monoxide
Anticholinergics	Phenothiazines	Ethanol
Arsenic (acute)	Salicylates	Hypoglycemic agents
Cocaine	Sedative-hypnotics	Opioids
Antidepressants	Theophylline	Phenothiazines
LSD	Thyroxine	Sedative-hypnotics

Mydriasis (pupillodilation)		Miosis (pupilloconstriction)	
Anticholinergics	Amphetamines	Anticholinesterase	Clonidine
Antihistamines	Cocaine	Opioids, nicotine	Coma from barbit-
Antidepressants	Sympathomimetics	Cholinergics	urates, benzodi-
Anoxia(any cause)	Drug withdrawal	(e.g. pilocarpine)	azepines, ethanol

Toxins that Cause Seizures

Antidepressants	Cocaine, camphor	INH, Lead, Lithium	Organophosphates
β blockers	Ethanol withdrawal	PCP, theophylline	Sympathomimetics

[1]All agents causing ↓BP, fever, hypoglycemia and CNS bleeding can cause seizures.

Toxidromes – _See specific toxins within text for treatment_

Syndrome	Toxin	Manifestations
anticho-linergic	_Natural:_ belladonna alkaloids, atropine, homatropine, amanita muscarina. _Synthetics:_ cyclopentolate, dicyclomine, tropicamide, antihistamines, tricyclics, phenothiazines	_Peripheral antimuscarinic:_ delirium, dry skin, thirst, blurred vision, clonus, mydriasis, ↑ HR,↑BP, red rash, ↑temperature, abdominal distention, urine retention. _Central symptoms:_ delirium, mumbling speech, ataxia, cardiovascular collapse, seizures
acetyl-cholines-terase inhibition	insecticides (organophosphates, carbamates)	_Muscarinic effects_ (SLUDGE): salivation, lacrimation, urination, defecation, GI upset, emesis. Also↓or↑ pulse and BP, miosis. _Nicotinic effects:_ ↑pulse, muscle fasciculations, weakness, paralysis, ↓RR, sympathetic stimulation. _Central effects:_ anxiety, ataxia, seizure, coma, ↓respirations, cardiovascular collapse
choli-nergic	acetylcholine, betelnut, bethanechol, Clitocybe, methacholine, pilocarpine	see _muscarinic_ and _nicotinic_ effects above
extra-pyramidal	haloperidol, phenothiazines	_Parkinsonism:_ dysphonia, rigidity, tremor, torticollis, opisthotonos
hemoglo-binopathy	carbon monoxide, methemoglobin	headache, nausea, vomiting, dizziness, coma, seizures, cyanosis, cutaneous bullae, "chocolate" blood with methemoglobinemia
narcotic	morphine, dextromethorphan, heroin, fentanyl, meperidine, propoxyphene, codeine,	CNS depression, miosis (except meperidine), ↓respirations, ↓BP, seizures (propoxyphene, meperidine)
sodium channel blockade	β-blockers _(not all)_, Benadryl, calcium channel blockers, carbamazepine, citalopram, class I antiarrhythmic, cocaine, cyclic antidepress, lamotrigine, loxapine, orphenadrine, phenothiazines, thioridazine	_SALT syndrome:_ Shock, Altered mental status, Long QRS (wide complex), Terminal R in aVR see page 183. Other ECG features: wide QRS with bradycardia, wide complex tachycardia (ventricular or supraventricular)
sympatho-mimetic	aminophylline, amphetamines, cocaine, ephedrine, caffeine, methylphenidate	CNS excitation, seizures, ↑pulse, ↑BP (↓BP with caffeine), mydriasis, diaphoresis.
withdraw syndromes	alcohol, barbiturates, benzodiazepines, opioids	diarrhea, mydriasis, piloerection, ↑BP, ↑pulse, tears, cramps, yawn,

Poisoning Antidotes and Treatments

Toxin	Antidote/Treatment	Other considerations
acetamino-phen	n-acetylcysteine see page 167, 168 for detail	very effective if used within 8h, may be helpful up to 72h
β-blockers	Glucagon 1-5 mg IV/SC/IM see page 168, 169 for detail	glucagon may help reverse ↓pulse and ↓BP
Ca+2channel blockers	CaCl2 (10%) 10 ml IV, gluca-gon 1-5 mg IV/SC/IM	glucagon may help reverse ↓ pulse and ↓BP, insulin/glucose
cyanide	(amyl nitrate, sodium nitrite, and sodium thiosulfate) or (hydroxocobalamin)	See *Cyanokit* and standard *Cyanide antidote kit* page 11
digoxin	digoxin Fab fragments	see page 173 for dose
ethylene glycol	fomepizole (*Antizol*) see page 181 for detail	If fomepizole not available. Ethanol: goal is level of 0.1 g/dl.
isoniazid	pyridoxine 4 g IV, then 1 g IM q 30 min if needed	reverses seizures
methanol	fomepizole, ethanol, dialysis	thiamine, folate – see page 182
nitrites	methylene blue (0.2 ml/kg of 1% solution IV over 5 min)	consider exchange transfusion if severe methemoglobinemia
opiates	naloxone 0.4-2.0 mg IV,	diphenoxylate and propoxyphene may require higher doses
organo-phosphates, carbamates	atropine 0.05 mg/kg IV pralidoxime (PAM) see page 176 for detail	exceptionally high antidote doses may be necessary; PAM doesn't work for carbamate toxicity
salicylates	dialysis, or sodium bicarbonate 1 mEq/kg IV	See page 177, 178 for detail
sodium channel block	sodium bicarbonate 1 mEq per kg IV	goal of narrowing QRS complex and reversing arrhythmias
tricyclic anti-depressants	NaHCO3 1 mEq per kg IV see page 183 for detail	goal is serum pH of 7.50-7.55 to alter protein binding

Radio-opaque ingestions (CHIPES)	Drugs Cleared by Hemodialysis[1]	
• **C**hloral hydrate,chlorinated hydrocarbon	• Bromide	• Isopropyl
• **H**eavy metals (arsenic, Pb, mercury)	• Salicylates	alcohol
• **H**ealth food (bone meal, vitamins)	• Lithium	• Chloral hydrate
• **I**odides, iron	• Methanol	• Ethylene glycol
• **P**otassium, psychotropics (e.g. phenothiazines, antidepressants)	**Drugs cleared by Hemoperfusion[1]**	
• **E**nteric coated tabs (KCl, salicylates)	• Barbiturates (e.g. phenobarbital)	
• **S**olvents (chloroform, CCl4)	• Theophylline, Phenytoin	
	• Possibly digoxin	

[1] Consult local poison center for more detail concerning latest indications

POISON HELP and HAZMAT (Hazardous Materials) Contacts

Poison Help" Number for nearest poison control center: 1-800 (222-1222)

Phone Numbers to Identify Hazardous Chemical Agents/Spills & their Management

• CDC/ (ATDSR). 404-488-7100 & (CHEMTREC) 800-424-9300

General Approach to Poisoning

- Treat airway, breathing and BP
- Insert IV and apply cardiac monitor
- Apply pulse oximeter, administer O_2
- Consider dextrose - 50 ml of D_{50}, naloxone 2 mg IV, and thiamine 100 mg IV

Charcoal

According to the American Academy of Clinical Toxicology & European Association of Poison Centres and Clinical Toxicologists, single-dose activated charcoal should not be administered routinely to poisoned patients. The greatest benefit is within the 1st hour of ingestion. Administration of charcoal may be considered if a patient has ingested a potentially toxic amount of a poison (which is known to be adsorbed to charcoal) up to 1 hour previously. There are insufficient data to support or exclude its use after 1 hour of ingestion. There is no evidence that the administration of activated charcoal improves clinical outcome. Unless a patient has an intact or protected airway, the administration of charcoal is contraindicated.

Dose: initial dose – 25-100 g PO or per NG mixed with cathartic such as sorbitol	
Contraindications	Drugs Cleared by Multi-dose Charcoal[1]
• Unprotected airway • Corrosives, caustics (acids, alkalis) • Ileus, bowel obstruction • Drugs bound poorly by charcoal (arsenic, bromide, K^+, toxic alcohols, heavy metals [iron, iodide, lithium])	chlorpropamide, dextropropoxyphene, diazepam, digoxin, nadolol, nonsteroidals, phenytoin, phenobarbital, salicylates, theophylline, and tricyclic antidepressants

[1] Administer repeat charcoal doses q 3-4 hours (use cathartic only for 1st dose).

www.aactox.org

Cathartics[1]

There are no definite indications for the use of cathartics in the management of the poisoned patient. If used, a cathartic should be limited to a single dose in order to minimize adverse effects.

Overview: Cathartics theoretically help by ↑ fecal elimination of charcoal-bound toxins, and preventing concretions. Monitor electrolytes closely with their use.

Contraindications	Cathartic choices
• Bowel injury, obstruction, perforation, or recent abdominal surgery • Lo BP, electrolyte abnormality (avoid magnesium if renal failure) • Corrosive or caustic ingestion	• Sorbitol (70%) – 1-2 g/kg PO or NG • Magnesium citrate 250 ml of 10% solution PO or NG • Na^+ or $MgSO_4$ – 30 g PO or NG

[1] Cathartics have never been shown to alter the clinical outcome in acute overdose.

www.aactox.org

Ipecac

There are no absolute indications for ED use. Ipecac (30 ml PO) delays charcoal administration, incompletely empties the stomach and has many side effects. Most experts do not use. (www.aactox.org)

Gastric lavage

Gastric lavage should not be considered unless a patient has ingested a potentially life-threatening amount of poison and the procedure can be performed < 60 min. after ingestion. Clinical benefit has not been confirmed in controlled studies and serious side effects (e.g. death, aspiration, esophageal trauma) can occur.

Directions for Lavage in Overdose	Indications
• Use 36-40 French *Ewald* tube	• Dangerous ingestion within 1 hour
• Lavage stomach with 250-300 ml NS or H_2O aliquots until the return is clear	• Toxins that slow GI transit
	• Toxins with possible rapid onset
• Protect the airway with endotracheal intubation if there is an absent gag reflex, or altered mental status	seizure, or ↓mental status
	• Toxins poorly bound by charcoal
	Contraindications
• Monitor the total input and output from the *Ewald* tube to ensure fluid overload does not occur.	• Caustics (acids, alkalis), solvents (hydrocarbons), nontoxic ingestions, coagulopathy, GI tract pathology.

www.aactox.org

Whole bowel irrigation (WBI)

There are no absolute indications for WBI. WBI is an option for potentially toxic ingestions of sustained-release or enteric-coated drugs. WBI has theoretical value for patients who have ingested substantial amounts of iron or for the removal of ingested packets of illicit drugs and in the management of patients who have ingested substantial amounts of poisons not adsorbed to activated charcoal.

Administration	Indications
• Administer PO or place NG tube	• Metals (iron, zinc)
• Administer polyethylene glycol (Go-Lytely) at 1-2 L/hour	• Lithium, borates
	• Ingested crack vials or drug packets
• Stop when objects are recovered if packet or vial ingestion	• Sustained release medications
• Stop when effluent is clear	• Toxic bezoars
	Contraindications
	• CNS or respiratory depression[1]
	• GI tract pathology (e.g. bleed, ileus, perforation, or obstruction)

[1] Unless intubated   www.aactox.org

Acetaminophen Toxicity

Phase	Time after ingestion	Signs and Symptoms
1	30 min to 24 hours	Asymptomatic, or minor GI irritant effects
2	24-72 hours	Relatively asymptomatic, GI symptoms resolve, possible mild elevation of LFT's or renal failure
3	72-96 hours	Hepatic necrosis with potential jaundice, hepatic encephalopathy, coagulopathy, and renal failure
4	4 days - 2 weeks	Resolution of symptoms or death

Acetaminophen

Ingestion of $\geq$ 140 mg/kg is potentially toxic. Obtain acetaminophen level $\geq$ 4h after acute ingestion and plot on the Rumack-Matthews nomogram. A 4h level $\geq$ 140 ug/ml indicates need for n-acetylcysteine. On nomogram (page 168), levels above dotted line (- - - - - - - -) indicates probable risk, while levels above the bottom solid line (_____) indicate possible risk of toxicity. If time from ingestion unknown, obtain level at time 0 and 4 h later to calculate half-life. If half-life is > 4 h, administer antidote.

Management	
Decontamination	• Charcoal is indicated only if toxic co-ingestants are present. • Increase oral *Mucomyst* dose by 20% if charcoal given.
N-acetylcysteine [NAC] *Mucomyst* (*Acetadote* – IV formulation)	• Assess toxicity based on nomogram. • If drug level will return in < 8 h post ingestion, treatment can be delayed until level known. NAC prevents 100% of toxicity if administered < 8 hours from ingestion. If level will return > 8 hours and $\geq$140 mg/kg ingested, administer 1st dose of *Mucomyst*. NAC is definitely useful $\leq$ 24 hours after ingestion and possibly up to 72 hours. • <u>PO Dose</u>: 140 mg/kg PO, then 70 mg/kg q4h X 17 doses. Shorter course (36 h) may be effective if no liver toxicity at 36 h. May dilute in cola to 5% solution. Contact poison center for short protocol specifics. • <u>IV Dose</u> - 150 mg/kg IV (in 200 ml D$_5$W) over 60 minutes, then 50 mg/kg (in 500 ml D$_5$W) over 4 hours, then 100 mg/kg (in 1000 ml D$_5$W) over 16 hours. Up to 18% develop anaphylactoid reaction (esp. if asthmatic or if prior NAC reaction). If this happens, discontinue and manage symptoms (e.g. antihistamines, epinephrine, inhaled ß agonists, IV fluids). If symptoms stop and were mild, consider restarting NAC. Otherwise, do not restart. Consult poison for assistance with management (1 800 222-1222).

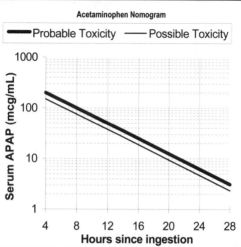

Acetaminophen Nomogram

━━━━━ Probable Toxicity   ─────── Possible Toxicity

Serum APAP (mcg/mL) vs. Hours since ingestion

Used with permission, Tarascon Internal Medicine & Critical Care Pocketbook, 4th ed. 2006

βeta-Blockers

<u>β1 stimulation</u> - ↑ contraction force + rate, AV node conduction, & renin secretion.
<u>β2 stimulation</u> - blood vessel, bronchi, GI, & GU smooth muscle relaxation. Propranolol is nonselective, blocking β1 and β2 receptors. Other nonselective β-blockers: nadolol, timolol, pindolol. Selective β1 blockers: metoprolol, atenolol, esmolol, + acebutolol. Pindolol + acebutolol have some β agonist properties.

System	Clinical Features
CNS	• Coma and seizures (esp. with lipid soluble agents – propranolol)
Cardiac	• ↓HR, AV block (1st, 2nd or 3rd), ↑QRS, ↑QT interval (sotalol), ↑ T waves, + ST changes
	• ↑HR possible with pindolol, practolol, sotalol. ↓BP is common.
	• Congestive heart failure can occur.
Pulmonary	• Bronchospasm and respiratory arrest can occur.
Metabolic	• Hypoglycemia is uncommon in adults.

Treatment of β-blocker Toxicity

Option	Recommendations
Gastrointestinal decontamination	• Charcoal ± preceded by gastric lavage if < 1 h from ingestion • Whole bowel irrigation if sustained release preparation
Glucagon	• Indications: ↓HR or BP. Administer 5 mg IV then 1-5 mg/h
Atropine	• Has no effect on BP and will only ↑HR in 25%. • No HR response to 1 mg is typical of β-blocker toxicity. Administer 0.5 mg IV prn (maximum of 2 mg).
Fluid/pressors	• If ↓BP does not respond to NS, administer α + β agonists (epinephrine/norepinephrine) or β agonists (dobutamine)
Other options	• High dose insulin: 1st bolus 1 U/kg insulin & 25 g D_{50}, then insulin infusion (0.5 – 1 U/kg/hour) with dextrose infusion (usually D_{10}W-D_{25}W) to maintain normal glucose • Use pacemaker if no response to above. Consider dialysis if atenolol, nadolol, sotalol, or acebutolol overdose. • Inamrinone–consult pharmacist, special dosing/monitoring

Calcium Channel Blockers

System	Clinical Features
CNS	• Lethargy, slurred speech, confusion, coma, seizure, ↓respirations
Cardiac	• ↓HR, ↓BP, AV block (1st, 2nd or 3rd), sinus arrest, asystole
GI	• Nausea, vomiting, ileus, obstruction, bowel ischemia/infarction
Metabolic	• Hyperglycemia (esp. verapamil), lactic acidosis

Option	Treatment Recommendations
Gastrointestinal decontamination	• Charcoal ± preceded by gastric lavage. • Whole bowel irrigation if sustained-release preparation
Calcium	• Primary indication is to reverse hypotension (not HR) • Administer calcium gluconate 3 g (30 ml of 10% solution) IV over 5 minutes, repeat prn. Alternatively, administer 10 ml of calcium chloride 10% IV over 5 minutes.
Glucagon	• Indications: ↓HR or BP. Administer 5 mg IV, then 1-5 mg/h
Atropine	• 0.5 mg IV if symptomatic↓HR (repeat X 3) – often ineffective
Fluids/pressors	• ↓BP primarily occurs from peripheral vasodilation, therefore administer fluids followed by vasoconstrictors (e.g. norepinephrine, phenylephrine or high dose dopamine).
Other options	• Use pacemaker if no response to medications. • High dose insulin: 1st bolus 1 U/kg insulin & 25 g D_{50}, then insulin infusion (0.5 – 1 U/kg/hour) with dextrose infusion (usually D_{10}W-D_{25}W) to maintain normal glucose

Carbon Monoxide

Carbon monoxide (CO) exposure can occur from fire, catabolism of heme compounds, cigarettes, pollution, ice-surfacing machines, & methylene chloride (inhaled or dermally-

FIO_2	CO half-life
room air	320 min
100% rebreather	80 min
3 ATM hyperbaric O_2	23 min

absorbed paint remover) degradation. CO displaces O_2 off Hb. O_2-Hb dissociation curve shifts to left. CO binds cytochrome-A, cardiac/skeletal muscle myoglobin.

CO-Hb level	Typical symptoms at given level of CO toxicity
0-10%	Usually none, $\pm\downarrow$exercise tolerance, $\uparrow$angina, and $\uparrow$claudication
10-20%	Frontal headache, dyspnea with exertion
20-30%	Throbbing headache, dyspnea with exertion, $\downarrow$concentration
30-40%	Severe headache, vomiting, visual changes
40-50%	Confusion, syncope on exertion, myocardial ischemia
50-60%	Collapse, seizures
> 60-70%	Coma and death
Variable	Cherry red skin, visual field defect, homonymous hemianopsia, papilledema, retinal bleed, hearing changes, pulmonary edema.

- CO poisoning may present with flu-like symptoms. Consider this diagnosis especially when multiple family members present with these complaints.
- *Delayed neuropsychiatric syndrome* (permanent neurological or psychiatric abnormalities 3 days to 3 weeks after exposure).

Assessment of CO Intoxication	
CO-Hb levels	Levels are unreliable & may be low in significant intoxication. Standard pulse oximetry is unreliable. CO specific coximeters are available for non-invasive bedside CO screening.
Anion gap	Cyanide and lactic acidosis may contribute to anion gap
Saturation gap	Calculated – directly measured arterial O_2 saturation. This gap also occurs with methemoglobin & sulfhemoglobin.
ECG	May show changes consistent with myocardial ischemia.
Cardiac markers	May be elevated from direct myocardial damage.

Management of CO Intoxication	
Criteria for Admission	Possible criteria for hyperbaric oxygen[1]
• All with CO-Hb > 15-20% • Pregnancy and CO-Hb > 10% • Acidosis, ECG changes, chest pain, abnormal neurologic exam or history of unconsciousness • Persistent symptoms following 100% O_2 X 3 hours	• Absolute: cyanide toxic, coma, un-conscious > 20 min, abnormal neuro. exam, abnormal ECG, arrhythmias, CO-Hb > 25%, pH < 7.20, neurologic symptoms after 100% O_2 X 3 • Relative: pregnancy, CO-Hb > 20%.

[1] Exact utility and indications for hyperbaric oxygen are controversial. ACEP Clinical Policy states that (1) Hyperbaric oxygen is a therapeutic option but its use cannot be mandated and (2) No clinical variables including CO level identifies a subgroup of CO patients for whom HBO is most likely to benefit or harm.   www.acep.org

Clonidine

Clonidine is an α-adrenergic agonist that lowers BP, and ameliorates opiate withdrawal. Clonidine tablets (*Catapres*), in combination with chlorthalidone (*Chlorpres*), and transdermal patches (*Catapres*-TTS) are available. Leftover patches may contain up to 2 mg of active drug. Clonidine is rapidly absorbed from GI tract lowering BP within 30-60 min peaking at 2-4 h. Serum half-life is 12 h (6-24 h). Clonidine lowers BP at the presynaptic α$_2$-agonist receptors resulting in ↓ sympathetic outflow. At high doses, it is a peripheral α-agonist + causes ↑ BP. It is also a CNS depressant.

Clinical Features of Clonidine Toxicity

CNS	• Lethargy, coma, recurrent apnea, miosis, hypotonia
Cardiac	• Sinus bradycardia, hypertension (transient), later hypotension
Other	• Hypothermia and pallor

Treatment

Monitor	• Apply cardiac monitor + pulse oximeter and observe closely for apnea. Apnea often responds to tactile stimulation.
Decontamination	• Charcoal ± gastric lavage. Avoid ipecac.
Atropine	• Indication: bradycardia. Dose: 0.5 mg IV.
Antihypertensives	• Hypertension is transient & usually no treatment is required. If needed, use short acting titratable agent (e.g. *Nipride*).
Fluids/pressors	• Treat hypotension with fluids and dopamine prn.
Naloxone	• 2 mg IV may reverse CNS but not cardiac/BP effects.

Cocaine

Cocaine is the HCl salt of the alkaloid extract of the *Erythroxylon coca* plant. It can be absorbed across all mucous membranes. It is a local anesthetic.

Route	Peak effect	Duration
Nasal	30 min	1 – 3 hr
GI	90 min	3 hr
IV/Inhaled	1 - 2 min	≤ 30 min

(ester-type) that blocks the reuptake of norepinephrine, dopamine, & serotonin

Clinical Features of Cocaine Toxicity

General	• Agitation, hyperthermia, sweating, rhabdomyolysis, GI perf./ischemia
Cardiac	• A direct myocardial depressant, prolongs QT with sympathetic hyperactivity, myocardial ischemia (often with atypical clinical features & ECG findings - acutely or during withdrawal), ↑BP, ↑HR, LVH, arrhythmias, ↑platelet aggregation, accelerated atherosclerosis
CNS	• Seizures, CNS infarct or bleed, CNS abscess, vasculitis, dystonia
Lung	• Pneumothorax/mediastinum, hemorrhage, pneumonitis, ARDS

Management of Cocaine Toxicity

General	• Apply cardiac monitor, oxygen, pulse oximeter and observe closely for arrhythmia, seizures, and hyperthermia. Benzodiazepines are drug of choice for agitation, while *Haldol* is also effective (without ↑ cocaine seizure threshold)
Hyperthermia & Rhabdomyolysis	• Benzodiazepines to reduce agitation and muscle activity. Cool with mist and fan. Continuous rectal probe temperature. Check serum CK/C0₂. Administer IV fluids & bicarbonate to prevent renal failure (page 63).
GI decontaminate	• *Body stuffers* (rapid ingestion to hide drugs) – charcoal & monitor for perforation/ischemia • *Body packer* (hidden packets for transportation)– Xray & whole bowel irrigation (page 166). If rupture, consider laparotomy to remove cocaine
Cardiovascular (*Arrhythmias & Hypertension*)	• Administer benzodiazepines for ↑BP, ↑HR. Treat according to standard ACLS protocols: Use sodium nitroprusside (*Nipride*) or phentolamine for severe HTN. In the past, experts have recommended avoiding β blockade (due to possible unopposed alpha effects). Limited studies suggest there may be a beneficial, protective effect of β blockade. Currently, clear cut recommendations cannot be given regarding their use. *Ann Emerg Med* 2008; 51: 117-134. • <u>Wide complex tachycardia</u> is due to quinidine-like effect. Administer sodium bicarbonate and cardiovert.
Cardiovascular (*Chest pain*)	• Administer benzodiazepines, aspirin, and IV NTG. Alternately, phentolamine IV may reverse coronary vasoconstriction. PCI/PTCA is preferred over thrombolytics as CNS bleed/vasculitis/HTN ↑ risk of CNS bleed.
Neurologic	• Treat status epilepticus with benzodiazepines. Barbiturates are 2ⁿᵈ line while phenytoin is not useful. Exclude coexisting pathology (CT, glucose, electrolytes, infection).

Digoxin

Natural sources: foxglove, oleander, lily of the valley, and the skin of toads.
Therapeutic range - 0.6-1.2 ng/ml. Severe poisoning may not demonstrate ↑levels.

Clinical Features – Acute Toxicity	
Digoxin level	Usually markedly elevated (obtain > 6 hours after ingestion)
GI and CNS	Nausea, vomiting, diarrhea, headache, confusion, coma
Cardiac	Supraventricular tachycardia, AV blocks, bradyarrhythmias
Metabolic	Hyperkalemia from inhibition of the Na^+/K^+ ATP pump

Clinical Features – Chronic Toxicity	
Digoxin level	May be normal
History	URI symptoms, on diuretics, renal insufficiency, yellow-green halos
Cardiac	Ventricular arrhythmias are more common than with acute toxicity
Metabolic	Potassium low or normal, magnesium is often low

Treatment of Digoxin Toxicity	
• Digoxin Fab fragments (*Digibind*) • Multi-dose charcoal ± lavage. • Atropine 0.5 mg for ↓HR • Ventricular arrhythmia: lidocaine 1 mg/kg IV ± MgSO₄ 20 mg/kg IV	• Acutely, treat ↑K⁺: page 51. Do not use calcium to treat in this instance. • Chronically, treat low K⁺. • Avoid cardioversion if possible (predisposes to ventricular fibrillation).

Indications for Digibind	Total body load digoxin - TBLD estimates
• Ventricular arrhythmias • Symptomatic bradyarrhythmias unresponsive to Rx • Ingestion of > 0.1 mg/kg • Digoxin level of > 5 ng/ml • Consider if K⁺ >5-5.5 mEq/l	TBLD (total body load of digoxin) in milligrams = • [digoxin level¹ (ng/ml) x weight (kg)] ÷ 100 • (Acute ingestion) - total mg ingested if digoxin capsules or elixir is ingested • (Acute ingestion) - total mg ingested X 0.8 if digitoxin ingested (due to 80% bioavailability)

¹ *Chronic ingestions may have normal to mildly elevated digoxin levels.*

Digibind Dosing
• Number of vials to administer = TBLD in mg divided by 0.5 (mg/vial)   • If ingested quantity unknown consider empiric administration of 10 vials   • One 38 mg *Digibind* vial can bind 0.5 mg of digoxin if amount ingested known   • Dilute *Digibind* to 10 mg/ml & administer IV over 30 min. Consider using 0.22 micron filter for infusion. Serum levels are useless after use assay measures bound + unbound digoxin. Once bound, digoxin-Fab complex is renally excreted.

Flunitrazepam - Rohypnol "Roofies"

Rohypnol is a benzodiazepine marketed outside the US for insomnia, sedation, & pre-anesthesia. It is 10 X as potent as diazepam. It potentiates and prolongs the effects of heroin, methadone, & alcohol and attenuates the withdrawal of cocaine. It produces disinhibition and amnesia and has been used as a "date rape" drug.

Onset/duration	• Maximal absorption is 0.5-1.5 hr with T½ of nearly 12 hours.
Major clinical effects	• <u>CNS</u> - sedation, incoordination, hallucinations. Paradoxical excitement, esp. with alcohol use. ↓DTRs, mid to small pupils. • <u>CV-Pulm</u> - Respiratory depression, hypotension, aspiration
Management	• NOT routinely detected in urine benzodiazepine screen • Lavage if < 1 hr from ingestion, otherwise administer charcoal • Protect airway and apply cardiac monitor, pulse oximeter • Admit if lethargic or unstable after 2-4 hr of observation. • Routine use of flumazenil to reverse this drug's effects cannot be recommended due to the possibility of seizures if current use of cyclic antidepressants, chronic benzodiazepine or flunitrazepam use, or underlying seizure disorder.

Gamma Hydroxybutyric acid (GHB)

Gamma hydroxybutyric acid (GHB) has been promoted as a steroid alternative, a weight control agent, and as a narcolepsy treatment.

Onset/duration	• Onset of symptoms is ~ 15 minutes, with spont. resolution from 2 to > 48 hours (depending on dose & co-ingestant).
Major clinical effects	• CNS Acts synergistically with ethanol to produce CNS and respiratory depression. At high serum levels patients are unresponsive to noxious stimuli and lose pharyngeal/laryngeal reflexes. Seizures, clonic arm/leg/face movements, vomiting, amnesia, ↓DTRs & vertigo occur. Nystagmus and ataxia occur. • CV-Pulm – ↓ HR, Irregular or ↓ respirations, ↓ BP.
Management	• Protect airway and apply cardiac monitor, pulse oximeter • Treat symptomatically (e.g. use atropine for persistent ↓ HR). • Exclude coingestant or alternate diagnosis (e.g. CNS trauma). • Admit if symptoms do not resolve after 6 hours of observation.

Hallucinogens

Common hallucinogens include LSD (lysergic acid diethylamide), mescaline (peyote plant), psilocybin (mushrooms – esp. from cow pastures), morning glory seeds (similar to LSD), nutmeg and toads (skin contains hallucinogenic *bufotoxins*).

Clinical Features of Hallucinogen Toxicity	
General	• Onset of symptoms is generally 30-60 minutes with 4-8 hr duration. • Sympathetic stimulation(↑pupils, diaphoresis, piloerection) • Hyperthermia, neuroleptic malignant syndrome, rhabdomyolysis (esp. if patient is restrained)
CNS	• Panic attacks with hallucinations that are often cross-sensory (tasting colors/seeing sounds), illusions, misperceptions. Seizures and coma are less common. ↑DTRs
Cardiac	• ↑ HR often with normal or mild ↑ BP.
GI	• Vomiting & diarrhea are more common with mescaline, psilocybin
Treatment	
Monitor	• Apply cardiac monitor + pulse oximeter and observe closely for seizures, agitation, hyperthermia, rhabdomyolysis
Decontamination	• Decontamination is usually not necessary. Charcoal ± lavage may bind peyote or psilocybin (not LSD), but effects are generally limited and side effects of this therapy may be more severe than toxic effects of agents.
Agitation	• Verbal reassurance may be useful. Benzodiazepines followed by haloperidol may be useful if severe agitation.

Neuroplectics

Side effects of neuroleptics OD:
(1) <u>anti-adrenergic</u> - ↓BP, ↑ HR
(2) <u>anticholinergic</u> - ↑ temp, dry, urine retention, ↑pupils (phenothiazines may cause ↓pupils), CNS and respiratory depression
(3) <u>anti-dopaminergic</u> – dystonia, akithisia, motor disorders,
(4) <u>quinidine effect</u> on heart (↑QT, ↑PR, torsades). Low potency drugs *Thorazine, Serentil* have more anticholinergic/anti-adrenergic effect, while ↑ potency butyrophenones & thioxanthenes have more antidopamine effects. Thioridazine & mesoridazine have most quinidine-like cardiac effect.

Class	Example Drugs
Atypical neuroleptics	aripiprazole, clozapine, olanzapine, quetiapine, risperidone, ziprasidone
Butyrophenone	droperidol *Inapsine*
	haloperidol *Haldol*
Dibenzazepine	loxapine *Loxitane*
Dihydroindolone	molindone *Moban*
Phenothiazines	chlorpromazine *Thorazine*
	fluphenazine *Prolixin*
	mesoridazine *Serentil*
	perphenazine *Trilafon*
	prochlorperazine *Compazine*
	promethazine *Phenergan*
	thioridazine *Mellaril*
	trifluoperazine *Stelazine*
Thioxanthenes	thiothixene *Navane*

Treatment	
Monitor	• Apply cardiac monitor + pulse oximeter and obtain ECG.
GI decontaminate	• Charcoal 1g/kg PO, consider lavage 1st if < 1 hour since ingestion and potentially lethal overdose
Hypotension	• NS IV, if unresponsive use α agonist (e.g. norepinephrine)
Ventricular Arrhythmias	• If wide QRS (SALT syndrome), IV NaHCO₃ 1-2 mEq/kg • Lidocaine or amiodarone– page 222 • Magnesium 2-4 g IV over 15 min (if no renal insufficiency) • Avoid Class IA anti-arrhythmics (e.g. procainamide)
Medically admit	• All who are symptomatic or become symptomatic over 6 h (e.g. ↓BP, altered mental status, arrhythmia, ECG changes) • All thioridazine or mesoridazine ingestions (delayed VF/VT)

Phencyclidine (PCP)

Three stages of intoxication include (1) acute organic brain syndrome with violent behavior (2) progressive stupor with intact pain response, and (3) deep coma.

Clinical features: <u>Mixed</u> adrenergic (↑BP,↑HR, hyperthermia, mydriasis), and cholinergic (miosis, sweating, wheezing, salivation) features. Nystagmus (any direction), with blank open-eyed stare and roving gave. Rhabdomyolysis, CNS bleed, stridor, DIC, respiratory depression, and seizures occur.

Management: Sedate (benzodiazepines ± haloperidol) and restraint patient for protection. Monitor neurologic, cardiac, and pulmonary status. Exclude life threats (e.g. hyperthermia, rhabdomyolysis). Consider repeat doses of charcoal.

Insecticides - Organophosphates and Carbamates

Organophosphates irreversibly bind and inhibit cholinesterases at CNS receptors, post-ganglionic parasympathetic nerves (muscarinic effects), and autonomic ganglia and skeletal myoneural junctions (nicotinic effects). Carbamates reversibly bind cholinesterases and are less toxic than organophosphates.

Clinical Features of Insecticide Toxicity	
Onset of symptoms	• Usually < 24h after exposure. Lipid-soluble organophosphates (e.g. fenthion) may take days to cause symptoms & last months
CNS	• Cholinergic excess: delirium, confusion, seizures, respiratory depression. Carbamates have less central effects.
Muscarinic	• SLUDGE (salivation, lacrimation, urination, defecation, GI upset, emesis), miosis, bronchoconstriction, bradycardia.
Nicotinic	• Fasciculations, muscle weakness, sympathetic ganglia stimulation (hypertension, tachycardia, pallor, rarely mydriasis)

Diagnostic Studies in Insecticide Poisoning	
Labs	• ↑glucose, ↑K⁺, ↑WBC, ↑amylase, glycosuria, proteinuria
ECG	• Early - ↑ in sympathetic tone (tachycardia) • Later - extreme parasympathetic tone (sinus bradycardia, AV block, and ↑QT).
Serum *(pseudo)* RBC *(plasma)* Cholinesterase	• Serum levels are more sensitive but less specific than RBC • Plasma levels return to normal before RBC levels • Mild cases: levels are < 50% of normal • Severe cases: levels are < 10% of normal

Treatment	
General	• Support airway, breathing and blood pressure. Respiratory depression is the most common cause of death. • Medical personnel should gown and glove if dermal exposure. • Wash toxin off patient if dermal exposure. • Administer charcoal if oral ingestion.
Atropine	• Competitively blocks acetylcholine at muscarinic (not nicotinic) receptors. Atropine may reverse CNS effects. • <u>Dose</u>: 1-2 mg (or >) q 5 min. Mix 50 mg in 500 ml NS + titrate. • <u>Goal</u>: titrate to mild anticholinergic signs (dry mouth, secretions) and not to pupil size or heart rate. • Treatment failure is usually due to not using enough atropine.
Pralidoxime (2-PAM)	• Reverses nicotinic & central effects, not carbamate toxicity. • <u>Dose</u>: 1-2 g in 100 ml IV over 15-30 minutes. May repeat in 1 hour then q 3-8 hours prn. Onset of effect is 10-40 minutes after administration.
Atrovent	• Ipratropium bromide 0.5 mg nebulized may dry secretions.

Salicylates

Methylsalicylate (oil of wintergreen) is the most toxic form. Absorption generally is within 1h of ingestion (delays $\geq$ 6h occur with enteric-coated and viscous preparations. At toxic levels, salicylates are renally metabolized. Alkaline urine promotes excretion. At different acidosis/alkalosis states, measurable salicylate levels change, therefore measure arterial pH at same time as drug level.

Ingestion	Severity	Signs and Symptoms
<150 mg/kg	mild	vomiting, tinnitus, and hyperpnea
150-300 mg/kg	moderate	vomiting, hyperpnea, diaphoresis, and tinnitus
>300 mg/kg	severe	acidosis, altered mental status, seizures, & shock

Clinical Features of Salicylate Toxicity

Direct	• Irritation of GI tract with reports of perforation
Metabolic	• <u>Early</u>: respiratory alkalosis from respiratory center stimulation • <u>Later</u>: metabolic acidosis - uncoupled oxidative phosphorylation • Hypokalemia, ↑or↓ glucose, ketonuria, and either ↑or↓ Na+
CNS	• <u>Early</u>: tinnitus, deafness, agitation, hyperactivity • <u>Later</u>: confusion, lethargy, coma, seizure, CNS edema
GI	• Vomiting, gastritis, pylorospasm, ↑ liver enzymes, perforation
Pulmonary	• Noncardiac pulmonary edema (esp. with chronic toxicity)

Indicators of Salicylate Toxicity

Clinical	• Features listed above are associated with toxicity
Ingestion	• Ingestion of > 150 mg/kg may be associated with toxicity
Ferric chloride	• Mix 2 drops $FeCl_3$+ 1 ml urine. Purple = salicylate ingestion but not salicylate toxicity.
Phenstix	• Dipstick test for urine. Brown indicates salicylate or phenothiazine ingestion (not toxicity). Adding 1 drop 20N H_2SO_4 bleaches out color for phenothiazines but not salicylates.
Salicylate Levels	• A level > 30 mg/dl drawn $\geq$ 6h after ingestion is toxic. Clinical findings are more important than serum levels. • Follow serial levels (q2-3h) until downward trend established • Arterial pH must be measured at same time, as acidemia increases CNS penetration and toxicity at lower levels. • *Done nomogram has been proven unreliable*
Nontoxic Ingestion	• If none of the following are present, acute toxicity is unlikely (1) < 150 mg/kg ingested, (2) absent clinical features (3) level < 30 mg/dl obtained $\geq$ 6h after ingestion (unless enteric coated preparation, viscous preparation, or chronic ingestion)

Treatment of Acute Salicylate Toxicity	
General	• Treat dehydration, electrolyte abnormalities. CSF hypoglycemia occurs with normal serum glucose – add D_5 or D_{10} to all fluids.
Decontaminate	• Multi-dose charcoal, Whole bowel irrigation (if enteric coated)
Alkalinization	• Add 100-150 mEq NaHCO$_3$ to 1 L D$_5$W (20-40 mEq/L K$^+$ if no renal failure since urine alkalinization often not possible until low K$^+$ corrected). Infuse at 200 ml/h. <u>Goal</u> – urine pH > 7.5
Hemodialysis	• <u>Indications</u>: renal failure, noncardiogenic pulmonary edema, CHF, persistent CNS disturbances, ↓BP, unable to correct acid-base or electrolyte imbalance, salicylate level > 100 mg/dl
Chronic Salicylate Toxicity	
Presentation	• Older, chronic salicylates, altered CNS, non-cardiogenic pulmonary edema. ± Misdiagnosed as infectious/neuro disease.
Drug levels	• Salicylate levels are often normal to therapeutic.
Treatment	• Supportive measures and urinary alkalinization. Dialyze if acidosis, confusion, or pulmonary edema even if level normal.

Selective Serotonin Reuptake Inhibitors & Non-Tricyclic antidepressants

Selective serotonin reuptake inhibitors (SSRIs) OD is relatively benign (morbidity related to co-ingestants) Most common symptoms: ↑ HR, tremor, vomiting, and drowsiness. ECG: ↑ HR, non-specific ST-T changes. Seizures and cardiotoxicity (wide QRS/QTc) can occur at high levels (esp. fluoxetine). ↓ HR is seen with fluvoxamine at high or low doses. *Treatment*: (1) exclude coingestants (2) observe for 6 hours (3) Charcoal 1g/kg (4) Sodium bicarbonate IV is useful if wide QRS tachycardia, (5) Observe for potentially lethal *Serotonin Syndrome* – see pg 179.	**SSRIs** citalopram (*Celexa*) escitalopram (*Lexapro*) fluoxetine (*Prozac*) fluvoxamine (*Luvox*) paroxetine (*Paxil*) sertraline (*Zoloft*)
MAOI OD may have onset up 12 h later. Excess α+β adrenergic symptoms: Headache, tremor, ↑BP,↑DTR rigidity, chest pain, ↑temp. Later ↓BP, ↓HR, seizures <u>*Treatment*</u>: (1) *Nipride* or phentolamine for ↑ BP [No β blockers] (2) NS + Norepi. for ↓ BP (3) Charcoal (4) benzodiazepines (5) treat hyperthermia with aggressive cooling (see malignant hyperthermia management) (6) treat rhabdomyolysis, (7) Admit all intentional OD & all ingestions > 2 mg/kg	**Monoamine oxidase inhibitors (MAOIs)** isocarboxazid (*Marplan*) phenelzine (*Nardil*) selegiline (*Eldepryl*) tranylcypromine (*Parnate*)

Other Non-Tricyclic antidepressants

Serotonin, Norepinephrine reuptake inhibitors – Venlafaxine (*Effexor*), duloxetine (*Cymbalta*) – OD causes ↑ HR and ↓ level of consciousness, brief and limited seizures, mild hypotension. Treat with supportive care, benzodiazepines if seizures, saline and vasopressors for hypotension.

Norepinephrine & Dopamine reuptake inhibitor – bupropion (*Wellbutrin*). OD causes lethargy (41%), tremors (24%), and seizures (21%). Mean onset of seizures is 3.7 hours and responds to benzodiazepines and phenytoin. Single case report of prolonged QRS/QTc. Treat supportively.

Noradrenergic & Serotoninergic antidepressants – mirtazapine (*Remeron*) inhibits presynaptic α2 receptors increasing serotonin and norepinephrine transmission. Serotonin-2 and 3 receptors are blocked diminishing anxiety and GI side effects. OD is rare - with sedation and drowsiness requiring rare intubation. No cardiac conduction effects or seizures have been noted to date.

Serotonin-2 receptor antagonists – nefazodone (*Serzone*) and trazodone (*Desyrel*) block serotonin reuptake and inhibit serotonin-2 receptors. Nefazodone also blocks norepinephrine reuptake and had minimal α1 receptor antagonism. Both (esp. trazodone) cause sedation, lightheadedness, GI upset, headaches. Trazodone has been associated with nonsustained ventricular tachycardia and other dysrhythmias. Treatment for OD of either agent is supportive.

Serotonin Syndrome

	Mild	Moderate	Severe
CNS	Confused, restless	Agitated, somnolent	Coma, seizures
Autonomic	Temp. (T) < 38°C, mydriasis, diarrhea, ↑ heart rate	T < 39.5°C, BP low or high, mydriasis	T > 39.5°C, dyspnea, diaphoresis, ↑heart rate
Neuromuscular	Clonus, ataxia, akithesia, ↑ DTRs	Myoclonus, clonus, ataxia	Muscle rigidity (rhabdomyolysis)

Select causes: Drug interactions between SSRIs, TCAs, MAOIs, meperidine, codeine, and dextromethorphan. Compared to neuroleptic malignant syndrome (see page 62), patients with serotonin syndrome have more rapid onset, more GI features (diarrhea, nausea), more hyperkiness (myoclonus, ↑DTR), and less muscle rigidity.

Treatment: Stop drug, manage complications (hyperthermia/rhabdomyolysis), administer benzodiazepines. Some experts recommend cyproheptadine (serotonin antagonist) 4-8 mg PO q 8 hours (one authors states that 30 mg is needed for efficacy). *Emerg Med Clin North Am* 2007; 25: 477.

Sympathomimetics (Amphetamines & Derivatives)

Effects of amphetamines are (1) sympathomimetic - α& β adrenergic - mydriasis, ↑HR, ↑BP, ↑temp., arrhythmias, MI, rhabdomyolysis, psychosis, CNS bleed, ↑sweat, seizures (2) dopaminergic - restless, anorexia, hyperactive, movement disorders, paranoia & (3) serotonergic – mood, impulse control, serotonin syndrome **Ice/crank** (crystal methamphetamine) 1 of most commonly confused illicit drugs. Onset is minutes, lasts 2-24 h. **MDMA – Ecstasy** – popular at "raves" and consumed orally. Low dose - euphoria, mild sympathomimetic symptoms last ~ 4-6 h. Potent serotonin releaser (no impulse control). High dose - effects (1-3) above in addition to hyponatremia.

Treatment (1) supportive care, cardiopulmonary & neuro monitoring, (2) anticipate complications, (3) benzodiazepines for agitation, (4) labetalol or *Nipride*– 1st line for ↑ BP. Some recommend phentolamine as 1st line anti-hypetensive agent, (5) If ↓ BP, dopamine or norepinephrine (6) charcoal if oral ingestion, (7) treat MI, dysrhythmias, hyperthermia and rhabdomyolysis in standard fashion.

Theophylline

Clinical Features	
Cardiovascular	• Tachycardia, atrial and ventricular dysrhythmias
Neurological	• Agitation, tremors, seizures
Metabolic	• ↑Glucose, ↑catecholamines, ↓potassium
Gastrointestinal	• Vomiting

Treatment	
General	• Monitor for seizures, arrhythmias. Correct dehydration, hypoxia, and electrolyte imbalances.
Charcoal	• Administer 25-100 g q2-4h. Repeat doses q4h.
Arrhythmias	• β-blockade is preferred for tachyarrhythmias. Do not use verapamil. It inhibits theophylline metabolism.
Seizures	• Use benzodiazepines and barbiturates (not phenytoin).
Hemoperfusion Indications	• (1) seizures, (2) poorly responsive arrhythmias, (3) level > 100 mcg/ml in acute overdose > 60 mcg/ml in chronic OD

TOXIC ALCOHOLS: Ethanol

Ethanol (EtOH) contributes 22 mOsm/L for every 100mg/dl to serum osmolality. Mean elimination of ethanol is 20 mg/dl/h (range 16-25) *Am J Emerg Med* 1995; 276.

Clinical Features	
CNS	• Euphoria, disinhibition, sedation, Wernicke-Korsakoff syndrome
Cardiac	• ↑HR, ↓BP, atrial (esp. atrial fibrillation) & ventricular arrhythmias
Respiratory	• Aspiration, bradypnea
GI	• Vomiting, bleeding, ulcer, gastritis, hepatitis, pancreatitis
Metabolic	• ↑or↓temperature, ↓glucose, ↓Mg, ketoacidosis

Alcoholic Ketoacidosis

	Laboratory values
Due to an ethanol binge in patient who has a decreased caloric intake. Keto-acids, β-hydroxybutyric acid (βHB) and acetoacetate (AcA) accumulate in blood.	• Anion gap metabolic acidosis • Positive Nitroprusside test (serum and urine) detecting acetoacetate • Low, normal or mildly ↑glucose
Clinical Features	Management
• Vomiting, anorexia, abdominal pain • Hypothermia, dehydration, • ↑HR,↓BP, dehydration,↓urination • Recently terminated alcoholic binge • Poor caloric intake for 24-72 hours prior to presentation	• Rehydration with dextrose solution (D₅NS or D₅½NS) • Thiamine 100 mg before glucose • Correct electrolyte disturbances • Do not administer bicarbonate

Ethylene Glycol

Source: coolants (anti-freeze),preservatives,lacquer, cosmetics,polishes, detergents.

Timing	Clinical Features
1-12 hours	• Early: inebriation, ataxia, slurring without ethanol on breath • Later: coma, seizures, and death
12-24 hours	• Cardiac deterioration occurs during this phase • Early: tachycardia, hypertension, tachypnea • Later: congestive heart failure, ARDS, and cardiovascular collapse • Myositis occasionally occurs during this phase
24-72 hours	• Nephrotoxicity with calcium oxalate crystal precipitation leading to flank pain, renal failure, and hypocalcemia

Diagnosis	Treatment
• Anion gap acidosis • Osmol gap[2] (measured – calculated osmol) > 10 mOsm/L (page 6) • Hypocalcemia (ECG - ↑QT interval) • Calcium oxalate crystals in urine • ↑BUN and creatinine • Serum ethylene glycol level > 20 mg/dl is toxic • Serious toxicity has been reported in the <u>absence</u> of anion gap/crystalluria	• Contact poison center • Gastric lavage (if < 1 hour from ingest) • NaHCO₃ 50 mEq IV to keep pH ~7.40 • Ca⁺² gluconate 10%, 10-20 ml IV if ↓Ca⁺², MgSO₄ 2g IV over 15-30 min • Pyridoxine/thiamine, each 100 mg IV • Fomepizole[1] (Antizol) – 15 mg/kg IV, + 10 mg/kg q12h X 4 doses, then ↑ to 15 mg/kg IV q12h until level < 20mg/dl. Begin immediately based upon clinical suspicion, or lab or exam evidence of ethylene glycol ingestion. • Ethanol – only if Antizol unavailable – see methanol dosing • Dialysis if (1) oliguria/anuria, (2) severe acidosis, or (3) level > 50 mg/dl (> 20 mg/dl if fomepizole not used)

[1] Administer slow IV over 15 min. If unavailable, load IV ethanol (see Methanol).

[2] Osmol gap may be normal in significant toxicity.

Isopropanol

Isopropanol sources: rubbing alcohol, skin and hair products, jewelry cleaners, paint thinners, and antifreeze. Toxicity occurs after ingestion, inhalation, or dermal exposure (e.g. sponge bath).

Clinical Features	Diagnosis
• Onset of symptoms within 1 hour	• Osmol gap (see page 6)
• Inebriation, CNS depression, coma	• Acetonemia (ketonemia), acetonuria
• Hypotension - peripheral vasodilation	• Normal or mild ↓ pH (no anion gap)
• Abdominal pain, vomiting, ↓glucose	• Isopropanol > 50 mg/dl – mild
• Hemorrhagic gastritis, renal failure	intoxication, > 150 mg/dl – severe
• Hemolysis, rhabdomyolysis	• ↓ or ↔ glucose, ↑BUN & creatinine

Treatment
• Gastric lavage and charcoal are generally ineffective
• Supportive care, IV fluids (maintaining BP, respirations) is all that is required.
• Consider hemodialysis if (1) hypotension refractory to conventional therapy or (2) predicted peak level > 400 mg/dl. Dialysis rarely required.

Methanol

Methyl alcohol sources: wood alcohol, solvents, paint removers, shellacs, windshield washing fluids, and antifreeze. Toxicity is from formaldehyde/formic acid. Death has been reported after ingestion of 15 ml of 40% solution.

Clinical Features		Treatment
0-12 hours	• Inebriation, drowsiness	• Contact poison center
	• Asymptomatic period	• Gastric lavage/charcoal are ineffective
12-36 hours	• Vomiting, hyperventilation	• $NaHCO_3$ 50 mEq IV to keep pH > 7.35
	• Abdominal pain, pancreatitis	• Folate 50 mg IV q 4 hours
	• Visual blurring, blindness with mydriasis & papilledema	• Fomepizole (*Antizol*) – Begin immediately, (see ethylene glycol
	• CNS depression	dosing, indications)
Diagnostic Studies		• Ethanol (10%) in D_5W if fomepizole
• Osmol gap[1] may occur before anion gap acidosis (see page 6)		unavailable – (1) IV loading dose 10 ml/kg over 1-2 h (2) then 100 mg/kg/h
• Anion gap and lactic acidosis		(3) ↑ dose 50% if chronic alcohol use,
• Hemoconcentration, hyperglycemia		(4) Goal: ethanol level: 100-150 mg/dl
• Methanol levels > 20 mg/dl are toxic		• Dialyze if (1) visual symptoms, (2)
(1) CNS symptoms occur > 20 mg/dl		CNS depression, (3) level > 50 mg/dl,
(2) Visual symptoms occur > 50 mg/dl		(4) severe metabolic acidosis, or (5) history of ingestion of > 30 ml.
		• Stop dialysis and ethanol when methanol levels fall to < 20 mg/dl.

[1] Osmol gap may be normal in significant toxicity.

Tricyclic Antidepressants (TCA)

Clinical features are due to α adrenergic block ($\downarrow$BP), anticholinergic effects (altered mentation, seizures, $\uparrow$HR, mydriasis, inhabitation of norepinephrine uptake ($\uparrow$ catecholamines), Na$^+$ channel blockade (quinidine like cardiac depression)

ECG findings in TCA overdose	
• Sinus tachycardia • $\uparrow$QRS > 100 ms[1], $\uparrow$PR interval, $\uparrow$QT interval, BBB[2] (esp. right BBB) • Right axis deviation of the terminal 40 ms of the QRS > 120° (prominent terminal R in AVR – see figure) • AV conduction blocks (all degrees) • Ventricular fibrillation or tachycardia	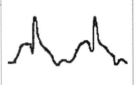

[1]ms – milliseconds; [2]bundle branch block

Treatment of TCA Toxicity

General	• Cardiac monitor, baseline ECG √ QRS width, QT interval.
Decontamination	• Administer charcoal 50 g PO or NG q 2-4h. Consider lavage if < 1 hour from ingestion (TCAs slow GI absorption) • Ensure patent airway & gag reflex prior to decontamination. • Avoid ipecac, as patients may have rapid mental status decline or develop seizures. (DO NOT use flumazenil)
NaHCO$_3$	• Indications: (1) acidosis, (2) QRS width > 100 milliseconds, (3) ventricular arrhythmias, or (4) hypotension. • Alkalinization enhances TCA protein binding and reverses Na$^+$ channel blockade and toxic cardiac manifestations. • <u>Dose</u>: 1-2 mEq/kg IV. May repeat. • <u>Goal</u>: Arterial pH of 7.50-7.55. • NaHCO$_3$ is ineffective for CNS side effects (e.g. seizures).
Fluids/pressors	• Administer 1-2 L NS for hypotension. Repeat 1-2 X. • If fluids are ineffective administer phenylephrine or norepinephrine (not dopamine) due to α-agonist effects.
Anti-seizure medications	• Use lorazepam followed by phenobarbital if seizure occurs. • Phenytoin is ineffective in TCA-induced seizures.
MgSO$_4$	• 25 mg/kg IV (over 15 min) may be useful for cardiac toxicity.
Disposition	*Transfer to a psychiatric facility if all of the following are present:* • no major evidence of toxicity during 6h ED observation • active bowel sounds and ≥ 2 charcoal doses are given • there is no evidence of toxic coingestant.

Initial Approach to Trauma Assessment and Management

PRIMARY SURVEY	
Assess **Airway** (*immobilize Cspine*)	• If poor/no air movement, perform jaw thrust or insert oral or nasal airway. Intubate if GCS ≤ 8, poor response to above, severe shock, flail chest or need to hyperventilate • Cricothyrotomy or laryngeal mask airway if unsuccessful
Assess **Breathing**	• Examine neck and thorax to detect deviated trachea, flail chest, sucking chest wound and breath sounds. • Needle chest for tension pneumothorax, apply occlusive dressing to 3 sides of sucking chest wound, reposition ET tube, or insert chest tubes (36-38 Fr) if needed. • Administer O_2, apply pulse oximeter, measure ET CO_2.
Assess **Circulation**	• Apply pressure to external bleeding sites. Insert 2 large IV lines, obtain blood for labs and type and crossmatch, administer 2L NS IV prn. ITIM[1] states normal mentation, skin signs, heart rate, respirations, and systolic BP of 80-90 mm Hg is goal (> 90 mm Hg if head injury) **if uncontrolled bleed & > 30 minutes to OR**. Others feel higher BP (systolic BP > 100-110 mm Hg) needed to ensure adequate resuscitation. Improvement in base deficit and lactate may guide adequacy of resuscitation. • Check pulses, listen for heart sounds, observe neck veins, assess cardiac rhythm & treat cardiac tamponade. • Apply cardiac monitor, obtain BP, HR (pulse quality)
Assess **Disability** (*neurologic status*)	• Measure Glasgow Coma Scale or assess if **A**lert, or respond to **V**erbal, **P**ainful, **U**nresponsive, check pupils
Patient **Exposure**	• Completely undress patient (but keep warm).
RESUSCITATION (Perform simultaneously during primary survey)	
Reassess **ABCD's**	• Reassess ABCs if patient deteriorates. Address abnormality as identified, place chest tube if needed. • Emergent thoracotomy if > 1.2-1.5 L of blood from initial chest tube, > 100-200 ml/h after 1st h, or persistent ↓ BP • Place NG tube + Foley catheter (unless contraindicated).
SECONDARY SURVEY – Consider NG and Foley at this step	
History & Exam	• **AMPLE** history (*Allergies, Meds, Past History, Last meal, & Events* causing injury), head to toe exam (FAST exam).
Xrays, CT scan, PAN-scan, FAST US exam (see page 143)	• Obtain cervical, chest, pelvic films, CT scans per decision rules. In multisystem trauma patient, <u>PAN-Scan</u> (head, cervical, chest, abdomen-pelvis CT) detects unsuspected injuries requiring management change in up to 19%.
Address injuries	• Reduce/splint fractures, call consultants, give analgesics, tetanus, + antibiotics prn, initiate admission or transfer
Disposition	• Initiate transfer, admit, or ready OR.

[1] Institute of Trauma and Injury Management 2007. www.itim.nsw.gov.au

Trauma Score (GCS=Glasgow coma score)

Respiratory rate	Systolic BP	GCS		Respiratory effort
2. ≥ 36/min	4. ≥ 90mmHg	5.	GCS 14-15	1. Normal
3. 25-35/min	3. 70-89 mm Hg	4.	GCS 11-13	0. Shallow
4. 10-24/min	2. 50-69 mm Hg	3.	GCS 8-10	0. Retractive
1. 0-9/min	1. 0-49 mm Hg	2.	GCS 5-7	Capillary refill
0. None	0. No pulse	1.	GCS 3-4	2. Normal

≤ 12 total points needs trauma center, > 14 < 1% mortality, 13-14 (1-2% risk), 11-12 (2-5% risk), ≤10 (> 10% risk).

			1. Delayed
			0. None

Revised Trauma Score

RTS – code	Glasgow Coma Scale	Systolic BP	Resp. rate
4	13-15	> 89 mm Hg	10-29
3	9-12	76-89	> 29
2	6-8	50-75	6-9
1	4-5	1-49	1-5
0	3	0	0

Coded RTS (insert RTS code 0 thru 4 above into following formula) = 0.9368GCS + 0.77326SBP + 0.2908RR. Coded RTS of 0 (97% mortality), 1 (93%), 2 (83%), 4 (39%), 5 (19%), 6 (8%), 7 (3%), 7.84 (1%)

Glasgow Coma Scale [Total - mild (13-15), mod (9-12), or severe (≤ 8) head injury]

Eye opening	Best verbal	Best motor	
4. spontaneous	5. oriented, converses	6. obeys	5. localize pain
3. to verbal command	4. disoriented, converses	4. withdrawal	
2. to pain	3. inappropriate words	3. abnormal flexion/decorticate	
1. no response	2. incomprehensible	2. extension/decerebrate	
	1. no response	1. no response	

*Total score indicates mild (13-15), moderate (9-12), or severe (≤ 8) head injury.

START (Simple Triage and Rapid Assessment) - Mass Casualty Incidents[1]

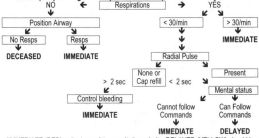

[1]IMMEDIATE (RED) patients are 1st resuscitation priority, DELAYED (YELLOW) should be reassessed for early transport care or change in triage class (after RED), DECEASED (BLACK) are not resuscitated unless resources become available, GREEN walking wounded are moved away from scene.

Management of Adults with Blunt Abdominal Trauma

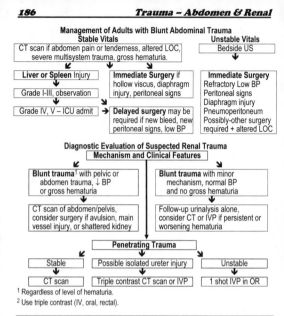

Stable Vitals		Unstable Vitals
CT scan if abdomen pain or tenderness, altered LOC, severe multisystem trauma, gross hematuria.		Bedside US

Liver or Spleen Injury	**Immediate Surgery** if hollow viscus, diaphragm injury, peritoneal signs	**Immediate Surgery** Refractory Low BP Peritoneal signs Diaphragm injury Pneumoperitoneum Possibly-other surgery required + altered LOC
Grade I-III, observation		
Grade IV, V – ICU admit →	**Delayed surgery** may be required if new bleed, new peritoneal signs, low BP	

Diagnostic Evaluation of Suspected Renal Trauma
Mechanism and Clinical Features

Blunt trauma[1] with pelvic or abdomen trauma, ↓ BP or gross hematuria	**Blunt trauma** with minor mechanism, normal BP and no gross hematuria
CT scan of abdomen/pelvis, consider surgery if avulsion, main vessel injury, or shattered kidney	Follow-up urinalysis alone, consider CT or IVP if persistent or worsening hematuria

Penetrating Trauma		
Stable	Possible isolated ureter injury	Unstable
CT scan	Triple contrast CT scan or IVP	1 shot IVP in OR

[1] Regardless of level of hematuria.

[2] Use triple contrast (IV, oral, rectal).

Penetrating Abdominal-Flank Trauma

- Consult Surgery for Penetrating Injuries of Abdomen or Flank

Indications for Laparotomy	
Unstable vital signs, peritoneal signs Diaphragm injury or GI bleeding.	Impaled, embedded weapon, gun shot Bowel protrusion or evisceration

[1]Debate exists as to need for laparotomy in stab wound entering peritoneum without peritoneal signs or evidence of organ, bowel injury.

Penetrating Flank or Back Injuries - Management
- Immediate celiotomy if shock, or obvious intraperitoneal or vascular injury.
- CT scan with triple contrast (oral, IV, and rectal) if no signs or symptoms of significant injury or gross hematuria alone in a hemodynamically stable patient.
- Angiography consider if significant retroperitoneal hematoma/bleeding

Trauma - Chest Injuries

Myocardial Contusion

Overview & ED Diagnosis	Features of Myocardial Contusion
The most common injuries are to (1) right ventricle (2) anterior septum, & (3) anterior apical left ventricle *Diagnosis*: CXR, ECG, & O₂ sat. CXR: pulmonary contusion, 1ˢᵗ or 2ⁿᵈ rib fractures, clavicle or sternal fractures, CHF. ECG findings may take 24 h to develop. Cardiac markers are elevated in ½ to 2/3 of cases.	Anginal pain (1-3 days after trauma) unrelieved by nitroglycerin External thoracic trauma (73%) Tachycardia (70%) Friction rub Beck's triad (cardiac tamponade) ↓BP, JVD, muffled HR (present in < 50% of cases)

Radiologic Studies	ECG in Myocardial Contusion	
(1) <u>Echo</u> - RV wall dyskinesia ± chamber dilation. Echo identifies most problems that require treatment.	Sinus tachycardia	70%
	Nonspecific ST-T changes	60%
(2) <u>Radionuclide angiography</u> - assesses ejection fraction (EF). LVEF < 50% or RVEF < 40% are abnormal.	Repolarization disturbances	61%
	Atrial arrhythmias (Afib) or conduction defect (RBBB)	12%
(3) <u>Single Photon Emission CT</u> (SPECT) – can detect contusions/ischemia.	Ventricular dysrhythmias	22%
	Normal ECG	12%
	Myocardial infarction	2%

Management
Consider admission for monitoring if ECG changes, cardiac disease, co-existing trauma or > 45-55 years. Consider Echo or other tests (1-3 above or cardiac markers) based on local protocols. Additional studies are only performed if problems/complications. (e.g. arrhythmia, hemodynamic instability). If < 45 years old, normal ECG & tachycardia resolves, consider discharge after 4 h observation/cardiac monitoring.

Traumatic Thoracic Aortic Rupture

Only 10-20% of patients survive to reach the ED. Rupture most frequently occurs at the fixed immobile ligamentum arteriosum due to a rapid deceleration injury.

Clinical Features	CXR in Thoracic Aortic Rupture
• Retrosternal or intra-scapular pain • Dyspnea, stridor, hoarse, dysphagia • ↑ or ↓BP (mean BP 152/98) • Depressed lower extremity BP • Systolic intrascapular/precordial murmur, swelling at base of neck • Sternal, scapula or multiple rib fractures (esp. 1ˢᵗ or 2ⁿᵈ rib • Chest tube with initial output > 750 ml	• ↑ mediastinal width[1,2] (52-90%) • Aborted aortic knob • Opacified aorticopulmonary window • NG tube > 2 cm to the right of T4 • Tracheal stripe > 5 mm from right lung • Left main stem bronchus 40° below horizontal • Left hemothorax/apical pleural cap • NORMAL CXR (up to 15%)

[1] MW on erect PA CXR > 6 cm, on supine AP > 8 cm, > 7.5 at aortic knob or MW at aortic knob/chest width > 0.25 all correlate with thoracic aortic rupture.

[2] Since a wide mediastinum is common on a supine chest Xray in major trauma patients (while ruptured aorta is not), an upright film, or plain Xray obtained in reverse Trendelenberg may be more specific for aortic injury (see diagnosis next page).

Diagnosis of Thoracic Aortic Rupture

- *Helical CT angiography* - nearly 100% sensitive for aortic rupture.
- Transesophageal echo- very accurate - best reserved for the unstable patient
- Intraarterial Digital Subtraction Angiography - 100% sensitive in 1 series

Management of Suspected Thoracic Aortic Rupture

- Perform resuscitation of ABC's as per resuscitation of all trauma patients.
- Most experts state that repair of life threatening cranial and abdominal injuries take precedence over aortic rupture.
- Keep systolic BP $\leq$ 120 mm Hg by controlling fluids, sedation, & pain. Consider short acting IV agents [β-blockade (esmolol)+ *Nipride*) See pg 79, 222
- Contact thoracic surgeon and prepare for possible surgery.

Genitourinary Trauma

Urethral Trauma

Overview	Retrograde Urethrogram Indications[1]
Pelvic fractures cause most proximal injuries while anterior injuries are usually due to falls, or straddle. Perform abdominal, perineal, & rectal exam, and obtain urethrogram if injury suspected	Penile, scrotal, perineal trauma Blood at urethral meatus High riding prostate on examination Suspected pelvis fracture (*controversial*) Inability to easily pass Foley catheter
Management	Retrograde Urethrogram Technique[1]
If a partial urethral disruption, a urologist may attempt to gently pass a 14-16 F catheter. If unsuccessful or a complete urethral disruption is found, a supra-pubic catheter will need to be placed.	Obtain preinjection KUB film Place Cooke adapter on 60 ml syringe. (Do not use Foley) Inject 10-15 ml of contrast in 60 seconds TAP/oblique xrays during last 10 sec

Bladder Trauma

Overview	Cystogram Indications
All with bladder trauma have pelvic fractures, abdominal trauma requiring CT, or gross hematuria (98%). If gross hematuria perform cystogram. Abdominal CT scan can miss this injury. CT abdomen before cystogram so dye does not obscure CT.	Penetrating injury to low abdomen/pelvis Blunt abdominal or perineal trauma with (1) gross hematuria, (2) blood at the urethral meatus, (3) pelvic fracture or (4) abnormal retrograde urethrogram or (5) inability to void or minimal urine from Foley catheter
Management	Cystogram Technique
<u>Intraperitoneal</u> rupture releases dye into abdomen,. Exploration of abdomen + repair often required. <u>Extraperitoneal</u> rupture dye is in perivesical tissues, while washout may show dye behind bladder. Treat with catheter (Foley if small, suprapubic if large) alone.	After urethrogram, insert Foley.Obtain baseline KUB, Instill dye[1] by gravity until 400 ml or bladder contraction Clamp Foley, Obtain (AP + oblique) Xrays, then empty bladder +/- wash out bladder with saline solution Then obtain final KUB with oblique film

[1]Use *Hypaque* 50%, *Cystografin* 40, or *Renografin* 60, or non-ionic dye (*Omnipaque* or *Isovue*) diluted to $\leq$ 10% solution with NS.

NEXUS II Criteria for Cranial CT in Trauma Patients

Study of 13,728 patients, ~ 10,5000 in minor head injury: GCS 13-15

Criteria	Utility of Criteria at Detecting Clinically Important[1,2] Intracranial Injury	
• Abnormal alertness, behavior	(All 13728 Patients)	
• Suspected skull fracture		
• Scalp hematoma	Sensitivity	98.3% (97.2-99%)
• Persistent vomiting	Specificity	13.7% (13.1-14.3%)
• Age > 64 years	NPV[3]	99.1% (98.5-99.5%)
• Persistent vomiting (recurrent, persistent, forceful)	Utility in Minor Head Injury Patients	
	Sensitivity[4]	95.2% (92.2-97.2%)
• Neurologic deficit	Specificity	17.3% (16.5-18%)
• Coagulopathy (e.g. on warfarin)	NPV[3]	99.1% (98.5-99.5%)

[1] Clinically important defined as mass effect/sulcal effacement, herniation, midline shift, basal cistern compressed, epidural/subdural hematoma (> 1 cm or more than one site), extensive subarachnoid bleed, posterior fossa blood, bilateral hemorrhage of any type, depressed or diastatic skull fracture, pneumocephalus, diffuse edema or axonal injury.

[2] Numbers in parenthesis = 95% confidence intervals

[3] NPV – negative predictive value

[4] Criteria detected 314 of 330 (95%) of minor head injury patients (GCS 13-15) with clinically important injury. Of the 16 "missed cases", only 1 required an intervention (ICP monitoring) [> 99% sensitivity and 99.9% negative predictive value for detecting injury requiring immediate intervention].

J Trauma 2005; 59: 954.

Canadian Criteria for Cranial CT in Trauma Patients with a GCS of 13-15

Major Risk Factors	Utility of Major Criteria in Predicting Need for Neurologic intervention[1]	
• Failure to reach GCS of 15 in 2h	Sensitivity	100% (92-100%)
• Suspected open skull fracture		
• Any sign of basal skull fracture	Specificity	68.7% (67-70%)
• Vomiting > 1 episode	Utility of Major + Minor Criteria in Predicting Clinically Important CNS Injury[2]	
• Age > 64 years		
Minor Risk Factors	Sensitivity	98.4% (96-99%)
• Amnesia before impact > 30 min	Specificity	49.6% (48-51%)
• Dangerous mechanisms (Pedestrian struck, assault by blunt object, fall > 3 feet/5 stairs, heavy object fall on head, vehicle ejection)	[1] death ≤ 7 days after accident, craniotomy, elevation of skull fracture, ICP monitor, intubation for head injury [2] any CT injury requiring admission and neurologic follow up	

Numbers in parentheses are 95% confidence intervals.

Lancet 2001, 357: 1391-1396; *JAMA* 2005; 294: 1511.

Management of Severe Head Injury (Glasgow Coma Scale ≤ 8)

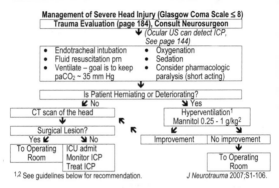

1,2 See guidelines below for recommendation.   *J Neurotrauma* 2007;S1-106.

Guidelines for Management of Severe Traumatic Brain Injury

Blood pressure/Oxygen – monitor & keep BP ≥ 90 mm Hg and O_2 ≥ 90%, pO_2 > 60 mm Hg
Hypertonic saline (3% NS) – limited studies show ICP reduction is similar to mannitol without rebound phenomenon. Due to limited data, guidelines cannot recommend its use routinely. Dose - 0.1 – 1 ml/kg/hour. (7.5% NS is also being evaluated for this purpose).
Hyperventilation – Only recommended as a temporizing measure for reducing ICP. Negative effects are more severe in early injury, so avoid if possible, in the 1st 24 hours after injury. If hyperventilation used, jugular venous O_2 saturation or brain tissue oxygen tensions measurements are recommended to monitor O_2 delivery.
Hypothermia – Pooled data indicated hypothermia not associated with decreased mortality, although it may have a higher chance of mortality reduction if maintained > 48 hours.
Mannitol - Prior to ICP monitor, restrict mannitol use to patients with signs of transtentorial herniation, or progressive neurological deterioration not due to extracranial cause. Keep systolic BP ≥ 90 mm Hg. Dose - 0.25 -1 g/kg.
Sedation & Analgesia – Prophylactic barbiturates not recommended. However, high dose barbiturates are recommended to control ↑ICP refractory to maximum standard medical and surgical therapy. Propofol is recommended for control of ICP. Both agents require close cardiopulmonary monitoring. Other recommended agents include morphine sulfate infusion, midazolam infusion, fentanyl/sufentanil infusion (NO bolus as this can raise ICP)
Seizures – Prophylactic anticonvulsants do not prevent late (> 7 days) post traumatic seizures. They prevent early (< 7 days) seizures esp. if cortical contusion, depressed fracture, subdural/epidural/intracerebral bleed, penetrating wound, seizure within 1st 24h. However, early post-traumatic seizures are not associated with worse outcome.

Guidelines have more detail regarding, ICP monitor, antibiotics, cerebral perfusion goals.
Brain Trauma Foundation *J Neurotrauma* 2007;S1-106. www.braintrauma.org

Trauma - Neck Injuries - Penetrating

Wounds through platysma muscle are of major concern.
(A) Some believe Zone I & III injuries require angiography (or CT angiography) to identify major vascular injury while Zone II injuries do not.
(B) Others manage penetrating injuries per the algorithm outlined below.

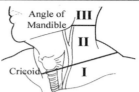

Initial Management of Patient with Penetrating Neck Injury

Airway	• Expanding hematomas, stridor, or other indicators of impending airway compromise mandate endotracheal intubation.
Breathing	• Obtain CXR to exclude pneumothorax. Chest tube prn.
Circulation	• Control bleeding by direct compression and give NS or blood.
Other Evaluation _See below algorithm_	• Contact consultants early. Exclude cervical, neuro-, vascular, airway, lung, GI injury clinically, via imaging, or exploration (see algorithm below). CT angiography may be used as first test in stable patients to evaluate larynx, trachea, major arteries of neck.

Management of the Penetrating Neck Injury

Severe or pulsatile bleed, shock, pulse deficit, expanding hematoma, air bubbling from wound, or deteriorating neurological status?	Yes →	Surgical Exploration

↓ No

Helical CT angiography if wound penetrates platysma
(observation alone appropriate if no platysma penetration)

↙   ↓   ↘

Negative	Possible airway, or GI tract injury	Vascular injury?
↓		↓ ↓
Observation	Endoscopy or esophogram	Positive Inconclusive

↙   ↘

Negative	Positive

↙   Diagnostic angiography

J Trauma 2005; 58: 413.   Surgery ←

Pelvis and Extremity Trauma

Criteria for Pelvic Radiography Following Blunt Trauma

• Glasgow coma scale < 14	• Pain, swelling, bruise to medial thigh, groin genitalia, suprapubic area, back
• Intoxication with drugs or alcohol	
• Hypotension or gross hematuria	• Instability of pelvis to anterior-posterior or lateral-medial pressure
• Lower extremity neurologic deficit	
• Femur fracture or painful/tender pelvis, symphysis pubis, or iliac spine	• Pain with abduction, adduction, rotation, or flexion of either hip

Criteria – 100% sensitive. _Ann Emerg Med_ 1988; 17: 488; and _J Trauma_ 1993; 34: 236.

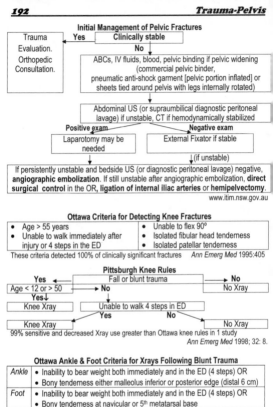

Initial Management of Pelvic Fractures

Trauma Evaluation. Orthopedic Consultation.

Yes ← **Clinically stable**

No ↓

ABCs, IV fluids, blood, pelvic binding if pelvic widening (commercial pelvic binder, pneumatic anti-shock garment [pelvic portion inflated] or sheets tied around pelvis with legs internally rotated)

↓

Abdominal US (or supraumbilical diagnostic peritoneal lavage) if unstable, CT if hemodynamically stabilized

Positive exam ↓   **Negative exam** ↓

Laparotomy may be needed   External Fixator if stable

↓ (if unstable)

If persistently unstable and bedside US (or diagnostic peritoneal lavage) negative, **angiographic embolization**. If still unstable after angiographic embolization, **direct surgical control** in the OR, **ligation of internal iliac arteries** or **hemipelvectomy**.

www.itim.nsw.gov.au

Ottawa Criteria for Detecting Knee Fractures

• Age > 55 years	• Unable to flex 90°
• Unable to walk immediately after injury or 4 steps in the ED	• Isolated fibular head tenderness
	• Isolated patellar tenderness

These criteria detected 100% of clinically significant fractures   *Ann Emerg Med* 1995:405

Pittsburgh Knee Rules

Yes ←   Fall or blunt trauma   → **No**

Age < 12 or > 50   **No**   No Xray

Yes↓

Knee Xray   Unable to walk 4 steps in ED

Yes   **No**

Knee Xray   No Xray

99% sensitive and decreased Xray use greater than Ottawa knee rules in 1 study

Ann Emerg Med 1998; 32: 8.

Ottawa Ankle & Foot Criteria for Xrays Following Blunt Trauma

Ankle	• Inability to bear weight both immediately and in the ED (4 steps) OR
	• Bony tenderness either malleolus inferior or posterior edge (distal 6 cm)
Foot	• Inability to bear weight both immediately and in the ED (4 steps) OR
	• Bony tenderness at navicular or 5th metatarsal base

Criteria - 100% sensitive in detecting clinically significant ankle/foot fractures.

Ann Emerg Med 1992; 21: 384-390.

Cervical, Thoracic, Lumbar Spine, Shoulder Injuries

NEXUS Cervical Spine Xray Criteria[1]

• Neck tenderness - midline	• Intoxication with drugs or alcohol
• Motor or sensory deficit	• Distracting painful injury
• Altered mental status	

[1] These criteria were 99% sensitive, with a 99.9% negative predictive value (*if features absent 0.1% probability of fracture*) in detecting clinically significant C spine fractures.
N Engl J Med 2000; 343: 94.

Canadian C-Spine Rule (CCR)

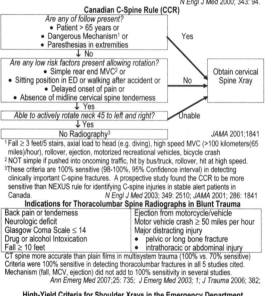

Are any of follow present?
- Patient > 65 years or
- Dangerous Mechanism[1] or
- Paresthesias in extremities

↓ No

Are any low risk factors present allowing rotation?
- Simple rear end MVC[2] or
- Sitting position in ED or walking after accident or
- Delayed onset of pain or
- Absence of midline cervical spine tenderness

↓ Yes

Able to actively rotate neck 45 to left and right?

↓ Yes

No Radiography[3]

Yes → / No → / Unable → Obtain cervical Spine Xray

JAMA 2001;1841

[1] Fall ≥ 3 feet/5 stairs, axial load to head (e.g. diving), high speed MVC (>100 kilometers(65 miles)/hour), rollover, ejection, motorized recreational vehicles, bicycle crash
[2] NOT simple if pushed into oncoming traffic, hit by bus/truck, rollover, hit at high speed.
[3] These criteria are 100% sensitive (98-100%, 95% Confidence interval) in detecting clinically important C-spine fractures. A prospective study found the CCR to be more sensitive than NEXUS rule for identifying C-spine injuries in stable alert patients in Canada. *N Engl J Med 2003; 349: 2510; JAMA 2001; 286: 1841*

Indications for Thoracolumbar Spine Radiographs in Blunt Trauma

Back pain or tenderness	Ejection from motorcycle/vehicle
Neurologic deficit	Motor vehicle crash ≥ 50 miles per hour
Glasgow Coma Scale ≤ 14	Major distracting injury
Drug or alcohol Intoxication	• pelvic or long bone fracture
Fall ≥ 10 feet	• intrathoracic or abdominal injury

CT spine more accurate than plain films in multisystem trauma (100% vs. 70% sensitive)
Criteria were 100% sensitive in detecting thoracolumbar fractures in all 5 studies cited. Mechanism (fall, MCV, ejection) did not add to 100% sensitivity in several studies.
Ann Emerg Med 2007;25: 735; J Emerg Med 2003; 1; J Trauma 2006; 382;

High-Yield Criteria for Shoulder Xrays in the Emergency Department

• Shoulder deformity or swelling	• History of fall (with age ≤ 43.5 years)
• Abnormal range of motion	*AJEM 1998;560; J Rheumatol 2000; 200*

These criteria were 100% sensitive in detecting clinically significant abnormal Xrays (fracture, 3rd AC joint, infection, cancer) in 2 studies.

Spinal Cord Injury Syndromes[1]

Anterior Cord Syndrome	Central Cord Syndrome
• Flexion or vertical compression injury to anterior cord or spinal artery • Complete motor paralysis • Hyperalgesia with preserved touch and proprioception (position sense) • Loss of pain and temperature sense • Most likely cord injury to require surgery	• Hyperextension injury in young trama victim or elderly with spondylosis • Motor weakness and paresthesias in hands > arms • Legs are unaffected or less affected • Variable bladder/sensory dysfunction • Prognosis is generally good and most do not require surgery

Complete Cord Injury	Brown-Sequard Syndrome
	• Hemisection of cord • Ipsilateral weakness • Ipsilateral loss of proprioception • Lose contralateral pain/temperature
• Flaccid below injury level • Warm skin ,↓BP,↓HR • Sensation may be preserved • ↓ Sympathetics ± priapism • Absent deep tendon reflexes • If lasts > 24 h will be permanent	Posterior Cord Syndrome
	• Pain, tingling, of neck and hands • 1/3 have upper extremity weakness • Mild form of central cord syndrome

[1] see page 129 for dermatomes, muscles, and reflexes.

Steroid Protocol for Treatment of Acute Spinal Cord Injury[1]

Indications	• Acute blunt spinal cord injury presenting within **8 hours** of injury.
Contra-indications	• Age < 13 y (*controversial*) • Isolated nerve root injury • Cauda equina syndrome • Penetrating cord trauma • Life-threatening illness/injury independent of spinal cord injury • Patients who were pregnant or on steroids were excluded from original study and may be relative contraindications
Protocol	• Methylprednisolone (*Solu-Medrol*) 30 mg/kg IV over 15 minutes, then wait 45 minutes • If < 3 hours since injury, *Solu-Medrol* 5.4 mg/kg/h over 23 hours • If 3-8 hours since injury, *Solu-Medrol* 5.4 mg/kg/h over 47 hours

[1] Debate exists as to the utility of steroids in acute spinal cord injury. Multiple American, Canadian, and European emergency medicine, trauma, and neurosurgical societies state that steroids are NOT the standard of care for acute spinal cord injury. Some experts consider this therapy experimental, while others consider it an unproven treatment option. www.aaem.org, www.caep.ca, www.trauma.org.

New Engl J Med 1990; 322: 1405 & *JAMA* 1997; 277: 1597.

Consensus Panel Recommendations for Wound Dressings

Definitions

Acute Wound - Wounds expected to heal in < 4 weeks with no local or general factor delaying healing including: burns, split skin donor graft, sacrococcygeal cyst, bites, frostbite, deep dermabrasion, or postoperative guided tissue regeneration.

Chronic Wounds – Wounds expected to take > 4-6 weeks to heal due to one of following: venous or pressure ulcer, diabetic foot ulcer, extended burn, amputation

Recommendations

Stage	Dressing type	Select Examples (Brands)
Debridement Chronic	Hydrogels	Flexigel Strands Absorbent Wound Dressing, GranuGel, Intrasite Gel, Sterigel, 2nd Skin, Tegagel Hydrogel wound filler, Vigilon Primary Wound Dressing
Debridement Acute	No consensus	No consensus
Epithelialzation Chronic	Hydrocolloid	Aquacel, Combiderm, Comfeel Plus, Cutinova Hydro or Cavity, Duoderm, Granuflex, Tegasorb
	Low adherence	N-A Ultra, Cutilin, Tricotex, Melolin, Melolite, Release, Skintact, Paraffin tulle dressings, Mepitel, Mepilex, Tegapor
Epithelialzation Acute	Low adherence	See examples for epithelialization, chronic above
Fragile Skin	Low adherence	See examples for epithelialization, chronic above
Granulation Chronic	Foam	Allevyn, Biatain, Cutinova, Lyofoam Extra, Mepilex, Optifoam, SOF Foam, Sorbacell, Tielle, Tegaderm
	Low adherence	N-A Ultra, Cutilin, Tricotex, Melolin, Melolite, Release, Skintact, Paraffin tulle dressings, Mepitel, Mepilex, Tegapor
Granulation Acute	No consensus	No consensus
Hemorrhagic wounds	Alginates	Algosteril, Kaltogel, Kaltostat, Comfeel, SeaSorb, Sorbsan, Tegagen
Malodorous wounds	Activated charcoal	Carbonet, CliniSorb, Lyofoam C, Actisorb Plus

The consensus panel DID NOT recommend any specific brands and brand names are only listed for convenience.

Arch Derm 2007; 143: 1291.

Urologic Disorders

The Painful Scrotum

Feature	Torsion of Testicle	Epididymitis & Orchitis	Torsion of Testicular Appendix
Frequency, age 0-20 yr	25-50%	10-25%	30-50%
Frequency, age 20-29	20%	80%	0%
Pain onset	acute onset	gradual onset	gradual onset
Pain location	testis, groin, or abdomen	testes, groin, epididymis	testis or upper pole
Prior similar episodes	often	occasional	rare
Fever	rare	up to 1/3	rare
Dysuria	rare	common	rare
Testicle/Scrotum	horizontal high riding testis	firm, red, warm epididymis or testis (>70%)	usually nontender, blue-dot upper testis
Cremasteric reflex	usually absent	may be present	may be present
Pyuria	up to 10%	25-60%	rare
Doppler/Nuclear scan	↓ flow	↑flow	normal flow

Accuracy of Diagnostic Tests for Testicular Torsion in Adults	Test	Sensitivity	Specificity
	Doppler ultrasound	80-90%	80-90%
	Color Doppler US	86-100%	100%
	Nuclear scan	80-90%	>95%

Urology Clin North Am 1996; Radiology Clin North Am 1997;

Management of Suspected Testicular Torsion

- In men under 40 with a painful testicle, assume torsion until proven otherwise.
- Contact a urologist immediately, as early surgical detorsion has the best chance of saving the testicle.
- If the clinical suspicion is low to moderate, consider diagnostic test above after consultation with urologist.
- An attempt to manually detorse the testicle may restore blood flow. To manually detorse, rotate the anterior aspect of the testicle towards the ipsilateral thigh (like opening a book). The testicle will need to be torsed at least 360 degrees. If successful, the patient will experience a marked relief of pain, and the testicle will develop a normal lie (position in scrotum).

Select Emergency Drugs & Infusions

ALLERGY	diphenhydramine (*Benadryl*): 50 mg IV/IM. epinephrine: 0.3-0.5 mg IM (1:1000) or 0.1 mg IV (1:10,000) repeat in 20 min methylprednisolone (*Solu-Medrol*): 125 mg IV/IM.
HYPERTENSION	enalapril (*Vasotec*): 1.25-5 mg IV over 5 minutes (avoid in acute MI) esmolol (*Brevibloc*): 500 mcg/kg IV over 1 min, then titrate 50-300mcg/kg/min fenoldopam (*Corlopam*): 0.1-0.3 mcg/kg/min, titrate up to 1.6 mcg/kg/min labetalol (*Normodyne*): 0.25 mg/kg IV, may double dose q 10-15 min prn (maximum cumulative total dose of 300 mg or 2 mg/kg – whichever is less) nicardipine (*Cardene*): start 2-4 mg/h IV, ↑ 1-2 mg/h q 15 min (Max 15 mg/h) nitroglycerin (*Tridil*): Start 5-20 mcg/min IV, titrate up to 100 mcg/min sodium nitroprusside (*Nipride*): 0.25-10 mcg/kg/minute
DYSRHYTHMIAS / CARDIAC ARREST	adenosine (*Adenocard*): SVT (not A-fib/flutter): 6 mg rapid IV & flush, pref- erably through a central line or proximal IV. If no response after 1-2 minutes then 12 mg. A third dose of 12 mg may be given prn. amiodarone (*Cordarone, Pacerone*): Life-threatening ventricular arrhythmia: Load 150 mg IV over 10 min, then 1 mg/min x 6h, then 0.5 mg/min x 18h. atropine: 0.5-1.0 mg IV or 2-3 mg (in 10 ml) via ET diltiazem (*Cardizem*): Rapid atrial fib: bolus 0.25 mg/kg or 20 mg IV over 2 min. May repeat 0.35 mg/kg or 25 mg IV 15 min later. Infuse 5-15 mg/h. epinephrine: 1 mg (2-2.5 mg in 10 ml ET) for cardiac arrest. [1:10,000] lidocaine (*Xylocaine*): 1 mg/kg, then 0.5 mg/kg q5-10min prn to max 3 mg/kg. Maintenance 2g in 250ml D5W (8 mg/ml) at 1-4 mg/min (7-30 ml/h) vasopressin (*Pitressin*, ADH): Ventricular fibrillation: 40 units IV once. May also be effective in asystolic cardiac arrest.
PRESSORS	dobutamine: 250 mg in 250ml D5W (1 mg/ml) at 2.5-20 mcg/kg/min dopamine: 400 mg in 250ml D5W (1600 mcg/ml) at 2-20 mcg/kg/min. Doses in mcg/kg/min: 2-5 = dopaminergic, 5-10 = beta, >10 = alpha. epinephrine: 0.1-4 mcg/minute norepinephrine (*Levophed*): 4 mg in 500 ml D5W (8 mcg/ml) at 0.5-10 mcg/min. (max 30 mcg/min) phenylephrine (*Neo-Synephrine*): 100-500 mcg boluses IV. Infusion for hypo- tension: 20 mg in 250ml D5W (80 mcg/ml), start at 100-180 mcg/min (75- 135 ml/h). Once BP stable, decrease to maintenance of 40-60 mcg/min
INTUBATION	etomidate (*Amidate*): 0.3-0.4 mg/kg IV. propofol (*Diprivan*): 2-2.5 mg/kg IV. *Ventilator sedation* = 5-50 mcg/kg/min rocuronium (*Zemuron*): 0.6-1.2 mg/kg IV. succinylcholine (*Anectine*): 1-1.5 mg/kg IV. thiopental (*Pentothal*): 3-5 mg/kg IV
SEIZURES	diazepam (*Valium*): 2-20 mg IV, or 0.2-0.5 mg/kg rectal gel up to 20 mg PR fosphenytoin (*Cerebyx*): 15-20 phenytoin equivalents/kg IM/IV ≤ 150 mg/min lorazepam (*Ativan*): 0.1 mg/kg up to 3-4 mg IV/IM phenobarbital: 200-320 mg IV at 60 mg/min; status epilepticus give 20 mg/kg phenytoin (*Dilantin*): 20 mg/kg up to 1000 mg IV no faster than 50 mg/min